The Pediatric Cerebellum

Editors

ANDREA PORETTI
THIERRY A.G.M. HUISMAN

NEUROIMAGING CLINICS
OF NORTH AMERICA

www.neuroimaging.theclinics.com

Consulting Editor
SURESH K. MUKHERJI

August 2016 • Volume 26 • Number 3

ELSEVIER

1600 John F. Kennedy Boulevard • Suite 1800 • Philadelphia, Pennsylvania, 19103-2899

http://www.neuroimaging.theclinics.com

NEUROIMAGING CLINICS OF NORTH AMERICA Volume 26, Number 3
August 2016 ISSN 1052-5149, ISBN 13: 978-0-323-45977-8

Editor: John Vassallo (j.vassallo@elsevier.com)
Developmental Editor: Casey Jackson

Neuroimaging Clinics of North America (ISSN 1052-5149) is published quarterly by Elsevier Inc., 360 Park Avenue South, New York, NY 10010-1710. Months of issue are February, May, August, and November. Business and editorial offices: 1600 John F. Kennedy Blvd., Suite 1800, Philadelphia, PA 19103-2899. Business and editorial offices: 6277 Sea Harbor Drive, Orlando, FL 32887-4800. Periodicals postage paid at New York, NY, and additional mailing offices. Subscription prices are USD 365 per year for US individuals, USD 564 per year for US institutions, USD 100 per year for US students and residents, USD 415 per year for Canadian individuals, USD 718 per year for Canadian institutions, USD 525 per year for international individuals, USD 718 per year for international institutions and USD 260 per year for Canadian and foreign students and residents. To receive student/resident rate, orders must be accompanied by name of affiliated institution, date of term, and the *signature* of program/residency coordinator on institution letterhead. Orders will be billed at individual rate until proof of status is received. Foreign air speed delivery is included in all *Clinics* subscription prices. All prices are subject to change without notice. POSTMASTER: Send address changes to *Neuroimaging Clinics of North America*, Elsevier Health Sciences Division, Subscription **Customer Service, 3251 Riverport Lane, Maryland Heights, MO 63043. Telephone: 1-800-654-2452 (U.S. and Canada); 314-447-8871 (outside U.S. and Canada). Fax: 314-447-8029. E-mail: journalscustomer service-usa@elsevier.com (for print support); journalsonlinesupport-usa@elsevier.com (for online support).**

Reprints. For copies of 100 or more of articles in this publication, please contact the Commercial Reprints Department, Elsevier Inc., 360 Park Avenue South, New York, NY 10010-1710. Tel.: 212-633-3874; Fax: 212-633-3820; E-mail: reprints@elsevier.com.

Neuroimaging Clinics of North America is covered by *Excerpta Medical/EMBASE,* the RSNA Index of Imaging Literature, *MEDLINE/PubMed (Index Medicus),* MEDLINE/MEDLARS, SciSearch, Research Alert, and Neuroscience Citation Index.

Printed in the United States of America.

PROGRAM OBJECTIVE
The goal of *Neuroimaging Clinics of North America* is to keep practicing radiologists and radiology residents up to date with current clinical practice in radiology by providing timely articles reviewing the state of the art in patient care.

TARGET AUDIENCE
Practicing radiologists, radiology residents, and other healthcare professionals who utilize neuroimaging findings to provide patient care.

LEARNING OBJECTIVES
Upon completion of this activity, participants will be able to:
1. Review normal cerebellar development and the role of the cerebellum in normal motor and cognitive functions.
2. Discuss neuroimaging in prenatal cerebellar disruptions and developmental malformations.
3. Recognize neuroimaging in vascular, neurodegenerative, and other disorders of the cerebellum.

ACCREDITATION
The Elsevier Office of Continuing Medical Education (EOCME) is accredited by the Accreditation Council for Continuing Medical Education (ACCME) to provide continuing medical education for physicians.

The EOCME designates this enduring material for a maximum of 15 *AMA PRA Category 1 Credit*(s)™. Physicians should claim only the credit commensurate with the extent of their participation in the activity.

All other health care professionals requesting continuing education credit for this enduring material will be issued a certificate of participation.

DISCLOSURE OF CONFLICTS OF INTEREST
The EOCME assesses conflict of interest with its instructors, faculty, planners, and other individuals who are in a position to control the content of CME activities. All relevant conflicts of interest that are identified are thoroughly vetted by EOCME for fair balance, scientific objectivity, and patient care recommendations. EOCME is committed to providing its learners with CME activities that promote improvements or quality in healthcare and not a specific proprietary business or a commercial interest.

The planning committee, staff, authors and editors listed below have identified no financial relationships or relationships to products or devices they or their spouse/life partner have with commercial interest related to the content of this CME activity:
Almundher Al-Maawali, MD; Alejandro Berenstein, MD; Susan I. Blaser, MD; Eugen Boltshauser, MD; Thangamadhan Bosemani, MD; Marie Brossard-Racine, PhD; Asim F. Choudhri, MD; Reade A. De Leacy, MBBS, BSc, FRANZCR; Thierry A.G.M. Huisman, MD, EQNR, FICIS; Paul Klimo Jr, MD, MPH; Catherine Limperopoulos, PhD; Carola Martinetti, MD; Giovanni Morana, MD; Suresh K. Mukherji, MD, MBA, FACR; Thomas P. Naidich, MD, FACR; Andrea Poretti, MD; Andrea Rossi, MD; Michael S. Salman, MBBS, MSc, PhD; Erin Scheckenbach; Mariasavina Severino, MD; Adeel Siddiqui, MD; Maja Steinlin, MD; Karthik Subramaniam; Domenico Tortora, MD; Peter Tsai, MD, PhD; John Vassallo; Grace Yoon, MD.

UNAPPROVED/OFF-LABEL USE DISCLOSURE
The EOCME requires CME faculty to disclose to the participants:
1. When products or procedures being discussed are off-label, unlabelled, experimental, and/or investigational (not US Food and Drug Administration [FDA] approved); and
2. Any limitations on the information presented, such as data that are preliminary or that represent ongoing research, interim analyses, and/or unsupported opinions. Faculty may discuss information about pharmaceutical agents that is outside of FDA-approved labelling. This information is intended solely for CME and is not intended to promote off-label use of these medications. If you have any questions, contact the medical affairs department of the manufacturer for the most recent prescribing information.

TO ENROLL
To enroll in the *Neuroimaging Clinics of North America* Continuing Medical Education program, call customer service at 1-800-654-2452 or sign up online at http://www.theclinics.com/home/cme. The CME program is available to subscribers for an additional annual fee of USD 235.

METHOD OF PARTICIPATION
In order to claim credit, participants must complete the following:
1. Complete enrolment as indicated above.
2. Read the activity.
3. Complete the CME Test and Evaluation. Participants must achieve a score of 70% on the test. All CME Tests and Evaluations must be completed online.

CME INQUIRIES/SPECIAL NEEDS
For all CME inquiries or special needs, please contact elsevierCME@elsevier.com.

NEUROIMAGING CLINICS OF NORTH AMERICA

ISSUE OF RELATED INTEREST

Radiologic Clinics of North America, May 2016 (Vol. 54, No. 3)
Imaging of Select Multisystem Disorders
Srinivasa R. Prasad, *Editor*
Available at: http://www.radiologic.theclinics.com

THE CLINICS ARE AVAILABLE ONLINE!
Access your subscription at:
www.theclinics.com

Contributors

CONSULTING EDITOR

SURESH K. MUKHERJI, MD, MBA, FACR
Professor and Chairman, Walter F. Patenge
Endowed Chair, Chief Medical Officer and
Director of Health Care Delivery, Michigan
State University Health Team, Department of
Radiology, Michigan State University, East
Lansing, Michigan

EDITORS

ANDREA PORETTI, MD
Assistant Professor of Radiology, Head of
Pediatric Neuroradiology Research, Section of
Pediatric Neuroradiology, Division of Pediatric
Radiology, Russell H. Morgan Department of
Radiology and Radiological Science, The
Johns Hopkins University School of Medicine,
The Johns Hopkins Hospital, Baltimore,
Maryland

**THIERRY A.G.M. HUISMAN, MD, EQNR,
FICIS**
Professor of Radiology, Pediatrics, Neurology,
and Neurosurgery, Director of Pediatric
Radiology and Pediatric Neuroradiology and
Co-Director of the Neurosciences Intensive
Care Nursery, Division of Pediatric Radiology,
and Chairman of the Department of Imaging
and Imaging Science, The Johns Hopkins
Bayview Medical Center, The Johns Hopkins
Hospital, Baltimore, Maryland

AUTHORS

ALMUNDHER AL-MAAWALI, MD
Consultant Medical Genetics, Department of
Genetics, Sultan Qaboos University Hospital,
Al Khoudh, Muscat, Oman

ALEJANDRO BERENSTEIN, MD
Director, Pediatric Cerebrovascular Program;
Professor, Department of Neurosurgery,
Radiology and Pediatrics, Cerebrovascular
Center, Mount Sinai Hospital, Mount Sinai
Medical Center, New York, New York

SUSAN I. BLASER, MD
Professor, Division of Paediatric
Neuroradiology, The Hospital for Sick Children,
University of Toronto, Toronto, Ontario,
Canada

EUGEN BOLTSHAUSER, MD
Department of Pediatric Neurology, University
Children's Hospital, Zurich, Switzerland

THANGAMADHAN BOSEMANI, MD
Section of Pediatric Neuroradiology,
Division of Pediatric Radiology, Russell H.
Morgan Department of Radiology and
Radiological Science, The Johns Hopkins
University School of Medicine, Baltimore,
Maryland

MARIE BROSSARD-RACINE, PhD
MRI Research of the Developing Brain,
Developing Brain Research Program,
Division of Neonatology, Children's National
Medical Center, Washington, DC; Assistant
Professor, School of Physical and
Occupational Therapy, Associate Member,
Department of Pediatrics and Department of
Neurology & Neurosurgery, McGill University,
Montréal, Canada

ASIM F. CHOUDHRI, MD
Departments of Radiology, Neurosurgery and Ophthalmology, University of Tennessee Health Science Center; Le Bonheur Neuroscience Institute, Le Bonheur Children's Hospital, Memphis, Tennessee

READE A. DE LEACY, MBBS, BSc, FRANZCR
Assistant Professor, Departments of Neurosurgery and Radiology, Cerebrovascular Center, Mount Sinai Hospital, Mount Sinai Medical Center, New York, New York

THIERRY A.G.M. HUISMAN, MD, EQNR, FICIS
Professor of Radiology, Pediatrics, Neurology, and Neurosurgery, Director of Pediatric Radiology and Pediatric Neuroradiology and Co-Director of the Neurosciences Intensive Care Nursery, Division of Pediatric Radiology, and Chairman of the Department of Imaging and Imaging Science, The Johns Hopkins Bayview Medical Center, The Johns Hopkins Hospital, Baltimore, Maryland

PAUL KLIMO Jr, MD, MPH
Department of Neurosurgery, University of Tennessee Health Science Center; Le Bonheur Neuroscience Institute, Le Bonheur Children's Hospital; Division of Neurosurgery, St. Jude's Children's Hospital; Semmes Murphey Neurologic & Spine Institute, Memphis, Tennessee

CATHERINE LIMPEROPOULOS, PhD
Associate Professor of Neurology, Radiology, and Pediatrics; Director, MRI Research of the Developing Brain, Director, Developing Brain Research Program, Co-Director of Research, Divisions of Neonatology and Diagnostic Imaging and Radiology, Children's National Medical Center, Washington, DC

CAROLA MARTINETTI, MD
Neuroradiology Unit, Istituto Giannina Gaslini, Genova, Italy

GIOVANNI MORANA, MD, PhD
Neuroradiology Unit, Istituto Giannina Gaslini, Genova, Italy

THOMAS P. NAIDICH, MD, FACR
Professor, Departments of Radiology, Neurosurgery and Pediatrics, Irving and Dorothy Regenstreif Research Professor of Neuroscience (Neuroimaging), Mount Sinai Medical Center, New York, New York

ANDREA PORETTI, MD
Assistant Professor of Radiology, Head of Pediatric Neuroradiology Research, Section of Pediatric Neuroradiology, Division of Pediatric Radiology, Russell H. Morgan Department of Radiology and Radiological Science, The Johns Hopkins University School of Medicine, The Johns Hopkins Hospital, Baltimore, Maryland

ANDREA ROSSI, MD
Neuroradiology Unit, Istituto Giannina Gaslini, Genova, Italy

MICHAEL S. SALMAN, MBBS, MSc, PhD
Section of Pediatric Neurology, Children's Hospital, Associate Professor, Department of Pediatrics and Child Health, College of Medicine, Faculty of Health Sciences, University of Manitoba, Winnipeg, Manitoba, Canada

MARIASAVINA SEVERINO, MD
Neuroradiology Unit, Istituto Giannina Gaslini, Genova, Italy

ADEEL SIDDIQUI, MD
Department of Radiology, University of Tennessee Health Science Center; Le Bonheur Neuroscience Institute, Le Bonheur Children's Hospital, Memphis, Tennessee

MAJA STEINLIN, MD
Professor, Division of Neuropaediatrics, Development and Rehabilitation, University Children's Hospital Inselspital, University of Bern, Bern, Switzerland

DOMENICO TORTORA, MD
Neuroradiology Unit, Istituto Giannina Gaslini, Genova, Italy

PETER TSAI, MD, PhD
Department of Neurology and Neurotherapeutics, Assistant Professor, University of Texas Southwestern Medical Center, Dallas, Texas

GRACE YOON, MD
Associate Professor of Paediatrics, Division of Clinical and Metabolic Genetics, The Hospital for Sick Children, University of Toronto, Toronto, Ontario, Canada

Contents

be caused by disruptive (acquired) causes. Starting from the neuroimaging pattern, this report describes a spectrum of prenatal cerebellar disruptions including cerebellar agenesis, unilateral cerebellar hypoplasia, cerebellar cleft, global cerebellar hypoplasia, and vanishing cerebellum in Chiari type II malformation. The neuroimaging findings, possible causative disruptive events, and clinical features of each disruption are discussed. Recognition of cerebellar disruptions and their differentiation from cerebellar malformations is important in terms of diagnosis, prognosis, and genetic counselling.

Evaluation of imaging studies of the cerebellum in inherited neurodegenerative disorders is aided by attention to neuroimaging patterns based on anatomic determinants, including biometric analysis, hyperintense signal of structures, including the cerebellar cortex, white matter, dentate nuclei, brainstem tracts, and nuclei, the presence of cysts, brain iron, or calcifications, change over time, the use of diffusion-weighted/diffusion tensor imaging and T2*-weighted sequences, magnetic resonance spectroscopy; and, in rare occurrences, the administration of contrast material.

Neurocutaneous syndromes encompasses a broad group of genetic disorders with different clinical, genetic, and pathologic features that share developmental lesions of the skin as well as central and peripheral nervous system. Cerebellar involvement has been shown in numerous types of neurocutaneous syndrome. It may help or be needed for the diagnosis and to explain the cognitive and behavioral phenotype of affected children. This article describes various types of neurocutaneous syndrome with cerebellar involvement. For each neurocutaneous disease or syndrome, clinical features, genetic, neuroimaging findings, and the potential role of the cerebellar involvement is discussed.

Key differences exist in the epidemiology, pathophysiology, and clinical presentation of vascular lesions of the cerebellum in children versus adults. An understanding of these differences and an appreciation of the distinct imaging features of these lesions aid in distinguishing normal vascular variations from pathology, in predicting lesion etiology, and in directing effective treatment strategies. This paper reviews the embryogenesis of the normal vascular system of the cerebellum and brainstem and then discusses the clinical and imaging features of the common vascular lesions affecting these structures in the pediatric population.

Cerebellar tumors are the most common group of solid tumors in children. MR imaging provides an important role in characterization of these lesions, surgical planning, and postsurgical surveillance. Preoperative imaging can help predict the histologic subtype of tumors, which can provide guidance for surgical planning. Beyond histology, pediatric brain tumors are undergoing new classification schemes based on genetic features. Intraoperative MR imaging has emerged as an important tool in the surgical management of pediatric brain tumors. Effective understanding of the imaging features of pediatric cerebellar tumors can benefit communication with neurosurgeons and neuro-oncologists and can improve patient management.

Andrea Rossi, Carola Martinetti, Giovanni Morana, Mariasavina Severino, and Domenico Tortora

Cerebellar involvement by infectious-inflammatory conditions is rare in children. Most patients present with acute ataxia, and are typically previously healthy, young (often preschool) children. Viral involvement is the most common cause and ranges from acute postinfectious ataxia to acute cerebellitis MR imaging plays a crucial role in the evaluation of patients suspected of harboring inflammatory-infectious involvement of the cerebellum and brainstem. Knowledge of the imaging features of these disorders and technical competence on pediatric MR imaging are necessary for a correct interpretation of findings, which in turn prompts further management.

Foreword
The Pediatric Cerebellum

 CrossMark

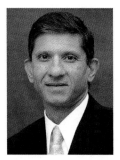

Suresh K. Mukherji, MD, MBA, FACR
Consulting Editor

This issue of the *Neuroimaging Clinics* is specifically devoted to the cerebellum and its disorders in children. There has been substantial progress in the understanding of the cerebellum over the last decade. This issue provides the reader with a comprehensive, yet concise update on the most recent advancements that will allow radiologists to play a larger role in management, prognosis, and counseling of the affected children and their families.

I would like to thank Drs Poretti and Huisman for creating such a unique and innovative issue. They have assembled a "world-class" group of authors whose contributions are outstanding. This issue discusses the important role of conventional and advanced neuroimaging techniques in the diagnosis of various cerebellar disorders in children. The articles cover the topics of embryogenesis, congenital malformations, metabolic disorders, vascular malformations, neoplasms, and infectious and inflammatory processes. There is also an article devoted to the role of the cerebellum in neurocognition and behavior.

Drs Poretti and Huisman have clearly succeeded in their goal of creating a detailed, up-to-date, and comprehensive body of information that can be used by both radiologists and clinicians for their daily practice and may stimulate scientific interest. This issue is already an instant "classic"!

Suresh K. Mukherji, MD, MBA, FACR
Department of Radiology
Michigan State University Health Team
Michigan State University
846 Service Road
East Lansing, MI 48824, USA

E-mail address:
mukherji@rad.msu.edu

Neuroimag Clin N Am 26 (2016) xi
http://dx.doi.org/10.1016/j.nic.2016.06.002
1052-5149/16/$ – see front matter © 2016 Published by Elsevier Inc.

Preface
The Pediatric Cerebellum

CrossMark

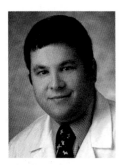

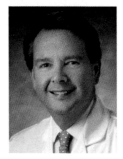

Andrea Poretti, MD   Thierry A.G.M. Huisman, MD, EQNR, FICIS

Editors

This issue of the *Neuroimaging Clinics* focuses on the cerebellum and its disorders in children. The cerebellum is a small part of the brain that is located within the posterior fossa. Although the cerebellum represents only about 10% of the weight of the whole brain, 50 billion granule cells are located in the cerebellum, representing about 75% of brain neuronal cells. 200 million mossy fibers connect the cerebellum with almost the entire brain, elucidating the key role of the cerebellum not only in motor but also in cognitive and behavioral functions in children.

In 2004, Professor Eugen Boltshauser[1] wrote a seminal review article with the title "Cerebellum—Small Brain but Large Confusion." Professor Boltshauser discussed the difficulties related to the correct definition and classification of the multiple morphological cerebellar abnormalities. He emphasized the role of a neuroimaging-based pattern recognition approach to improve our knowledge, understanding, and the final diagnosis of pediatric cerebellar disorders.

In the last decade, progress in conventional and advanced neuroimaging techniques has significantly improved the visualization, delineation, and evaluation of the various anatomical posterior fossa structures and, hence, helps to solve the "confusion." Cerebellar abnormalities have been anatomically characterized in better detail, and neuroimaging-based diagnostic criteria have been defined for several cerebellar diseases in children, particularly malformations and disruptions. Awareness and application of

specific criteria in daily practice will allow neuroradiologists to make specific diagnoses, which are important not only from an academic point of view but also (and more important) for management, prognosis, and counseling of the affected families. In the current era of precision medicine, nonspecific and confusing terms such as "Dandy-Walker variant" and "Dandy-Walker complex" should be avoided, or even better: abandoned. In neuroscience, precision in the use of language, whether verbal or written, does matter and is a reflection of precision in scientific thought and patient care.[2]

The outstanding contributions in this issue discuss the key role of conventional and advanced neuroimaging techniques in the diagnosis of various cerebellar disorders in children. In addition, the articles in this issue highlight the important role of neuroimaging in the elucidating the pathogenesis, establishing a phenotype (neuroimaging)-genotype correlation, and predicting the neurological outcome of cerebellar diseases in children. We aim to present a detailed, up-to-date, comprehensive body of information that can be used by both radiologists and clinicians for their daily practice and may stimulate scientific interest.

For a better and complete understanding of cerebellar diseases in children, a multidisciplinary approach is mandatory, involving experts from neuroembryology, neurogenetics, neurochemistry,

Neuroimag Clin N Am 26 (2016) xiii–xiv
http://dx.doi.org/10.1016/j.nic.2016.06.001
1052-5149/16/$ – see front matter © 2016 Published by Elsevier Inc.

pediatric neurosurgery, pediatric neurology, and last but not least, pediatric neuroradiology. The significance of an interdisciplinary approach is also reflected by the specialty training of the two guest editors of this special collection, who combine pediatric neuroradiology (T.A.G.M.H.) with pediatric neurology (A.P.).

We are thankful to Suresh K. Mukherji, MD, MBA, FACR, Consulting Editor of the *Neuroimaging Clinics* for inviting us to be guest editors for this special issue on the pediatric cerebellum. We are particularly grateful to John Vassallo, Associate Publisher of Elsevier, and Casey Jackson, Developmental Editor of Elsevier, for their support in the conceptualization, preparation, and realization of this issue. Last but not least, as guest editors we have been very fortunate that multiple world-renowned experts in the field accepted our invitation to share their knowledge and expertise with us. We are sincerely grateful to all the authors for the invaluable excellent contributions.

We hope that this issue will be interesting, helpful, informative, and educational for all colleagues who deal with cerebellar disorders in children on an occasional or frequent basis and that it will be as enjoyable for readers as its preparation was for us.

Andrea Poretti, MD
Division of Pediatric Radiology
Russell H. Morgan Department of Radiology and
Radiological Science
The Johns Hopkins University School of Medicine
Zayed Building, Room 4174
1800 Orleans Street
Baltimore, MD 21287, USA

Thierry A.G.M. Huisman, MD, EQNR, FICIS
Division of Pediatric Radiology
Russell H. Morgan Department of Radiology and
Radiological Science
The Johns Hopkins University School of Medicine
Zayed Building, Room 4174
1800 Orleans Street
Baltimore, MD 21287, USA

E-mail addresses:
aporett1@jhmi.edu (A. Poretti)
thuisma1@jhmi.edu (T.A.G.M. Huisman)

REFERENCES

1. Boltshauser E. Cerebellum-small brain but large confusion: a review of selected cerebellar malformations and disruptions. Am J Med Genet A 2004;126A:376–85.
2. Sarnat HB. Semantics do matter! Precision in scientific communication in pediatric neurology. J Child Neurol 2007;22:1245–51.

The Role of the Pediatric Cerebellum in Motor Functions, Cognition, and Behavior: A Clinical Perspective

Michael S. Salman, MBBS, MSc, PhD[a],*, Peter Tsai, MD, PhD[b],*

KEYWORDS

- Cerebellum • Motor coordination • Eye movements • Speech articulation • Language
- Attention deficit hyperactivity disorder • Schizophrenia • Autism

KEY POINTS

- The pediatric cerebellum is important for processing, controlling, and modulating movement, cognition, and behavior.
- Pediatric cerebellar dysfunction causes poor coordination, increased variability, impaired accuracy, and tremor manifesting during limbs movements, walking, stance, talking, and eye movements.
- Pediatric cerebellar dysfunction results in cognitive and behavioral dysregulation.
- Cognitive and behavioral disorders, such as developmental dyslexia, attention deficit hyperactivity disorder, autism spectrum disorder, and schizophrenia, display cerebellar abnormalities/dysfunction.

INTRODUCTION

The cerebellum, Latin for small brain, weighs only about 10% of the adult human brain; however, it contains four times as many cerebral neurons. The cerebellum has undergone a rapid size increase in humans and apes that has been even faster than the rapid change in neocortex size.[1] This disproportionate increase in size is unlike that seen in other anthropoid primates where the neocortex and the cerebellum underwent similar expansion rates. Such expansion underscores the relative importance of the cerebellum in humans. Nevertheless, despite more than 100 years of scientific research, the function of the cerebellum remains elusive, but there is no shortage of possible theories on how the cerebellum works.

The anatomy of the cerebellum is discussed elsewhere in this issue. For the interested reader, physiologic cerebellar anatomy has been reviewed recently.[2] Basically, mossy fibers and climbing fibers provide excitatory inputs to the cerebellum via the superior, middle, and inferior cerebellar peduncles. Mossy fibers form synapses with granule cells, whereas climbing fibers synapse on Purkinje cells. Both fibers also send collaterals to the deep cerebellar nuclei. Granule cells form synaptic contacts with Purkinje cells via parallel fibers. Inhibitory outputs from Purkinje cells innervate the vestibular nuclei and the deep cerebellar nuclei. The latter constitutes the main output of the

Disclosure and Conflict of Interest: None.
[a] Section of Pediatric Neurology, Children's Hospital, Department of Pediatrics and Child Health, College of Medicine, Faculty of Health Sciences, University of Manitoba, AE 308, 820 Sherbrook Street, Winnipeg, Manitoba R3A 1R9, Canada; [b] Department of Neurology and Neurotherapeutics, University of Texas Southwestern Medical Center, 6000 Harry Hines Boulevard, Dallas, TX 75390-8813, USA
* Corresponding authors.
E-mail addresses: msalman@hsc.mb.ca; Peter.Tsai@UTSouthwestern.edu

Neuroimag Clin N Am 26 (2016) 317–329
http://dx.doi.org/10.1016/j.nic.2016.03.003

cerebellum and makes excitatory synapses on their targets. Other cells in the cerebellar cortex include Golgi cells, Lugaro cells, unipolar brush cells, stellate cells, and basket cells. They form interneurons within the cerebellar cortex.[2]

Different cerebellar regions have important roles in voluntary control of limb movements, ocular motor control, balance, walking, and nonmotor higher cognitive functions.[3] How does the cerebellum provide these functions?

The answer to this question has been addressed indirectly based on studies in patients with cerebellar damage. Computational modeling and experimental animal studies using pharmacologic, lesion, and genetic manipulations have also contributed further important insights. More recently, cerebellar transcranial direct current stimulation has provided a noninvasive approach to investigating cerebellar functions in health and disease.[4]

Movement abnormalities resulting from cerebellar impairment include poor coordination, increased variability, impaired accuracy, and tremor manifesting during limbs movements, walking, stance, talking, and eye movements.[5]

Two popular proposals on how the cerebellum functions are actively debated.[6,7] The first proposal states that the cerebellum contributes to motor and nonmotor control by acting as a timer. The second proposal states that the cerebellum functions by updating and/or storing an internal model of body dynamics.[8,9] In this model, the cerebellum essentially predicts the consequences of motor command on the body and its surroundings (eg, how a motor command will change the state of a limb or object position and velocity). A feedforward (ie, predictive and planned in advance) signal provides a fast response instead of relying on a visual or peripheral sensory feedback system with its attending long delay to ensure a real-time, correct, and appropriate motor response.[6] In addition, the cerebellum improves proprioception (ie, sensing the position of a limb in space in the absence of visual input) during active but not passive limb movement, through prediction.[10]

Other theories on cerebellar function include temporal and spatial sequence detection within the feedforward control mechanism,[11] tonic facilitation providing fine tuning of downstream target structures, and the initiation of coordinated compound movements.[12]

LIMBS MOTOR CONTROL

Parallel fibers link Purkinje cells and deep cerebellar nuclei, where single muscles are represented, thus providing a way of linking movements involving many muscles (ie, complex sequence of movements).[12] It is not known what signal the cerebellum uses to exert its modulatory control on movements. Candidate signals that may be used by the cerebellum include sensory information from the periphery or copies of the movement commands (efference copy) from the primary motor cortex. Another possibility that has not been proven is that the cerebellum is capable of generating motor commands that could lead a limb toward a desired target.[5]

Smooth and accurate execution of voluntary movements and adaptation to changing motor tasks depend on a healthy cerebellum.[13] Through trial and error, the cerebellum can learn and store different combinations needed for precise compound movements. Motor learning in children is not similar to adults.[14] Prior experience but not error size improves motor learning in young children. Various types of motor learning are achieved at different ages. In children up to 11 years of age, spatial adaptation matured at a slower rate than temporal adaptation in locomotion tasks that demanded walking on a split-belt treadmill with each leg's speed controlled independently.[15] Temporal adaptation (learning a new timing change) of a locomotor task matures by the age of 3 years.

Patients with cerebellar lesions can perform simple motor tasks, with incoordination and impaired initiation of movement appearing when compound complex movements are performed, especially at a rapid pace.[12] Cerebellar impairment cause greater dysfunction in predictive movements than in movements that require feedback (ie, visual or somatosensory feedback information).[5] However, the mechanism uses peripheral feedback functions suboptimally as the demand on it increases. Patients with cerebellar disorders have been shown to have proprioceptive deficits during active but not passive limb movements.[10] Cerebellar dysfunction affects fast movements to a greater extent than slow movements. In addition, the ability to adapt to novel changes in movements is impaired. Imprecise movements and errors in perception during active predictable movements following cerebellar impairment have been attributed to a malfunction in the internal models of body dynamics.[7] **Table 1** shows a list of signs seen in patients with cerebellar impairment.

OCULAR MOTOR CONTROL

The cerebellum is important for all types of eye movements and for ensuring fixation stability. The vestibulocerebellum is essential for gaze

Table 1
Cerebellar signs causing abnormal control of voluntary movement

Sign	Comment
Dysmetria	Inaccurate movement trajectory with undershooting or overshooting a target. It can be observed during finger-nose-finger examination
Intention (kinetic) tremor	Oscillation of a limb especially when approaching a target during voluntary movements
Dysdiadochokinesia	Irregular and slow movements observed during rapid alternating movements of the hand involving successive pronation and supination
Action tremor	Oscillations observed during postural tasks, for example, maintaining the heel of one foot over the contralateral knee for a few seconds
Essential tremor	Oscillations of a body part, for example, the head or outstretched arms during a maintained posture
Palatal tremor	Rhythmic oscillations of the palate
Dysrhythmokinesia	Abnormal rhythm observed during tapping of a limb
Hypotonia	Decreased resistance to passive stretch
Motor delay	Slow acquisition of motor milestones
Rebound	Abnormally large displacement of an outstretched arm following a tap on the wrist with overshooting followed by few oscillations around the primary position
Ataxia of stance	Swaying of the body while standing up
Ataxia of gait	Wide-based gait with staggering and swaying
Head tilt	Lateral displacement of the head
Titubation	Involuntary rhythmic oscillations of a body part, for example, head or trunk
Pendular reflexes	Excessive oscillations of a limb (like the swing of a pendulum) observed after eliciting a deep tendon jerk

stability, vestibulo-ocular reflex, and smooth ocular pursuit. Various types of nystagmus, for example, gaze-evoked nystagmus and saccadic intrusions, which are abnormal fast eye movements that take the fovea off the target, occur following cerebellar damage and result in fixation instability. The oculomotor cerebellum, which includes the fastigial nuclei and dorsal vermis lobules VI and VII, is mostly important for saccade processing; however, it also participates in smooth ocular pursuit initiation, horizontal alignment of the 2 eyes, and vergence processing.[16,17]

The cerebellum fine-tunes eye movements and reduces their baseline variability to ensure that the 2 eyes are stable and working together. These actions are important for bringing and maintaining objects of interest on the fovea, which in turn leads to the best visual acuity whether the person is moving or not. This fine-tuning occurs online and also over time by a process called adaptation.

Adaptation ensures the best calibration of the ocular motor responses, for example, the amplitude and direction of the vestibulo-ocular reflex, the velocity of smooth ocular pursuit relative to target velocity. In addition, the amplitude of saccades can undergo adaptation (ie, change in size), for which the cerebellum provides an essential role.[16] **Table 2** shows a list of ocular motor signs seen in patients with cerebellar diseases.

SPEECH CONTROL

Spoken language broadly consists of 2 different neurologic functions with different anatomic correlates. Language is discussed in a separate section of this article. Here, the production of speech is focused on, which is a complex process that involves several networks located in the cerebrum and cerebellum.[18] The cerebellar contribution to speech control is likely similar to its control of limb movements. The production of speech involves the coordination of a large number of muscles, in particular the tongue and orofacial muscles.[19] Specifically, the cerebellum plays an important role in speech articulation, prosody (ie, characteristics of speech style including rhythm, speed, emphasis, and pitch), and planning and processing of speech and language.[19,20] Inputs from premotor, auditory, and somatosensory areas to the cerebellum provide important information for choosing motor commands for speech.

Table 2
Cerebellar ocular motor signs

Sign	Comment
Gaze-evoked nystagmus	Ocular oscillations observed while trying to hold gaze eccentrically (ie, off center), horizontally, and/or vertically. The fast phase of the nystagmus is toward the direction of gaze
Downbeat nystagmus	Ocular oscillations observed with the eyes in central position (ie, the eyes are located in the primary mid orbital position). The fast component beats downward. The nystagmus is exacerbated in downgaze and lateral gaze
Upbeat nystagmus	Ocular oscillations observed with the eyes in central position. The fast component beats upward. The nystagmus is exacerbated in upgaze
Rebound nystagmus	Transient ocular oscillations observed with the eyes in central position after returning from a maintained eccentric gaze
Periodic alternating nystagmus	Horizontal ocular oscillations observed with the eyes in central position that change direction gradually after a silent phase. It occurs in a periodic manner, usually every 1–2 min
Opsoclonus	Conjugate, random, involuntary, and multidirectional back-to-back fast eye movements observed during attempted fixation or movement of the eyes
Ocular flutter	Conjugate, random, involuntary, and horizontal back-to-back fast eye movements observed during attempted fixation or movement of the eyes
Ocular bobbing	Fast downward displacement of the eyes followed by slow return back to the central orbital position
Square wave jerks/ macrosaccadic oscillations	Fast, intruding, unwanted, involuntary, and conjugate eyes movements, which take the eyes off fixation. They may occur repetitively
Saccadic dysmetria	Inaccurate fast eye movement that either undershoot (hypometria) or overshoot (hypermetria) a visual target
Saccade initiation delay (ocular motor apraxia)	Increased latency of fast eye movements that can usually be overcome with a head thrust or a blink
Slowing of smooth pursuit velocity (especially initiation)	Jerky (instead of smooth) eye movements that are observed during visual tracking
Impaired vestibulo-ocular reflex cancellation	The ability to fixate objects moving in the same direction of the head requires cancellation of the vestibulo-ocular reflex, which normally drives the eyes contralateral to the direction of the head movement. Patients with cerebellar disease may not be able to cancel the vestibulo-ocular reflex
Abnormal optokinetic nystagmus	Fast ocular oscillations (jerk nystagmus) are normally observed while tracking a rotating drum with alternating white and black stripes. The nystagmus generated with such a stimulus may be exaggerated with chronic cerebellar disease or dampened with acute cerebellar lesions
Impaired adaptation of eye movements	Motor learning (adaptation) of the ocular motor system usually occurs physiologically or following disease to repair and improve the accuracy or velocity of eye movements. Adaptation may be impaired in cerebellar disease.
Skew deviation	Vertical misalignment of the eyes (ie, one eye is higher than the fellow eye), which changes as a function of horizontal gaze position
Abnormalities in the control of torsion	Abnormal rotational control of the eye around an axis perpendicular to the center of the pupil

Cerebellar impairment can cause ataxic dysarthria.[18] **Box 1** shows the characteristics of speech abnormalities in patients with cerebellar disorders. Abnormalities in speech motor programming through impaired timing and deficits in speech execution are implicated in ataxic dysarthria.[20] It is hypothesized that processing abnormalities in the feedforward motor commands result in abnormal speech production because it becomes more reliant on sensory feedback with its attendant delays. Such a delay may slow speech, produce pauses, and disrupt speech rhythm.

There is some evidence for specific sites within the cerebellum that are important for speech articulation. Increased signal intensity on functional MR imaging over the medial parts of the anterior lobe of the cerebellum has been described in association with tongue and lip movements in healthy volunteers. Lesions caused by stroke involving the superior paravermal area of the right cerebellar hemisphere may lead to dysarthria.[19]

A ROLE BEYOND MOTOR SYSTEMS

With the transition from the nineteenth to the twentieth century, work from such distinguished neurologists as Babinski and Holmes postulated exclusive roles for the cerebellum in motor control with isolated cerebellar lesions resulting in deficits of motor coordination, motor speech output, and ocular motor function.[21–23] Over the next three-quarters of a century, as cerebellar circuitry was further elucidated and theories postulated regarding its mechanisms of actions, few studies challenged this view of a motor cerebellum.

The first challenge to this idea of a strictly motor cerebellum was postulated by Leiner and colleagues,[24] after examination of the development of the dentate nucleus during evolution. From more primitive species to primates, dentate nuclear development occurred most dramatically in the ventral dentate, an expansion mirrored by growth in the prefrontal cortex. By comparing dentate-thalamic and thalamic-cortical projections, they postulated that these newly expanded areas of the dentate were connected to nonmotor areas of the cortex and thus were likely to have roles outside of strict motor constructs.

These hypotheses were supported over the next decade by the work of Schmahmann and Pandya[25,26] and Middleton and Strick.[27,28] These 2 groups used new developments in anterograde and retrograde tracing methodologies to define afferent and efferent circuits connecting the cerebellum to the cortex. Although these studies detailed connections to cortical motor areas as expected, these studies also identified extensive connections to nonmotor cortical areas.

These tracing studies have since been supported by imaging studies examining both anatomic and functional connectivity of the human cerebellum. From functional MR imaging and resting state connectivity studies, extensive connections between nonmotor cortex and cerebellum have been established.[29–33] In fact, these studies have remarkably demonstrated that most of cerebellum appears to be connected, not to motor, but to nonmotor cortical areas.

In addition, cerebellar abnormalities and dysfunction have been identified in cognitive and neuropsychiatric disorders. Moreover, clinical evidence, functional imaging, and targeted preclinical studies further support nonmotor roles for the cerebellum in multiple areas of cognition and behavior, which are detailed in later discussion with a specific emphasis on the pediatric population.

LANGUAGE

Roles for the cerebellum in speech initially revolved around motor control of speech. However, a role for the cerebellum in nonmotor aspects of language has emerged.[18,34–36] Initial functional imaging studies demonstrated activation of the cerebellum, predominantly in lateral cerebellum on the opposite side to cortical language domains, in tasks of verbal fluency.[37] Moreover, cerebellar lesions have been demonstrated to result in verbal fluency deficits.[38,39] The cerebellum has also been implicated in production and comprehension of syntax, prosody, and grammar,[40] with cerebellar dysfunction resulting in disturbances in these domains. Furthermore, clinical case studies have produced a picture of a cerebellar aphasia with difficulties in syntax, anomia, perseveration, reduced

---

Box 1
Speech abnormalities in cerebellar diseases

Scanning speech (eg, hesitation, accentuation of some syllables, omission of appropriate pauses, addition of inappropriate pauses)

Explosive speech

Slowness of speech

Syllables or words are not understandable with lack in speech clarity

Slurring of speech

Loss of intonation (abnormal rhythm and emphasis)

Voice tremor

speech output, and speed. Although these deficits again correlate mostly with cerebellar lesions localized to the opposite side of the dominant language cortex, evidence has emerged for a more complicated role and involvement for both lateral cerebellar hemispheres.[41,42]

Most of these studies, however, have involved adult patients. In the pediatric population, a role for the cerebellum in language has been postulated since the initial description by Daly and Love,[43] of posterior fossa syndrome, a syndrome characterized by mutism, behavioral, and affective disturbance, and executive dysfunction in children after posterior fossa surgery. Although the mutism often improves, children frequently continue to have persistent language dysfunction.[44,45] This syndrome has since been shown to involve disruption of afferent and efferent tracts of the cerebellum.[46] Similar findings have been identified in patients with acute disseminated encephalomyelitis involving the cerebellum,[47,48] while residual language disturbance has also been identified in pediatric multiple sclerosis in patients with cerebellar lesions.[49] Similar to adults, in pediatric patients with epilepsy, language appears to localize mostly to the cerebellar hemisphere contralateral to cortical language areas.[50]

Cerebellar language involvement has also been implicated in reading. The cerebellum has been implicated in brain networks critical for reading on functional MR imaging.[51–54] Furthermore, abnormalities in structural cerebellar (volumetric and diffusion) imaging have been found in individuals with developmental dyslexia with functional MR imaging demonstrating significant differences between children with dyslexia and age matched controls.[52,55] In addition, motor deficits have been identified in individuals with dyslexia, prompting the generation of a cerebellar developmental dyslexia hypothesis.[56] Further supporting a role for the cerebellum in reading, individuals with cerebellar disorders demonstrate significant reading impairments.[57–60]

COGNITION

As with language, studies investigating cortical-cerebellar connections support roles for the cerebellum in cognitive processes. Functional imaging has revealed cerebellar activation during numerous cognitive tasks. One of the more consistent processes associated with cerebellar activation involves tasks related to working memory or executive function.[31,61–66] Cerebellar activation has also been identified with tasks of attention and timing.[67–70] As with the cerebellar role in language, studies on a cerebellar contribution to

cognition largely support a role for the lateral cerebellar hemispheres in supporting cognitive processes.[31] Clinical and preclinical studies have corroborated these findings from imaging studies. Preclinical models and individuals with cerebellar lesions display diverse cognitive deficits: executive function deficits; deficiencies in procedural memory, declarative memory, and associative memory such as eye blink conditioning; and deficits in timing/attention.[71–76]

In the pediatric population, a similar picture emerges with significant cognitive disruption associated with pediatric cerebellar disruptions ranging from cerebellar developmental abnormalities to inflammatory insults, ischemic injury, and oncologic and postsurgical injury.[45,47–49,77–82] These cognitive deficits involve disruptions in executive dysfunction, working memory, procedural memory, and processing abilities in addition to impacting intellectual quotient and visuospatial abilities.

BEHAVIOR

In addition to cognitive and language processes, the cerebellum has been proposed to play roles in regulating behavior. Schmahmann and Sherman,[40] in their initial description of cerebellar cognitive affective syndrome described significant behavioral disruption in 20 patients with cerebellar disruption with behaviors ranging from affective changes to disinhibited behaviors. In fact, Daly and Love,[43] in their initial description of the posterior fossa syndrome in 1958, described a similar dysfunction with loss of affective responses, marked apathy, social disinterest, and emotional blunting. Subsequent studies of cerebellar lesions have supported these initial descriptions with numerous associated behavioral disruptions, including affective disruption, alterations in attention, anxious behaviors, emotional and social blunting, and obsessive and compulsive behaviors.[40,44,77,83] Conversely, examination of behavioral disorders has further supported a contributory role for the cerebellum in behavioral regulation with significant cerebellar abnormalities identified in several neurodevelopmental and behavioral disorders. Here, cerebellar involvement in 3 such disorders: attention deficit hyperactivity disorder (ADHD), schizophrenia, and autism spectrum disorders (ASD), are highlighted.

Attention Deficit Hyperactivity Disorder

ADHD is estimated to affect 5% of the pediatric population, with estimates approaching 50% of these individuals having persistent symptoms into adulthood.[84] Cerebellar lesions as noted previously are often accompanied by impaired attention and disinhibited behavior.[85,86]

As in developmental dyslexia, children with ADHD manifest high rates of motor abnormalities of up to 50% with motor deficits correlating with worse outcomes.[87,88] Multiple studies have reported decreased size of the cerebellum in patients with ADHD, with many studies demonstrating decreases in the posterior cerebellum (lobules VIII–X).[89–93] Reductions in the posterior cerebellar volumes themselves correlated with severity of illness.[85,94,95] Longitudinal studies of ADHD demonstrated persistent reductions in cerebellar size, whereas initial changes in the caudate resolved with time.[96] Compared with typically developing siblings, individuals with ADHD demonstrated reductions in right cerebellar volumes, whereas prefrontal regions showed changes in both individuals with ADHD and their typical developing siblings.[97] White matter abnormalities have also been identified in ADHD with involvement of bilateral middle cerebellar peduncles, whereas functional connectivity is also significantly disrupted.[98–100] As further evidence of cerebellar involvement, changes in cerebellar activation was visualized after just a single dose of the stimulant methylphenidate, one of the mainstays of ADHD therapy, whereas cerebellar volumes in patients receiving methylphenidate therapy were significantly larger than volumes in untreated cohorts.[95,101,102]

Schizophrenia

Schizophrenia is a devastating psychiatric disorder characterized by a constellation of symptoms including hallucinations, delusions, impaired judgment, disorganized speech and behavior, motor disruptions, and negative symptoms (decrease/absence of thoughts, actions, affect). The disorder is associated with impairment in cognitive domains, including memory, learning, and executive function.

The cerebellum has been implicated in the pathogenesis of schizophrenia. Cerebellar lesions result in psychiatric disturbances applicable to schizophrenia, including both positive and negative symptoms.[103] As with ADHD and developmental dyslexia, schizophrenia is also accompanied by elevated rates of motor abnormalities.[104,105] Studies have revealed numerous structural changes in the cerebellum of patients with schizophrenia, including reduced posterior vermis size, reductions in Purkinje cell size, and abnormal white matter connectivity, whereas reduction in cerebellar size correlates with symptom severity.[106–109] Functional studies also have revealed disruptions in corticocerebellar connections, with alterations in cerebellar-cortical activity during performance of many cognitive tasks, including memory, executive function, and working memory,[110–113] with other studies demonstrating abnormalities in cerebellar activity with theory of mind tasks.[114,115] Intriguingly, treatment of a small cohort of treatment-resistant patients with cerebellar vermal theta burst stimulation demonstrated significant improvement in mood and negative symptoms in addition to improvements in cognitive measures.[116] The exact mechanism underlying these benefits is not understood, although modulation of cortico-cerebellar loops has been postulated.[117]

Although onset of the schizophrenia occurs mostly in adolescence or early adulthood, less commonly, symptoms will emerge in childhood. Childhood-onset schizophrenia tends to portend a more severe diagnosis and is often accompanied by more severe premorbid symptoms, such as language, social, and motor disturbance.[118–120] In this pediatric population, studies have documented reductions in cerebellar volume as seen in adult-onset schizophrenia.[121,122] Longitudinal studies demonstrated that volumes were initially comparable to controls with volume decreases noted only on subsequent studies.[121,123] Disruptions in functional connectivity have also been identified in the cerebellum during a verbal working memory task in childhood-onset schizophrenia.[124]

Autism Spectrum Disorders

ASDs are prevalent neurodevelopmental disorders (affecting 1 in 68 children in the United States from latest estimates) that are characterized by social dysfunction and repetitive behaviors/restricted interests.[125] Numerous studies have implicated the cerebellum in the pathogenesis of the disorder. As documented earlier, cerebellar activation is demonstrated in social paradigms.[126,127] As with the above disorders, motor dysfunction is prominent in ASDs with prevalent motor apraxias, alterations in tone, and abnormalities in eye movements affecting most patients (reviewed recently by Mosconi and colleagues[128]).

Pathologic findings have also implicated the cerebellum in these disorders. In fact, the most consistent pathologic feature identified in postmortem tissue from individuals with ASD is cerebellar Purkinje cell loss and/or reductions in Purkinje cell size.[129–132] ASD pathologic specimens also reveal evidence of increased oxidative stress in the cerebellum.[133–135] Abnormal gene networks associated with ASD have also been identified in the cerebellum in animal models.[136]

Structural changes have also been demonstrated in ASD with initial studies focused on alterations in vermis volume.[137,138] Subsequent studies have been able to narrow that focus to more specific areas, most localized to the posterior cerebellum.[139–141] Abnormalities in structural connectivity have also been identified in patients with ASD,[142,143] while studies have also revealed abnormalities in functional connectivity.[144] In addition, studies demonstrate reduced function in the cerebellum in patients with ASD.[145,146]

Supporting a critical role for the cerebellum in ASDs, isolated cerebellar injury also significantly increases the risk of developing ASD symptoms. Limperopoulos and colleagues[147] demonstrated that approximately 37% of children with isolated cerebellar hemorrhage demonstrated autistic behaviors. When location of hemorrhage was considered, involvement of cerebellar vermis resulted in an increased rate ranging from 80% to 100%. Furthermore, in children with developmental malformations of the cerebellum, rates of social dysfunction and positive autism screening are elevated and associated with vermian involvement.[77,78,148] Children with posterior fossa syndrome also demonstrate increased rates of autistic behavior.[44]

Preclinical models similarly suggest cerebellar dysfunction in ASDs. Cerebellar abnormalities have been identified in multiple rodent models of ASD.[149,150] The cerebellar-mediated associative learning paradigm, eye blink conditioning, was also found to be abnormal in multiple ASD rodent models.[73] Moreover, in mouse models of tuberous sclerosis complex, a neurodevelopmental disorder with high rates of ASD, genetic disruption limited to cerebellar Purkinje cells[151,152] resulted in these mice displaying autistic-like behaviors with social impairments, repetitive behaviors, and behavioral inflexibility. These models also displayed abnormality consistent with clinical abnormality with ASD loss, increased markers of oxidative stress, and abnormalities in dendritic spines,[152,153] while also displaying on electrophysiology studies, impaired Purkinje cell function and excitability, consistent with functional imaging in ASD.[145,146,152] Thus, whereas previous studies were unable to address whether cerebellar dysfunction can result in ASD behaviors or whether cerebellar abnormalities are secondary to other distal processes, these studies demonstrated that cerebellar dysfunction by itself was sufficient to generate abnormal behaviors seen in patients with ASD.

Other Disorders

In addition, the cerebellum has been implicated in a diverse array of additional behavioral disorders,

---

> **Box 2**
> **Cognitive and behavioral abnormalities in cerebellar diseases**
>
> Language (nonmotor speech, reading, writing)
>
> Executive function and working memory
>
> Autistic behavior (repetitive/restricted, social impairment)
>
> Attention deficit hyperactivity disorder
>
> Schizophrenia
>
> Anxiety behavior
>
> Mood disorders

including bipolar disorder, depression, and anxiety (reviewed by Phillips and colleagues[154]).

However, for the purposes of this review, the authors have tried to focus on those disorders that affect the pediatric population and for which sufficient data generated from children were available.

SUMMARY

Roles for the cerebellum beyond traditional roles in motor coordination continue to emerge (**Box 2**). Clear roles for the pediatric cerebellum have been identified in motor functions, cognition, and behavior in both normal development and in disease. With a significant portion of cerebellar development extending from the third trimester into the initial postnatal years, disruptions of cerebellar function from diverse causes may contribute to the pathogenesis of neurodevelopmental disorders. Attainment of a better understanding of the cerebellar involvement in these disorders should not only lead to a better mechanistic understanding of cerebellar function but should also lead to development of targeted therapies for neurodevelopmental disorders of childhood.

REFERENCES

1. Barton RA, Venditti C. Rapid evolution of the cerebellum in humans and other great apes. Curr Biol 2014;24(20):2440–4.
2. Roostaei T, Nazeri A, Sahraian MA, et al. The human cerebellum: a review of physiologic neuroanatomy. Neurol Clin 2014;32(4):859–69.
3. Morton SM, Bastian AJ. Cerebellar control of balance and locomotion. Neuroscientist 2004;10(3):247–59.
4. Grimaldi G, Argyropoulos GP, Bastian A, et al. Cerebellar transcranial direct current stimulation (ctDCS): a novel approach to understanding cerebellar function in health and disease. Neuroscientist 2014;22(1):83–97.

5. Bastian AJ. Learning to predict the future: the cerebellum adapts feedforward movement control. Curr Opin Neurobiol 2006;16(6):645–9.

6. Bastian AJ. Moving, sensing and learning with cerebellar damage. Curr Opin Neurobiol 2011; 21(4):596–601.

7. Bhanpuri NH, Okamura AM, Bastian AJ. Predicting and correcting ataxia using a model of cerebellar function. Brain 2014;137(Pt 7):1931–44.

8. Ito M. Control of mental activities by internal models in the cerebellum. Nat Rev Neurosci 2008;9(4):304–13.

9. Popa LS, Hewitt AL, Ebner TJ. The cerebellum for jocks and nerds alike. Front Syst Neurosci 2014; 8:113.

10. Bhanpuri NH, Okamura AM, Bastian AJ. Predictive modeling by the cerebellum improves proprioception. J Neurosci 2013;33(36):14301–6.

11. Leggio M, Molinari M. Cerebellar sequencing: a trick for predicting the future. Cerebellum 2015; 14(1):35–8.

12. Thach WT. Does the cerebellum initiate movement? Cerebellum 2014;13(1):139–50.

13. Morton SM, Bastian AJ. Mechanisms of cerebellar gait ataxia. Cerebellum 2007;6(1):79–86.

14. Patrick SK, Musselman KE, Tajino J, et al. Prior experience but not size of error improves motor learning on the split-belt treadmill in young children. PLoS One 2014;9(3):e93349.

15. Vasudevan EV, Torres-Oviedo G, Morton SM, et al. Younger is not always better: development of locomotor adaptation from childhood to adulthood. J Neurosci 2011;31(8):3055–65.

16. Kheradmand A, Zee DS. Cerebellum and ocular motor control. Front Neurol 2011;2:53.

17. Manto M, Bower JM, Conforto AB, et al. Consensus paper: roles of the cerebellum in motor control–the diversity of ideas on cerebellar involvement in movement. Cerebellum 2012;11(2):457–87.

18. Marien P, Ackermann H, Adamaszek M, et al. Consensus paper: language and the cerebellum: an ongoing enigma. Cerebellum 2014;13(3):386–410.

19. Urban PP, Marx J, Hunsche S, et al. Cerebellar speech representation: lesion topography in dysarthria as derived from cerebellar ischemia and functional magnetic resonance imaging. Arch Neurol 2003;60(7):965–72.

20. Spencer KA, Slocomb DL. The neural basis of ataxic dysarthria. Cerebellum 2007;6(1):58–65.

21. Holmes G. The Croonian Lectures on the clinical symptoms of cerebellar disease and their interpretation (reprinted from The Lancet, vol 1, pg 1232, 1922). Cerebellum 2007;6(2):148–53.

22. Holmes G. The Croonian Lectures on the clinical symptoms of cerebellar disease and their interpretation (reprinted from The Lancet, vol 1, pg 1178, 1922). Cerebellum 2007;6(2):142–7.

23. Babinski J. The role of the cerebellum in voluntary acts, necessitating a rapid succession of movements (Diadochokinesia). Rev Neurol 1902;10: 1013–5.

24. Leiner HC, Leiner AL, Dow RS. Does the cerebellum contribute to mental skills? Behav Neurosci 1986;100(4):443–54.

25. Schmahmann JD, Pandya DN. Projections to the basis pontis from the superior temporal sulcus and superior temporal region in the rhesus monkey. J Comp Neurol 1991;308(2):224–48.

26. Schmahmann JD, Pandya DN. Anatomic organization of the basilar pontine projections from prefrontal cortices in rhesus monkey. J Neurosci 1997; 17(1):438–58.

27. Middleton FA, Strick PL. Anatomical evidence for cerebellar and basal ganglia involvement in higher cognitive function. Science 1994; 266(5184):458–61.

28. Middleton FA, Strick PL. Cerebellar projections to the prefrontal cortex of the primate. J Neurosci 2001;21(2):700–12.

29. Buckner RL, Krienen FM, Castellanos A, et al. The organization of the human cerebellum estimated by intrinsic functional connectivity. J Neurophysiol 2011;106(5):2322–45.

30. O'Reilly JX, Beckmann CF, Tomassini V, et al. Distinct and overlapping functional zones in the cerebellum defined by resting state functional connectivity. Cereb Cortex 2010;20(4):953–65.

31. Stoodley CJ, Schmahmann JD. Functional topography in the human cerebellum: a meta- analysis of neuroimaging studies. NeuroImage 2009;44(2): 489–501.

32. Stoodley CJ, Schmahmann JD. Evidence for topographic organization in the cerebellum of motor control versus cognitive and affective processing. Cortex 2010;46(7):831–44.

33. Stoodley CJ, Valera EM, Schmahmann JD. Functional topography of the cerebellum for motor and cognitive tasks: an fMRI study. NeuroImage 2012; 59(2):1560–70.

34. De Smet HJ, Paquier P, Verhoeven J, et al. The cerebellum: its role in language and related cognitive and affective functions. Brain Lang 2013;127(3): 334–42.

35. Murdoch BE. The cerebellum and language: historical perspective and review. Cortex 2010;46(7): 858–68.

36. Stoodley CJ, Schmahmann JD. The cerebellum and language: evidence from patients with cerebellar degeneration. Brain Lang 2009;110(3): 149–53.

37. Petersen SE, Fox PT, Posner MI, et al. Positron emission tomographic studies of the cortical anatomy of single-word processing. Nature 1988; 331(6157):585–9.

38. Leggio MG, Silveri MC, Petrosini L, et al. Phonological grouping is specifically affected in cerebellar patients: a verbal fluency study. J Neurol Neurosurg Psychiatr 2000;69(1):102–6.

39. Schweizer TA, Alexander MP, Susan Gillingham BA, et al. Lateralized cerebellar contributions to word generation: a phonemic and semantic fluency study. Behav Neurol 2010;23(1–2):31–7.

40. Schmahmann JD, Sherman JC. Cerebellar cognitive affective syndrome. Int Rev Neurobiol 1997; 41:433–40.

41. Marien P, Engelborghs S, Fabbro F, et al. The lateralized linguistic cerebellum: a review and a new hypothesis. Brain Lang 2001;79(3):580–600.

42. Murdoch BE, Whelan BM. Language disorders subsequent to left cerebellar lesions: a case for bilateral cerebellar involvement in language? Folia Phoniatr Logop 2007;59(4):184–9.

43. Daly DD, Love JG. Akinetic mutism. Neurology 1958;8(3):238–42.

44. Catsman-Berrevoets CE, Aarsen FK. The spectrum of neurobehavioural deficits in the Posterior Fossa Syndrome in children after cerebellar tumour surgery. Cortex 2010;46(7):933–46.

45. De Smet HJ, Baillieux H, Wackenier P, et al. Long-term cognitive deficits following posterior fossa tumor resection: a neuropsychological and functional neuroimaging follow-up study. Neuropsychology 2009;23(6):694–704.

46. Miller NG, Reddick WE, Kocak M, et al. Cerebello-cerebral diaschisis is the likely mechanism of post-surgical posterior fossa syndrome in pediatric patients with midline cerebellar tumors. AJNR Am J Neuroradiol 2010;31(2):288–94.

47. McAndrew S, Listernick R, Kuntz N. Cerebellar mutism in acute disseminating encephalomyelitis. Pediatr Neurol 2014;50(5):511–4.

48. Parrish JB, Weinstock-Guttman B, Yeh EA. Cerebellar mutism in pediatric acute disseminated encephalomyelitis. Pediatr Neurol 2010;42(4):259–66.

49. Weier K, Till C, Fonov V, et al. Contribution of the cerebellum to cognitive performance in children and adolescents with multiple sclerosis. Mult Scler 2015;22(5):599–607.

50. Gelinas JN, Fitzpatrick KP, Kim HC, et al. Cerebellar language mapping and cerebral language dominance in pediatric epilepsy surgery patients. Neuroimage Clin 2014;6:296–306.

51. Gizewski ER, Timmann D, Forsting M. Specific cerebellar activation during Braille reading in blind subjects. Hum Brain Mapp 2004;22(3):229–35.

52. Stoodley CJ, Stein JF. Cerebellar function in developmental dyslexia. Cerebellum 2013;12(2):267–76.

53. Turkeltaub PE, Gareau L, Flowers DL, et al. Development of neural mechanisms for reading. Nat Neurosci 2003;6(7):767–73.

54. Wood AG, Harvey AS, Wellard RM, et al. Language cortex activation in normal children. Neurology 2004;63(6):1035–44.

55. Fernandez VG, Stuebing K, Juranek J, et al. Volumetric analysis of regional variability in the cerebellum of children with dyslexia. Cerebellum 2013;12(6):906–15.

56. Nicolson RI, Fawcett AJ. Developmental dyslexia, learning and the cerebellum. J Neural Transm Suppl 2005;(69):19–36.

57. Merchant TE, Sharma S, Xiong X, et al. Effect of cerebellum radiation dosimetry on cognitive outcomes in children with infratentorial ependymoma. Int J Radiat Oncol Biol Phys 2014;90(3):547–53.

58. Moretti R, Bava A, Torre P, et al. Reading errors in patients with cerebellar vermis lesions. J Neurol 2002;249(4):461–8.

59. Moretti R, Torre P, Antonello RM, et al. Peculiar aspects of reading and writing performances in patients with olivopontocerebellar atrophy. Percept Mot Skills 2002;94(2):677–94.

60. Scott RB, Stoodley CJ, Anslow P, et al. Lateralized cognitive deficits in children following cerebellar lesions. Dev Med Child Neurol 2001;43(10):685–91.

61. Chen SH, Desmond JE. Cerebrocerebellar networks during articulatory rehearsal and verbal working memory tasks. NeuroImage 2005;24(2):332–8.

62. Desmond JE, Fiez JA. Neuroimaging studies of the cerebellum: language, learning and memory. Trends Cogn Sci 1998;2(9):355–62.

63. Durisko C, Fiez JA. Functional activation in the cerebellum during working memory and simple speech tasks. Cortex 2010;46(7):896–906.

64. Hayter AL, Langdon DW, Ramnani N. Cerebellar contributions to working memory. NeuroImage 2007;36(3):943–54.

65. Marvel CL, Desmond JE. The contributions of cerebro-cerebellar circuitry to executive verbal working memory. Cortex 2010;46(7):880–95.

66. Pope PA. Modulating cognition using transcranial direct current stimulation of the cerebellum. J Vis Exp 2015;(96).

67. Akshoomoff NA, Courchesne E. A new role for the cerebellum in cognitive operations. Behav Neurosci 1992;106(5):731–8.

68. Kim SG, Ugurbil K, Strick PL. Activation of a cerebellar output nucleus during cognitive processing. Science 1994;265(5174):949–51.

69. Salman MS. The cerebellum: it's about time! But timing is not everything–new insights into the role of the cerebellum in timing motor and cognitive tasks. J Child Neurol 2002;17(1):1–9.

70. Xu D, Liu T, Ashe J, et al. Role of the olivocerebellar system in timing. J Neurosci 2006;26(22):5990–5.

71. Dimitrova A, Gerwig M, Brol B, et al. Correlation of cerebellar volume with eyeblink conditioning in

healthy subjects and in patients with cerebellar cortical degeneration. Brain Res 2008;1198:73–84.

72. Gerwig M, Esser AC, Guberina H, et al. Trace eyeblink conditioning in patients with cerebellar degeneration: comparison of short and long trace intervals. Exp Brain Res 2008;187(1):85–96.

73. Kloth AD, Badura A, Li A, et al. Cerebellar associative sensory learning defects in five mouse autism models. Elife 2015;4:e06085.

74. Koziol LF, Budding D, Andreasen N, et al. Consensus paper: the cerebellum's role in movement and cognition. Cerebellum 2014;13(1):151–77.

75. Ravizza SM, McCormick CA, Schlerf JE, et al. Cerebellar damage produces selective deficits in verbal working memory. Brain 2006;129(Pt 2): 306–20.

76. Schmahmann JD, Sherman JC. The cerebellar cognitive affective syndrome. Brain 1998;121(Pt 4):561–79.

77. Bolduc ME, Du Plessis AJ, Sullivan N, et al. Spectrum of neurodevelopmental disabilities in children with cerebellar malformations. Dev Med Child Neurol 2011;53(5):409–16.

78. Bolduc ME, Limperopoulos C. Neurodevelopmental outcomes in children with cerebellar malformations: a systematic review. Dev Med Child Neurol 2009;51(4):256–67.

79. Hennes E, Zotter S, Dorninger L, et al. Long-term outcome of children with acute cerebellitis. Neuropediatrics 2012;43(5):240–8.

80. Hoang DH, Pagnier A, Guichardet K, et al. Cognitive disorders in pediatric medulloblastoma: what neuroimaging has to offer. J Neurosurg Pediatr 2014;14(2):136–44.

81. Hoche F, Frankenberg E, Rambow J, et al. Cognitive phenotype in ataxia-telangiectasia. Pediatr Neurol 2014;51(3):297–310.

82. Riva D, Cazzaniga F, Esposito S, et al. Executive functions and cerebellar development in children. Appl Neuropsychol Child 2013;2(2):97–103.

83. Tavano A, Grasso R, Gagliardi C, et al. Disorders of cognitive and affective development in cerebellar malformations. Brain 2007;130(Pt 10): 2646–60.

84. Biederman J, Faraone SV. Attention-deficit hyperactivity disorder. Lancet 2005;366(9481):237–48.

85. Mackie S, Shaw P, Lenroot R, et al. Cerebellar development and clinical outcome in attention deficit hyperactivity disorder. Am J Psychiatry 2007;164(4):647–55.

86. Townsend J, Courchesne E, Covington J, et al. Spatial attention deficits in patients with acquired or developmental cerebellar abnormality. J Neurosci 1999; 19(13):5632–43.

87. Rasmussen P, Gillberg C. Natural outcome of ADHD with developmental coordination disorder at age 22 years: a controlled, longitudinal, community-based study. J Am Acad Child Adolesc Psychiatry 2000;39(11):1424–31.

88. Watemberg N, Waiserberg N, Zuk L, et al. Developmental coordination disorder in children with attention-deficit-hyperactivity disorder and physical therapy intervention. Dev Med Child Neurol 2007;49(12):920–5.

89. Berquin PC, Giedd JN, Jacobsen LK, et al. Cerebellum in attention-deficit hyperactivity disorder: a morphometric MRI study. Neurology 1998;50(4): 1087–93.

90. Castellanos FX, Giedd JN, Marsh WL, et al. Quantitative brain magnetic resonance imaging in attention-deficit hyperactivity disorder. Arch Gen Psychiatry 1996;53(7):607–16.

91. McAlonan GM, Cheung V, Cheung C, et al. Mapping brain structure in attention deficit-hyperactivity disorder: a voxel-based MRI study of regional grey and white matter volume. Psychiatry Res 2007;154(2):171–80.

92. Mostofsky SH, Reiss AL, Lockhart P, et al. Evaluation of cerebellar size in attention-deficit hyperactivity disorder. J Child Neurol 1998;13(9):434–9.

93. Valera EM, Faraone SV, Murray KE, et al. Meta-analysis of structural imaging findings in attention-deficit/hyperactivity disorder. Biol Psychiatry 2007;61(12):1361–9.

94. Bledsoe JC, Semrud-Clikeman M, Pliszka SR. Neuroanatomical and neuropsychological correlates of the cerebellum in children with attention-deficit/hyperactivity disorder–combined type. J Am Acad Child Adolesc Psychiatry 2011;50(6): 593–601.

95. Ivanov I, Murrough JW, Bansal R, et al. Cerebellar morphology and the effects of stimulant medications in youths with attention deficit-hyperactivity disorder. Neuropsychopharmacology 2014;39(3): 718–26.

96. Castellanos FX, Lee PP, Sharp W, et al. Developmental trajectories of brain volume abnormalities in children and adolescents with attention-deficit/hyperactivity disorder. JAMA 2002; 288(14):1740–8.

97. Durston S, Hulshoff Pol HE, Schnack HG, et al. Magnetic resonance imaging of boys with attention-deficit/hyperactivity disorder and their unaffected siblings. J Am Acad Child Adolesc Psychiatry 2004;43(3):332–40.

98. Bechtel N, Kobel M, Penner IK, et al. Decreased fractional anisotropy in the middle cerebellar peduncle in children with epilepsy and/or attention deficit/hyperactivity disorder: a preliminary study. Epilepsy Behav 2009;15(3):294–8.

99. Kucyi A, Hove MJ, Biederman J, et al. Disrupted functional connectivity of cerebellar default network areas in attention-deficit/hyperactivity disorder. Hum Brain Mapp 2015;36(9):3373–86.

100. van Ewijk H, Heslenfeld DJ, Zwiers MP, et al. Diffusion tensor imaging in attention deficit/hyperactivity disorder: a systematic review and meta-analysis. Neurosci Biobehav Rev 2012;36(4): 1093–106.

101. Bledsoe J, Semrud-Clikeman M, Pliszka SR. A magnetic resonance imaging study of the cerebellar vermis in chronically treated and treatment-naive children with attention-deficit/hyperactivity disorder combined type. Biol Psychiatry 2009; 65(7):620–4.

102. Czerniak SM, Sikoglu EM, King JA, et al. Areas of the brain modulated by single-dose methylphenidate treatment in youth with ADHD during task-based fMRI: a systematic review. Harv Rev Psychiatry 2013;21(3):151–62.

103. Baldacara L, Borgio JG, Lacerda AL, et al. Cerebellum and psychiatric disorders. Rev Bras Psiquiatr 2008;30(3):281–9.

104. Hirjak D, Wolf RC, Stieltjes B, et al. Neurological soft signs and subcortical brain morphology in recent onset schizophrenia. J Psychiatr Res 2012; 46(4):533–9.

105. Thomann PA, Wustenberg T, Santos VD, et al. Neurological soft signs and brain morphology in first-episode schizophrenia. Psychol Med 2009; 39(3):371–9.

106. Kyriakopoulos M, Vyas NS, Barker GJ, et al. A diffusion tensor imaging study of white matter in early-onset schizophrenia. Biol Psychiatry 2008;63(5):519–23.

107. Nopoulos PC, Ceilley JW, Gailis EA, et al. An MRI study of cerebellar vermis morphology in patients with schizophrenia: evidence in support of the cognitive dysmetria concept. Biol Psychiatry 1999;46(5):703–11.

108. Tran KD, Smutzer GS, Doty RL, et al. Reduced Purkinje cell size in the cerebellar vermis of elderly patients with schizophrenia. Am J Psychiatry 1998; 155(9):1288–90.

109. Wassink TH, Andreasen NC, Nopoulos P, et al. Cerebellar morphology as a predictor of symptom and psychosocial outcome in schizophrenia. Biol Psychiatry 1999;45(1):41–8.

110. Andreasen NC, O'Leary DS, Cizadlo T, et al. Schizophrenia and cognitive dysmetria: a positron-emission tomography study of dysfunctional prefrontal-thalamic-cerebellar circuitry. Proc Natl Acad Sci U S A 1996;93(18):9985–90.

111. Andreasen NC, Pierson R. The role of the cerebellum in schizophrenia. Biol Psychiatry 2008; 64(2):81–8.

112. Crespo-Facorro B, Wiser AK, Andreasen NC, et al. Neural basis of novel and well-learned recognition memory in schizophrenia: a positron emission tomography study. Hum Brain Mapp 2001;12(4): 219–31.

113. Walter H, Vasic N, Hose A, et al. Working memory dysfunction in schizophrenia compared to healthy controls and patients with depression: evidence from event-related fMRI. NeuroImage 2007;35(4): 1551–61.

114. Andreasen NC, Calarge CA, O'Leary DS. Theory of mind and schizophrenia: a positron emission tomography study of medication-free patients. Schizophr Bull 2008;34(4):708–19.

115. Pedersen A, Koelkebeck K, Brandt M, et al. Theory of mind in patients with schizophrenia: is mentalizing delayed? Schizophr Res 2012;137(1–3):224–9.

116. Demirtas-Tatlidede A, Freitas C, Cromer JR, et al. Safety and proof of principle study of cerebellar vermal theta burst stimulation in refractory schizophrenia. Schizophr Res 2010;124(1–3):91–100.

117. Parker KL, Narayanan NS, Andreasen NC. The therapeutic potential of the cerebellum in schizophrenia. Front Syst Neurosci 2014;8:163.

118. Alaghband-Rad J, McKenna K, Gordon CT, et al. Childhood-onset schizophrenia: the severity of premorbid course. J Am Acad Child Adolesc Psychiatry 1995;34(10):1273–83.

119. Hollis C. Child and adolescent (juvenile onset) schizophrenia. A case control study of premorbid developmental impairments. Br J Psychiatry 1995;166(4):489–95.

120. Rapoport JL, Addington A, Frangou S. The neurodevelopmental model of schizophrenia: what can very early onset cases tell us? Curr Psychiatry Rep 2005;7(2):81–2.

121. Greenstein D, Lenroot R, Clausen L, et al. Cerebellar development in childhood onset schizophrenia and non-psychotic siblings. Psychiatry Res 2011;193(3):131–7.

122. Jacobsen LK, Giedd JN, Berquin PC, et al. Quantitative morphology of the cerebellum and fourth ventricle in childhood-onset schizophrenia. Am J Psychiatry 1997;154(12):1663–9.

123. Keller A, Castellanos FX, Vaituzis AC, et al. Progressive loss of cerebellar volume in childhood-onset schizophrenia. Am J Psychiatry 2003; 160(1):128–33.

124. White T, Schmidt M, Kim DI, et al. Disrupted functional brain connectivity during verbal working memory in children and adolescents with schizophrenia. Cereb Cortex 2011;21(3):510–8.

125. Wingate M, Kirby RS, Pettygrove S, et al. Prevalence of autism spectrum disorder among children aged 8 years—autism and developmental disabilities monitoring network, 11 sites, United States, 2010. MMWR Surveill Summ 2014;63(2):1–21.

126. Jack A, Morris JP. Neocerebellar contributions to social perception in adolescents with autism spectrum disorder. Dev Cogn Neurosci 2014;10:77–92.

127. Van Overwalle F, Marien P. Functional connectivity between the cerebrum and cerebellum in social

cognition: a multi-study analysis. NeuroImage 2015;124(Pt A):248–55.

128. Mosconi MW, Wang Z, Schmitt LM, et al. The role of cerebellar circuitry alterations in the pathophysiology of autism spectrum disorders. Front Neurosci 2015;9:296.

129. Carper RA, Courchesne E. Inverse correlation between frontal lobe and cerebellum sizes in children with autism. Brain 2000;123(Pt 4):836–44.

130. Fatemi SH, Halt AR, Realmuto G, et al. Purkinje cell size is reduced in cerebellum of patients with autism. Cell Mol Neurobiol 2002;22(2):171–5.

131. Skefos J, Cummings C, Enzer K, et al. Regional alterations in Purkinje cell density in patients with autism. PLoS One 2014;9(2):e81255.

132. Whitney ER, Kemper TL, Bauman ML, et al. Cerebellar Purkinje cells are reduced in a subpopulation of autistic brains: a stereological experiment using calbindin-D28k. Cerebellum 2008;7(3):406–16.

133. Rose S, Melnyk S, Pavliv O, et al. Evidence of oxidative damage and inflammation associated with low glutathione redox status in the autism brain. Transl Psychiatry 2012;2:e134.

134. Sajdel-Sulkowska EM, Xu M, Koibuchi N. Increase in cerebellar neurotrophin-3 and oxidative stress markers in autism. Cerebellum 2009;8(3):366–72.

135. Sajdel-Sulkowska EM, Xu M, McGinnis W, et al. Brain region-specific changes in oxidative stress and neurotrophin levels in autism spectrum disorders (ASD). Cerebellum 2011;10(1):43–8.

136. Menashe I, Grange P, Larsen EC, et al. Co-expression profiling of autism genes in the mouse brain. PLoS Comput Biol 2013;9(7):e1003128.

137. Courchesne E. Brainstem, cerebellar and limbic neuroanatomical abnormalities in autism. Curr Opin Neurobiol 1997;7(2):269–78.

138. Courchesne E, Saitoh O, Yeung-Courchesne R, et al. Abnormality of cerebellar vermian lobules VI and VII in patients with infantile autism: identification of hypoplastic and hyperplastic subgroups with MR imaging. AJR Am J Roentgenol 1994; 162(1):123–30.

139. Becker EB, Stoodley CJ. Autism spectrum disorder and the cerebellum. Int Rev Neurobiol 2013;113:1–34.

140. D'Mello AM, Crocetti D, Mostofsky SH, et al. Cerebellar gray matter and lobular volumes correlate with core autism symptoms. Neuroimage Clin 2015;7:631–9.

141. Stoodley CJ. Distinct regions of the cerebellum show gray matter decreases in autism, ADHD, and developmental dyslexia. Front Syst Neurosci 2014;8:92.

142. Brito AR, Vasconcelos MM, Domingues RC, et al. Diffusion tensor imaging findings in school-aged autistic children. J Neuroimaging 2009;19(4):337–43.

143. Jeong JW, Tiwari VN, Behen ME, et al. In vivo detection of reduced Purkinje cell fibers with diffusion MRI tractography in children with autistic spectrum disorders. Front Hum Neurosci 2014;8:110.

144. Khan AJ, Nair A, Keown CL, et al. Cerebro-cerebellar resting-state functional connectivity in children and adolescents with autism spectrum disorder. Biol Psychiatry 2015;78(9):625–34.

145. Asano E, Chugani DC, Muzik O, et al. Autism in tuberous sclerosis complex is related to both cortical and subcortical dysfunction. Neurology 2001; 57(7):1269–77.

146. Ryu YH, Lee JD, Yoon PH, et al. Perfusion impairments in infantile autism on technetium-99m ethyl cysteinate dimer brain single-photon emission tomography: comparison with findings on magnetic resonance imaging. Eur J Nucl Med 1999;26(3): 253–9.

147. Limperopoulos C, Bassan H, Gauvreau K, et al. Does cerebellar injury in premature infants contribute to the high prevalence of long-term cognitive, learning, and behavioral disability in survivors? Pediatrics 2007;120(3):584–93.

148. Bolduc ME, du Plessis AJ, Sullivan N, et al. Regional cerebellar volumes predict functional outcome in children with cerebellar malformations. Cerebellum 2012;11(2):531–42.

149. Ellegood J, Anagnostou E, Babineau BA, et al. Clustering autism: using neuroanatomical differences in 26 mouse models to gain insight into the heterogeneity. Mol Psychiatry 2015;20(1):118–25.

150. Steadman PE, Ellegood J, Szulc KU, et al. Genetic effects on cerebellar structure across mouse models of autism using a magnetic resonance imaging atlas. Autism Res 2014;7(1):124–37.

151. Reith RM, McKenna J, Wu H, et al. Loss of Tsc2 in Purkinje cells is associated with autistic-like behavior in a mouse model of tuberous sclerosis complex. Neurobiol Dis 2013;51:93–103.

152. Tsai PT, Hull C, Chu Y, et al. Autistic-like behaviour and cerebellar dysfunction in Purkinje cell Tsc1 mutant mice. Nature 2012;488(7413):647–51.

153. Reith RM, Way S, McKenna J 3rd, et al. Loss of the tuberous sclerosis complex protein tuberin causes Purkinje cell degeneration. Neurobiol Dis 2011; 43(1):113–22.

154. Phillips JR, Hewedi DH, Eissa AM, et al. The cerebellum and psychiatric disorders. Front Public Health 2015;3:66.

Normal Cerebellar Development by Qualitative and Quantitative MR Imaging
From the Fetus to the Adolescent

Marie Brossard-Racine, PhD[a,b], Catherine Limperopoulos, PhD[a,c,*]

KEYWORDS

- Cerebellum • Normal development • MR imaging • DTI • Fetus • fMR Imaging • Children
- Adolescent

KEY POINTS

- This article summarizes normal cerebellar development as described by conventional and advanced MR imaging techniques.
- Advanced MR imaging techniques are providing critical insights into important developmental and maturational processes that occur in the normal cerebellum throughout the pediatric lifespan.
- Ongoing prospective studies using multimodal MR imaging are needed to better evaluate/explore emerging functional and microstructural development of the cerebellum.

INTRODUCTION

The cerebellum is increasingly recognized for its critical role not only in motor coordination and balance but in cognition, language, and social-emotional functioning as well. This expanding repertoire of cerebellar functions has captured the attention of the scientific community and the number of published reports on the cerebellum continues to grow rapidly. Although numerous studies have used MR imaging to characterize developmental cerebellar abnormalities in clinical populations (see Poretti A, Boltshauser E, Huisman TAGM: Prenatal cerebellar disruptions: Neuroimaging spectrum of findings in correlation with likely mechanisms and etiologies of injury, in this issue), available literature on normal cerebellar development across the pediatric lifespan is limited. An understanding of typical cerebellar developmental processes and maturational trajectories is essential in order to identify aberrant cerebellar development that is often associated with wide-ranging, long-term neurodevelopmental impairments.

This article first provides a detailed summary of published MR imaging studies describing typical cerebellum development in healthy, typically developing fetuses, children, and adolescents as currently described by different MR imaging modalities (eg, three-dimensional [3D] volumetric analyses, diffusion tensor imaging [DTI]). For each of the MR imaging modalities, we then appraised the available literature, highlighting areas where

[a] MRI Research of the Developing Brain, Developing Brain Research Program, Division of Neonatology, Children's National Medical Center, 1001 Décarie Boulevard, ES1.5066.1 Montréal, QC, H4A3J1 Canada; [b] School of Physical and Occupational Therapy, Department of Pediatrics and Department of Neurology & Neurosurgery, McGill University, Montreal, Canada; [c] MRI Research of the Developing Brain, Developing Brain Research Program, Division of Diagnostic Imaging and Radiology, Children's National Medical Center, 111 Michigan Avenue Northwest, Washington, DC 20010, USA
* Corresponding author. MRI Research of the Developing Brain, Developing Brain Research Program, Division of Neonatology, Children's National Medical Center, 1001 Décarie Boulevard, ES1.5066.1 Montréal, QC, H4A3J1 Canada.
E-mail address: climpero@childrensnational.org

Neuroimag Clin N Am 26 (2016) 331–339
http://dx.doi.org/10.1016/j.nic.2016.03.004

knowledge is currently lacking, emphasizing both opportunities and limitations of currently used MR imaging methods to study cerebellar development. In addition, potential targets for future research are reviewed.

EMBRYOLOGIC DEVELOPMENT OF THE CEREBELLUM

Delineating the histogenesis of the developing cerebellum is beyond the current resolution of conventional MR imaging. The timing of the first appearance of many developmental features of the cerebellum as detected by MR imaging is often delayed with respect to the true timing in the embryologic developmental time course.[1,2] Although a comprehensive discussion of the complex cellular processes of the developing cerebellum is beyond the scope of this article, an abbreviated overview of normal cerebellar morphogenesis is warranted.

During the fourth week of development, the cerebellum initially emerges from the bilateral thickening of the lateral portions of the alar plates that are facing the fourth ventricle.[3,4] About 2 weeks later, this increasing thickening forms the limbs of the cerebellar tubercle, and as it continues to grow rapidly it protrudes into the fourth ventricle. During the 12th week of development, growth of the midline area of the alar plates accelerates such that it eventually fills the gap between the limbs and forms the precursor of the vermis.[5] Around the 12th week of development, multidirectional growth is occurring laterally, rostrally, and outwardly, reshaping the cerebellum so that it achieves its specific lateral orientation.[3,5] Around the 20th week of gestation, the cerebellar cortex begins its rapid and exponential growth foliation, which corresponds with the timing of its increased visibility on fetal MR imaging.[4]

IN VIVO STRUCTURAL DEVELOPMENT OF THE CEREBELLUM BY CONVENTIONAL MR IMAGING

The detailed anatomic delineation of the brain, and particularly of the developing cerebellum, is extremely difficult to characterize by MR imaging in the fetus younger than 20 weeks of gestation because of the small size of the structures.[6] However, starting at around 20 weeks gestational age (GA), using T2-weighted (T2w) imaging during fetal MR imaging (1.5-T MR imaging), it is possible to visualize the perpendicular orientation of the tentorium, the equilateral triangular shape of the fourth ventricle, and the smooth and regular cerebellar hemispheres (Fig. 1).[7,8] After 21 weeks, the homogeneity of the hemispheres is interrupted by the

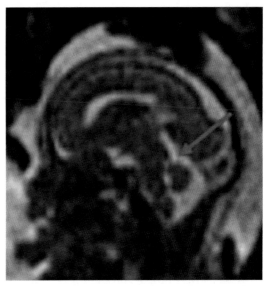

Fig. 1. Sagittal view of a 20-week-old fetus on T2w image showing perpendicular orientation of the tentorium (*arrow*) and the equilateral triangular shape of the fourth ventricle.

progressive appearance of early folia and tissue differentiation that becomes increasingly visible.[8] By about 27 weeks, the thin layer of hypointense signal on T2w images of the cerebellar cortical gray matter, and the adjacent thicker white matter layer seen as high signal intensity, can consistently be observed. Bounded by the white matter and the fourth ventricle, it is also possible to clearly delineate the hypointense T2w signal of the dentate nuclei (Fig. 2).[7,8] The signal changes specific to

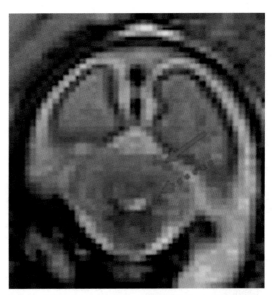

Fig. 2. Axial view of a 28-week-old fetus on T2w image showing cerebellar cortex (*solid arrow*), the dentate (*dotted arrow*), and the white matter in between.

the dentate nuclei are thought to reflect the high cellularity in these areas of deep gray matter.[7] At approximately 25 to 26 weeks, the separation between the anterior and posterior lobes of the vermis occurs; at the same time, the primary fissure of the vermis becomes more apparent on a sagittal plane and is typically consistently seen by 28 weeks (**Fig. 3**).[7] Although the cerebellar tonsils are observed by 27 weeks,[8] it is only after 32 weeks that the prepyramidal and the secondary fissures of the vermis become distinguishable (**Fig. 4**).[7]

On in vivo fetal MR imaging, the middle cerebellum peduncles can be first seen in 24-week fetuses and the superior cerebellar peduncles at 28 weeks.[8,9] On postnatal MR imaging, within the first few weeks of life, the superior and inferior peduncles are apparent. As the cerebellum enlarges during childhood, the fissures and folia increase in depth, and they become increasingly distinguishable (**Fig. 5**). The available evidence from quantitative MR imaging studies that capture and characterize unique features of normal cerebellar development are summarized below.

IN VIVO CEREBELLAR VOLUMETRIC AND SHAPE DEVELOPMENT OBSERVED BY QUANTITATIVE MR IMAGING

From 20 to 31 weeks, in parallel with an important volumetric expansion of the cerebellum, the surface of the cerebellum undergoes a dramatic change in structure. Scott and colleagues[10] performed shape analyses on manual cerebellar fetal segmentations and described important regional differences in surface curvature. Specifically, the inferior portion of the vermis and the

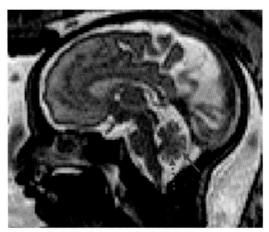

Fig. 4. Sagittal view of a 34-week-old fetus on T2w image showing the prepyramidal (*solid arrow*) and secondary fissure (*dotted arrow*).

anterior lobe of the hemispheres increased in concavity, whereas the apex of the vermis and the adjacent inferior-posterior lobe of the hemispheres increased in convexity. Notably, we and others have described an exponential increase in cerebellar volumetric growth in utero. Specifically, total cerebellar volume increases by 600% from 20 to 31 weeks,[10] whereas a 4-fold increase (384%) is observed between 25 and 37 weeks.[11] Between birth (term equivalent age) and the end of the first year of life, total cerebellum volume further increases by 240%,[12] with 108% of this volume gain occurring during the first 3 months of life.[13]

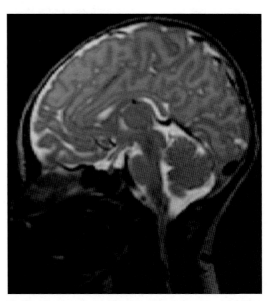

Fig. 5. Sagittal view of a 43-week-old newborn on T2w image showing the multiple folia of the cerebellar vermis.

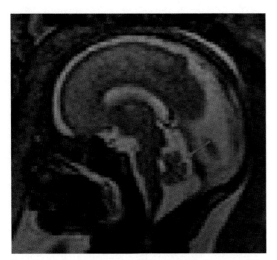

Fig. 3. Sagittal view of a 28-week-old fetus on T2w image showing the primary fissure (*arrow*).

By the end of the first year, the most active and impressive volumetric expansion is completed and only a 15% volume increase is reported to occur between the ages of 1 and 2 years.[12]

The total volume of the cerebellum and its cortex continue to change through childhood and adolescence and follows a similarly inverted U-shaped (ie, quadratic) trajectory.[14–17] This global cerebellar volume increase seems to be driven by the gain in cerebellar white matter compared with the cerebellar cortical gray matter, which tends to decrease with age through adolescence.[15,18,19] Sex differences are also observed with boys, consistently showing larger total and regional cortical cerebellar volumes than girls, with a gap that increases with age.[14,17,18,20] For both the cerebellar cortex and total cerebellar volume, growth peaks appear significantly earlier in girls than in boys. In boys, the cerebellar cortex and total volumes peak around 15.5 years of age. In contrast, in girls, the total cerebellar volume is at its highest point at 11.8 years and seems to peak even earlier with respect to cerebellar cortical volume.[14,18] Sex differences in cerebellar volumetric growth have not been reported in fetuses or children younger than 3 years of age.

Regional cerebellar growth trajectories have also been described. The cerebellar hemispheres of fetuses from 20 to 31 weeks mimic a quadratic growth trajectory.[10] This trajectory is maintained in the anterior and the superior lobes of the hemispheres during childhood and adolescence but not in the inferior-posterior lobe, which instead follows a cubic trajectory.[14] In contrast, vermian growth maintains a linear trajectory during antenatal and postnatal development.[10,14] Note that the volume gain of the vermis is more pronounced during the late second to early third trimester of pregnancy, during which it increases 3.5-fold.[10] Volumetric gain of the vermis and of its subregions during childhood and adolescence is minimal when compared to the volumetric expansion.[14,21]

Overall, the quadratic volumetric expansion of the cerebellum is well documented by converging evidence from the 3D quantitative MR imaging analyses performed by different groups. The seminal study of cerebellar surface analyses from Scott and colleagues[10] quantified for the first time changes in cerebellar curvature during the second trimester of pregnancy. Notably, shape analyses of the cerebellum have not been performed beyond 31 weeks of gestation and would be worth exploring during the third trimester as well as during postnatal development to better delineate potential critical periods of regional cerebellar maturation during this exuberant developmental stage.

CEREBELLAR MICROSTRUCTURE ORGANIZATION OBSERVED BY DIFFUSION TENSOR IMAGING

Using DTI, it is now possible to quantify both the diffusion rate and the directionality (ie, anisotropy) of the water molecules within the brain tissue, which in turn allows clinicians to make inferences about the degree and extent of microstructural organization. An increase in fractional anisotropy (FA) and a decrease in overall diffusion in bidirectional white matter fiber bundles is thought to be reflective of normal maturation processes (ie, increase of cell packing and reduction of water content as well as ongoing myelin formation).[22,23]

In vivo diffusion-weighted MR imaging studies of fetuses between 17 and 37 weeks have collectively reported a strong negative linear relationship between increasing GA and average diffusion coefficient (ADC) values in the cerebellar hemispheres.[24–26] Compared with the cerebral white and deep gray matter, the cerebellar hemispheres show the fastest and most pronounced decrease in ADC.[24–26] However, cerebellar ADC decline is less dramatic when evaluated during the early third trimester (26–33 weeks).[27] The overall decreasing diffusion in the cerebellum during pregnancy is thought to reflect the water content reduction that accompanies normal advancing gestation.

Because of poor contrast and maternal and fetal motion, the very small regions of interest are particularly challenging to characterize with DTI in utero. To date, only 2 studies have described the microstructure of the cerebellar cortex in postmortem fetuses without central nervous system anomalies. The first, by Saksena and colleagues,[28] used a region-of-interest approach to study FA in the cerebellar cortex and in the middle cerebellar peduncle of 24 newly aborted fetuses between 20 and 37 weeks GA. In the second, Takahashi and colleagues[29] collected high-angular-resolution diffusion imaging on a 4.7-T scanner in 6 fetuses between 17 and 38 weeks GA to visualize the organization of the fiber pathways in the cerebellar white and gray matter. Saksena and colleagues[28] described an FA increase in the cerebellar cortex from 20 to 28 weeks and then a gradual decrease until 37 weeks. Takahashi and colleagues[29] reported that, at 17 weeks, the cerebellar cortex is predominantly composed of radially orientated pathways that gradually disappeared with age and cortical thickening (**Fig. 6**). In contrast to the study by Saksesa and colleagues,[28] the cortical FA measured by Takahashi and colleagues[29] was stable across specimens. However, this discrepancy between studies could also stem from the small study

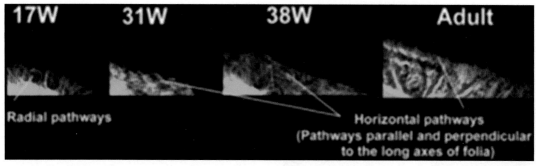

Fig. 6. Sagittal views of pathways in cerebellar cortex. 17W, 17 weeks; 31W, 31 weeks; 38W, 38 weeks. (*From* Takahashi E, Hayashi E, Schmahmann JD, et al. Development of cerebellar connectivity in human fetal brains revealed by high angular resolution diffusion tractography. Neuroimage 2014;96:329; with permission.)

sample as well as differences in image acquisition and processing. Nevertheless, both studies report low FA values in the cerebellar cortex closer to term, which is in line with the increasing number of crossing pathways found in the cerebellum between 31 and 38 weeks.[29] Both studies documented maturation of the white matter in the middle cerebellar peduncles. Saksena and colleagues[28] reported a steady increase between 20 and 37 weeks GA with probable early signs of hemispheric lateralization as shown by greater FA in the right peduncle compared with the left.[28] Takahashi and colleagues[29] similarly showed a thickening of the middle cerebellar pathways with increasing age and branching to the cerebellar cortex after 31 weeks.

Using a region-of-interest approach in 21 children between birth and 11 years of age, Saksena and colleagues[30] found that FA continues to increase in the middle, superior, and inferior cerebellar peduncles, and is accompanied by a corresponding decrease in mean diffusivity (MD). FA in the 3 pairs of cerebellar peduncles greatly increased during the first 36 months of life, compared with 24 months in the corpus callosum and in the posterior limb of the internal capsule, and followed a slower gradual enhancement after that point and until 132 months. In contrast, MD declined abruptly in the 3 pairs of cerebellar peduncles between birth and 6 months and stabilized thereafter, whereas the abrupt MD decline continued until 24 months in the cerebrum.[30] This change in growth trajectories is likely reflective of the dramatic increase in myelin formation within these white matter bundles that occurs soon after birth. This later stabilization in FA and MD is in line with the findings by Leitner and colleagues[31] who, using a deterministic tractography approach, reported no significant change in FA and MD in the cerebellar peduncles between the ages of 9 and 17 years.

Together these studies described age-dependent changes in diffusion properties of the cerebellum from fetal life to adolescence. Importantly, available information with respect to the developing cerebellar cortex comes exclusively from postmortem fetuses. In vivo imaging studies corroborating these postmortem observations are currently lacking. Moreover, diffusion MR imaging studies describing regional cerebellar nuclear organization are also lacking. The cerebellar white matter tracts of the cerebellum have been the regions most described with DTI and preliminary studies are converging to reflect the acute maturation processes that occur around birth and within the first few years of life.[28,30]

CEREBELLAR MYELINATION DESCRIBED BY CONVENTIONAL AND QUANTITATIVE MR IMAGING

Although most of the myelin of the brain develops postnatally, cerebellar myelination starts during fetal life but remains difficult to visualize on in vivo fetal MR imaging because of the limited contrast and size of the fetal brain. Developmentally, myelin appears first in the superior and inferior cerebellar peduncles.[32] However, the myelin in the middle cerebellar peduncles is first observed on conventional fetal MR imaging toward the middle to end of the third trimester of gestation.[7,21] At term and on postnatal MR imaging, the hypointense signal seen on T2w imaging caused by myelination is clearly visible in all 3 cerebellar peduncles (ie, superior, middle, and inferior cerebellar peduncles) (**Fig. 7**) as well as the floccule, the nodulus, the superior vermis, and the vestibular nuclei. Cerebellar myelination continues to develop rapidly during the first few months of life and by the end of the fourth month myelin is readily visible in the deep cerebellar white matter.[21,33]

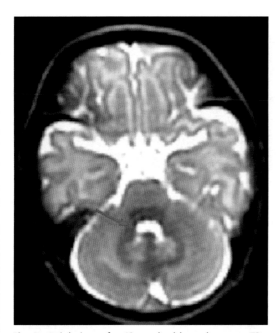

Fig. 7. Axial view of a 43-week-old newborn on T2w image showing the myelination in the middle cerebellar peduncle (*arrow*).

Using a novel approach to combine multicomponent-driven equilibrium single-pulse observation of T1 and T2 images, myelin estimation can be reliably measured in vivo using a calculation of the myelin water fraction.[34] In a study of myelin development in normally developing boys between 3 and 11 months, Deoni and colleagues[35] showed that the cerebellar hemispheric white matter is among the first regions of the brain to myelinate and has the greatest quantity of myelin at 3 months of age. These quantitative results are in line with the previously reported qualitative MR imaging studies that describe the myelination appearance based on change in signal intensity.[33]

Compared with other myelinated regions of the brain, the postnatal cerebellar myelin growth trajectory between the third and the eleventh month of age follows a slower increase over time than most supratentorial regions, such as the corpus callosum and optic radiations, which begin myelinating only after the fourth month following a term birth.[35] During the first year of life, the myelin of the right cerebellar hemisphere develops at a slower rate than that of the left hemisphere.[35] Extensions of this work show that after the early and rapid myelin increase in the cerebellar hemispheres, the cerebellar myelin continues to grow, but less drastically, between 2 and 5 years of age.[36] Using a contrast-based semiautomated tissue segmentation to estimate the myelinated white matter volume in the cerebellum, Wu and

colleagues[19] found that this steady increase continues up to 12 years of age. No other quantitative report on cerebellar myelin development is currently available beyond this age, and this is worth exploring in future studies.

Available imaging studies on cerebellar myelin show that the myelination in the cerebellum develops exponentially during the first year of life and continues during childhood but at a slower and steadier pace. These results overlap in part with the previously reported trends in diffusion characteristics of the cerebellar peduncles. However, myelin development only explains a portion of the histologic processes that affect the tissue's anisotropy and diffusion and this probably explains the plateauing age variations between the two techniques.

At present, in utero documentation of the cerebellar myelin development relies uniquely on qualitative MR imaging observations or from indirect inferences drawn from diffusion and anisotropy data. Although cerebellar myelin appears soon before birth, the limited resolution of fetal MR imaging and the diminished ability to obtain good high-resolution images in utero due to fetal and maternal motion have hindered the application of these techniques to living fetuses for myelin quantification/maturation. These techniques are currently under development and these data are likely to become available in the near future.

CEREBELLAR FUNCTIONAL NETWORK ORGANIZATION AND DEVELOPMENT OBSERVED BY FUNCTIONAL MR IMAGING

Studies of task-based functional MR (fMR) imaging in adults have been instrumental in delineating the functional topography of the mature cerebellum.[37] Preliminary data from emerging, innovative studies of resting-state fMR imaging in healthy fetuses and neonates suggests that cerebellar functional connectivity is already present at a very early age.[38] In fetuses between 31 and 39 weeks GA, Blood-oxygen-level dependent (BOLD) signal in the sensorimotor cortex highly correlated with areas in the left cerebellum. These strong correlations were not observed in fetuses younger than 31 weeks, which suggests that this cerebrocerebellar sensorimotor functional connectivity only appears in the late third trimester of pregnancy.[38] At term, neonates continue to show strong cerebellar connectivity with the sensorimotor cortex, and demonstrate prominent connections in the vermis.[39] However, these early-life observations conflict with available data from the mature cerebellar functional network reports, in which the right cerebellar hemisphere has been shown to be involved in the sensorimotor functional networks of adults.[37] Developmentally, the first functional networks to reflect existing structural connections and the primary networks are usually thought to develop before the associative networks.[40] Therefore, this lack of topographic specificity observed early in life most likely reflects the lack of maturity of these networks. Likewise, at birth, a cerebellar functional network with strong interhemispheric connectivity within homotopic regions but with little intrahemispheric connectivity can be observed and is thought to be an example of the undeveloped functional organization of what will later be a structured adult network.[39] Similarly, a nonspecific strong BOLD signal in the vermis is also observed during the first year of life, with stronger connectivity at 4 months than at 9 months.[41]

Although there has been no comprehensive investigation of how the cerebrocerebellar connectivity typically develops, information regarding normal cerebellar functional connectivity can be extrapolated from cross-sectional observations in healthy children and adolescents assessed in the context of high-risk group comparative studies. A recent study of resting-state functional connectivity successfully identified clear cerebrocerebellar connections in motor and nonmotor functional networks in typically developing children and adolescents between 8 and 17 years old.[42] Namely, cortical areas of the sensorimotor networks (ie, premotor, primary motor, somatosensory, superior temporal, and occipital cortexes) were highly correlated with the anterior (lobules I–V), superior (lobules IV–VI), and inferior (lobule VII) cerebellar regions (Fig. 8). Similarly supramodal regions, known to be involved in cognitive and emotional processing (ie, prefrontal and posterior parietal cortexes as well as the inferior and middle gyri), were found to be highly correlated with the posterolateral neocerebellum (lobule VII,

cru I and II) (see Fig. 8).[42] Overall, the observed resting-state functional connectivity networks in children and adolescents were similar to the networks observed in adults.[43]

Emerging evidence from resting-state fMR imaging studies are describing cerebrocerebellar motor and nonmotor functional connectivity at different ages during typical childhood development. However, there currently is a lack of longitudinal and serial designs describing how these networks appear, consolidate, and refine during development.

CEREBELLAR METABOLITE PROFILES DESCRIBED BY PROTON SPECTROSCOPY

Proton magnetic resonance spectroscopy (^{1}H-MRS) has been shown to be a valuable technique to assess brain metabolites and diagnose central nervous system anomalies.[44] Although cerebral age-related metabolite concentration profiles have been described in detail in healthy volunteers, cerebellar chemical profiles, as a function of age, have received far less attention to date. A preliminary quantitative study that performed single-voxel ^{1}H-MRS acquired with moderate/long echo time (TE = 135 milliseconds) in the cerebellar hemisphere of 31 healthy children aged between 3 and 18 years reported progressive increase in levels of N-acetyl-aspartate (NAA) and choline.[45] When comparing regional differences in metabolites and parieto-occipital white matter, this study found increased levels of NAA, choline, and creatine in the cerebellum.

These regional differences emphasize the need for additional metabolic studies to better delineate subtle but important changes in cerebellar metabolic profiles across the fetal and pediatric lifespan. Future studies in healthy participants using short echo times would be particularly valuable in providing a larger repertoire of metabolites (eg,

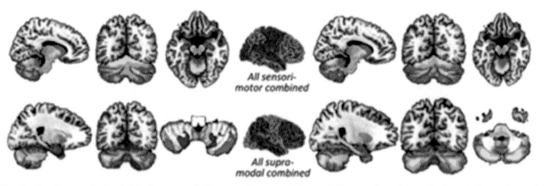

Fig. 8. Cerebrocerebellar intrinsic connectivity maps from partial correlation analyses by cortical seeds for regions of interest combined. (*From* Khan AJ, Nair A, Keown CL, et al. Cerebro-cerebellar resting-state functional connectivity in children and adolescents with autism spectrum disorder. Biol Psychiatry 2015;78(9):627; with permission.)

glutamate, glutamine) to better define cerebellar tissue properties and their evolution as a function of normal maturation.

SUMMARY

This article provides a current overview of normal cerebellar development as described by conventional and advanced MR imaging techniques. The qualitative (conventional) MR imaging studies reviewed in this article outnumber the MR imaging quantitative analyses. Collectively, both qualitative and quantitative reports of anatomic MR imaging have delineated important landmarks of fetal and postnatal cerebellar morphometric and volumetric development. A growing number of 3D volumetric MR imaging studies continue to corroborate the exuberant and accelerated period for cerebellar development taking place in the third trimester, at which time the cerebellum undergoes its most rapid growth, which is unparalleled to any other cerebral structure. In contrast, microarchitectural (using DTI) and functional connectivity (using resting-state fMR imaging) of the immature cerebellum prenatally and in the early postnatal period represent an important knowledge gap. Quantitative markers of emerging structural and functional maturation and connectivity are needed in healthy fetuses and newborns to better understand the timing and developmental consequences of acquired and developmental disorders of the cerebellum. To accomplish this, a greater focus on novel and sophisticated high-resolution fetal-neonatal MR imaging methodologies is needed in addition to the development of MR imaging spatio-temporal cerebellar-specific atlases.

In addition, there is an urgent need for prospective longitudinal studies that use a multimodal approach across the lifespan to adequately bridge information from structure to function. Serial measurements will inform clinicians about critical periods of cerebellum development, given its protracted developmental course, and pave the way for potential future therapeutic and rehabilitative interventions for pediatric cerebellar disorders.

ACKNOWLEDGMENTS

The authors thank Manouchka Jean-Gilles, PhD, for her assistance with article review/editing.

REFERENCES

1. Chong BW, Babcook CJ, Pang D, et al. A magnetic resonance template for normal cerebellar development in the human fetus. Neurosurgery 1997;41(4): 924–8 [discussion: 928–9].

2. Liu F, Zhang Z, Lin X, et al. Development of the human fetal cerebellum in the second trimester: a post mortem magnetic resonance imaging evaluation. J Anat 2011;219(5):582–8.

3. ten Donkelaar HJ, Lammens M, Wesseling P, et al. Development and developmental disorders of the human cerebellum. J Neurol 2003;250(9):1025–36.

4. Volpe JJ. Cerebellum of the premature infant: rapidly developing, vulnerable, clinically important. J Child Neurol 2009;24(9):1085–104.

5. ten Donkelaar HJ, Lammens M. Development of the human cerebellum and its disorders. Clin Perinatol 2009;36(3):513–30.

6. Levine D, Barnes PD, Sher S, et al. Fetal fast MR imaging: reproducibility, technical quality and conspicuity of anatomy. Radiology 1998;206:549–54.

7. Adamsbaum C, Moutard ML, Andre C, et al. MRI of the fetal posterior fossa. Pediatr Radiol 2005;35(2): 124–40.

8. Stazzone MM, Hubbard AM, Bilaniuk LT, et al. Ultra-fast MR imaging of the normal posterior fossa in fetuses. AJR Am J Roentgenol 2000;175(3):835–9.

9. Girard N, Raybaud C, Poncet A. In vivo MR study of brain maturation in normal fetuses. AJNR Am J Neuroradiol 1995;16:407–13.

10. Scott JA, Hamzelou KS, Rajagopalan V, et al. 3D morphometric analysis of human fetal cerebellar development. Cerebellum 2012;11(3):761–70.

11. Clouchoux C, Guizard N, Evans AC, et al. Normative fetal brain growth by quantitative in vivo magnetic resonance imaging. Am J Obstet Gynecol 2012; 206(2):173.e1–8.

12. Knickmeyer RC, Gouttard S, Kang C, et al. A structural MRI study of human brain development from birth to 2 years. J Neurosci 2008;28(47): 12176–82.

13. Holland D, Chang L, Ernst TM, et al. Structural growth trajectories and rates of change in the first 3 months of infant brain development. JAMA Neurol 2014;71(10):1266–74.

14. Tiemeier H, Lenroot RK, Greenstein DK, et al. Cerebellum development during childhood and adolescence: a longitudinal morphometric MRI study. Neuroimage 2010;49(1):63–70.

15. Ostby Y, Tamnes CK, Fjell AM, et al. Heterogeneity in subcortical brain development: a structural magnetic resonance imaging study of brain maturation from 8 to 30 years. J Neurosci 2009;29(38): 11772–82.

16. Lange N, Travers BG, Bigler ED, et al. Longitudinal volumetric brain changes in autism spectrum disorder ages 6-35 years. Autism Res 2015;8(1):82–93.

17. Brain Development Cooperative Group. Total and regional brain volumes in a population-based normative sample from 4 to 18 years: the NIH MRI Study of Normal Brain Development. Cereb Cortex 2012;22(1):1–12.

18. Wierenga L, Langen M, Ambrosino S, et al. Typical development of basal ganglia, hippocampus, amygdala and cerebellum from age 7 to 24. Neuroimage 2014;96:67–72.

19. Wu KH, Chen CY, Shen EY. The cerebellar development in Chinese children–a study by voxel-based volume measurement of reconstructed 3D MRI scan. Pediatr Res 2011;69(1):80–4.

20. Giedd JN, Snell JW, Lange N, et al. Quantitative magnetic resonance imaging of human brain development: ages 4-18. Cereb Cortex 1996;6:551–60.

21. Triulzi F, Parazzini C, Righini A. MRI of fetal and neonatal cerebellar development. Semin Fetal Neonatal Med 2005;10:411–20.

22. Beaulieu C. The basis of anisotropic water diffusion in the nervous system - a technical review. NMR Biomed 2002;15(7–8):435–55.

23. Murakami JW, Weinberger E, Shaw DW. Normal myelination of the pediatric brain imaged with fluid-attenuated inversion-recovery (FLAIR) MR imaging. AJNR Am J Neuroradiol 1999;20(8):1406–11.

24. Cannie M, De Keyzer F, Meersschaert J, et al. A diffusion-weighted template for gestational age-related apparent diffusion coefficient values in the developing fetal brain. Ultrasound Obstet Gynecol 2007;30(3):318–24.

25. Schneider JF, Confort-Gouny S, Le Fur Y, et al. Diffusion-weighted imaging in normal fetal brain maturation. Eur Radiol 2007;17(9):2422–9.

26. Schneider MM, Berman JI, Baumer FM, et al. Normative apparent diffusion coefficient values in the developing fetal brain. AJNR Am J Neuroradiol 2009;30(9):1799–803.

27. Hoffmann C, Weisz B, Lipitz S, et al. Regional apparent diffusion coefficient values in 3rd trimester fetal brain. Neuroradiology 2014;56(7):561–7.

28. Saksena S, Husain N, Das V, et al. Diffusion tensor imaging in the developing human cerebellum with histologic correlation. Int J Dev Neurosci 2008; 26(7):705–11.

29. Takahashi E, Hayashi E, Schmahmann JD, et al. Development of cerebellar connectivity in human fetal brains revealed by high angular resolution diffusion tractography. Neuroimage 2014;96:326–33.

30. Saksena S, Husain N, Malik GK, et al. Comparative evaluation of the cerebral and cerebellar white matter development in pediatric age group using quantitative diffusion tensor imaging. Cerebellum 2008; 7(3):392–400.

31. Leitner Y, Travis KE, Ben-Shachar M, et al. Tract profiles of the cerebellar white matter pathways in children and adolescents. Cerebellum 2015;14(6): 613–23.

32. Brody BA, Kinney HC, Kloman AS, et al. Sequence of central nervous system myelination in human infancy. I. An autopsy study of myelination. J Neuropathol Exp Neurol 1987;46(3):283–301.

33. Barkovich AJ, Kjos BO, Jackson DE, et al. Normal maturation of the neonatal and infant brain: MR imaging at 1.5 T. Radiology 1988;166:173–80.

34. Spader HS, Ellermeier A, O'Muircheartaigh J, et al. Advances in myelin imaging with potential clinical application to pediatric imaging. Neurosurg Focus 2013;34(4):E9.

35. Deoni SC, Mercure E, Blasi A, et al. Mapping infant brain myelination with magnetic resonance imaging. J Neurosci 2011;31(2):784–91.

36. Dean DC 3rd, O'Muircheartaigh J, Dirks H, et al. Modeling healthy male white matter and myelin development: 3 through 60 months of age. Neuroimage 2014;84:742–52.

37. Stoodley CJ, Schmahmann JD. Functional topography in the human cerebellum: a meta-analysis of neuroimaging studies. Neuroimage 2009;44(2): 489–501.

38. Thomason ME, Brown JA, Dassanayake MT, et al. Intrinsic functional brain architecture derived from graph theoretical analysis in the human fetus. PLoS One 2014;9(5):e94423.

39. Smyser CD, Inder TE, Shimony JS, et al. Longitudinal analysis of neural network development in preterm infants. Cereb Cortex 2010;20(12):2852–62.

40. Smyser CD, Snyder AZ, Neil JJ. Functional connectivity MRI in infants: exploration of the functional organization of the developing brain. Neuroimage 2011;56(3):1437–52.

41. Damaraju E, Caprihan A, Lowe JR, et al. Functional connectivity in the developing brain: a longitudinal study from 4 to 9months of age. Neuroimage 2014; 84:169–80.

42. Khan AJ, Nair A, Keown CL, et al. Cerebro-cerebellar resting-state functional connectivity in children and adolescents with autism spectrum disorder. Biol Psychiatry 2015;78(9):625–34.

43. O'Reilly JX, Beckmann CF, Tomassini V, et al. Distinct and overlapping functional zones in the cerebellum defined by resting state functional connectivity. Cereb Cortex 2010;20(4):953–65.

44. Dezortova M, Hajek M. (1)H MR spectroscopy in pediatrics. Eur J Radiol 2008;67(2):240–9.

45. Costa MO, Lacerda MT, Garcia Otaduy MC, et al. Proton magnetic resonance spectroscopy: normal findings in the cerebellar hemisphere in childhood. Pediatr Radiol 2002;32(11):787–92.

Cerebellar and Brainstem Malformations

Andrea Poretti, MD[a,b,*], Eugen Boltshauser, MD[b], Thierry A.G.M. Huisman, MD, EQNR, FICIS[a]

KEYWORDS

• Malformation • Cerebellum • Brain stem • Neuroimaging • Diffusion tensor imaging • Children

KEY POINTS

• Progress in neuroimaging and genetics in the last decades has led to a significant improvement/refinement in the definition of cerebellar and brainstem malformations.

• Neuroimaging plays a key role in the diagnostic work-up of children with cerebellar and brainstem malformations.

• Diagnostic criteria of cerebellar and brainstem malformations are mostly based on neuroimaging findings.

• Neuroimaging findings may elucidate the role of the cerebellum for neurocognitive functions in children with cerebellar malformations and serve as predictive biomarkers for cognitive outcome.

• Advanced neuroimaging techniques such as diffusion tensor imaging may provide additional information that is helpful to better understand the pathogenesis of selected cerebellar and brainstem malformations.

INTRODUCTION

In the last few decades, progress in neuroimaging techniques, genetic analysis, and mouse model research has led to a significant improvement in the definition of cerebellar and brainstem malformations as well as in the recognition of novel disorders. Classifications based on neuroimaging, molecular genetic criteria, and developmental biological criteria have been proposed and include both inherited (developmental) and acquired (disruptive) anomalies.[1–4]

Malformations are defined as nonprogressive, congenital morphologic anomalies of a single organ or body part caused by an alteration of the primary developmental program.[5] Malformations result from intrinsic developmental processes, which refer to the cellular and molecular pathways involved in organogenesis. The molecules in these pathways can be altered by gene mutations, teratogens, or combined effects. The complex development of the cerebellum and brainstem and the high number of involved genes result in a high number of malformations.

Neuroimaging plays a key role in the diagnostic work-up of posterior fossa malformations.[2–4] Diagnostic criteria for posterior fossa malformations are based on neuroimaging findings. For some posterior fossa malformations, the spectrum of neuroimaging findings has been shown to explain the cognitive outcome (eg, in Dandy-Walker malformation [DWM] and rhombencephalosynapsis).[6,7] In addition, the spectrum of neuroimaging findings may suggest the

Disclosure: The authors have nothing to disclose.
[a] Section of Pediatric Neuroradiology, Division of Pediatric Radiology, The Russell H. Morgan Department of Radiology and Radiological Science, Charlotte R. Bloomberg Children's Center, The Johns Hopkins School of Medicine, Sheikh Zayed Tower, Room 4174, 1800 Orleans Street, Baltimore, MD 21287-0842, USA;
[b] Department of Pediatric Neurology, University Children's Hospital, Steinwiesstrasse 75, Zurich 8032, Switzerland
* Corresponding author. Section of Pediatric Neuroradiology, Division of Pediatric Radiology, The Russell H. Morgan Department of Radiology and Radiological Science, Charlotte R. Bloomberg Children's Center, The Johns Hopkins School of Medicine, Sheikh Zayed Tower, Room 4174, 1800 Orleans Street, Baltimore, MD 21287-0842.
E-mail address: aporett1@jhmi.edu

Neuroimag Clin N Am 26 (2016) 341–357
http://dx.doi.org/10.1016/j.nic.2016.03.005
1052-5149/16/$ – see front matter © 2016 Elsevier Inc. All rights reserved.

underlying genotype (eg, in pontocerebellar hypoplasias [PCHs]).[8] Conventional magnetic resonance (MR) imaging, including two-dimensional and three-dimensional T1-weighted, T2-weighted, and fluid attenuated inversion recovery (FLAIR) sequences, plays a key role in the evaluation/characterization of posterior fossa malformations and many diagnostic criteria have been based on conventional MR imaging findings.[2,3] In the last decade, advanced MR imaging techniques became increasingly available in the clinical setting and have been applied to explore posterior fossa malformations in more detail.[4,9] Diffusion tensor imaging (DTI) has been shown to provide noninvasive detailed qualitative and quantitative information on white matter tracts in children with brain malformations.[4,9] In addition, the detailed internal neuroarchitectural exploration of the brain by DTI has allowed clinicians to elucidate certain aspects of the pathogenesis of selected posterior fossa malformations, such as Joubert syndrome (JS) and pontine tegmental cap dysplasia (PTCD).[10,11]

This article discusses the normal anatomy of the posterior fossa followed by a discussion of the characteristic neuroimaging features of a variety of cerebellar and brainstem malformations. In this context, we classify posterior fossa malformations based on the neuroimaging pattern into (1) predominantly cerebellar, (2) cerebellar and brainstem, and (3) predominantly brainstem malformations as previously suggested.[2,3]

NORMAL ANATOMY OF THE POSTERIOR FOSSA

Conventional MR imaging sequences allow detailed evaluation of the anatomy of the posterior fossa and its contents.[2,3] A midline sagittal T1-weighted or T2-weighted sequence is ideal for showing the size of the posterior fossa, the shape and size of the vermis, and the size and morphology of the fourth ventricle and brainstem (Fig. 1). The vermis is divided into 3 parts by the primary and prepyramidal fissures. The rostrocaudal length of the ventral pons should be approximately twice that of the midbrain from the isthmus (ventral midbrain-pons junction) to the third ventricle, whereas the rostrocaudal length of the midbrain should be roughly the same as that of the medulla (from the level of the obex to the level of the ventral pontomedullary junction).[2,3] The posterior margin of the brainstem extending from the caudal sylvian aqueduct to the obex should be a straight line. The fastigium, or summit of the fourth ventricle, should lie just below the midpoint of the ventral pons on sagittal images. The cerebellar hemispheres and peduncles can be well assessed on parasagittal images, whereas the size and morphology of the vermis, cerebellar hemispheres, dentate nuclei, and superior and middle cerebellar peduncles can be best evaluated on axial images. In addition, the cerebellar folia run parallel to the calvaria (onionlike configuration) (see Fig. 1). Coronal images show fissures

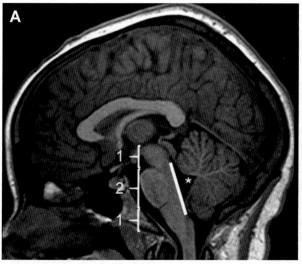
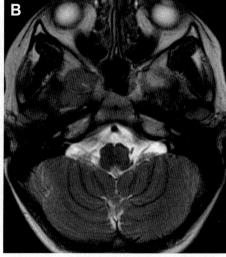

Fig. 1. Normal anatomy of the posterior fossa in a 12-year-old boy. (A) Midsagittal T1-weighted MR image shows a normal-sized posterior fossa, a normal vermis, an appropriate-sized pons (the rostrocaudal length of the pons is approximately twice [2] that of the midbrain [1] and medulla [1]), a flat dorsal surface of the brainstem (line), and a normal position of the fastigium just below the midpoint of the ventral pons (asterisk). (B) Axial T2-weighted MR image of the posterior fossa shows normal orientation of the cerebellar folia, which run parallel to the calvaria (onionlike orientation).

radiating toward the cerebellar nuclei. In addition, the superior, middle, and inferior cerebellar peduncles can be assessed in terms of size, symmetry, contour, and location.

PREDOMINANTLY CEREBELLAR MALFORMATIONS
Dandy-Walker Malformation

DWM is the most common posterior fossa malformation, and occurs mainly sporadically, with a low overall risk of recurrence (1%–5%).[2] DWM may be isolated or may be part of numerous chromosomal anomalies or well-defined mendelian disorders. Recently, genetic studies suggested that mutations resulting in dysgenesis of both the cerebellum and its overlying mesenchyme are likely to be needed to cause a DWM.[12]

Most children with DWM present before 1 year of age with signs and symptoms of increased intracranial pressure.[13] Macrocephaly is the most common manifestation, affecting 90% to 100% of children during the first months of life. Nowadays the diagnosis of DWM is made by fetal MR imaging in an increasing number of children.

The key neuroimaging features of DWM are (1) hypoplasia (or, rarely, agenesis) of the cerebellar vermis (of which the inferior portion is typically affected, possibly in combination with its superior portion), which is elevated and counterclockwise rotated; and (2) dilatation of the cystic-appearing

fourth ventricle, which may fill most of the posterior fossa (Fig. 2).[14] The cerebellar hemispheres are typically hypoplastic and displaced anterolaterally. The posterior fossa is usually enlarged, and the tentorium, the torcular Herophili, and transverse sinuses are elevated. Additional malformations, including callosal dysgenesis or agenesis, occipital encephalocele, polymicrogyria, and heterotopia, are present in 30% to 50% of patients. Hydrocephalus is associated with DWM in about 90% of children.

Neuroimaging allows the differentiation of DWM from other cystic posterior fossa malformations, such as Blake pouch cyst (BPC), posterior fossa arachnoid cyst (PFAC), and mega cisterna magna (MCM) (Fig. 3, Table 1).[15] BPC is characterized by a retrocerebellar or infraretrocerebellar cyst that directly communicates with the fourth ventricle, likely secondary to a deficient opening of the foramen of Magendie during development. The choroid plexus is displaced inferior to the vermis, and is best visualized in a sagittal T1-weighted postcontrast image. The absence of communication between the fourth ventricle and subarachnoid space results in a tetraventricular hydrocephalus. Mild mass effect may cause indentation of the inferior vermis and cerebellar hemispheres, but these are globally normal. PFAC may be located inferior or posterior to the vermis (retrocerebellar), cranial to the vermis (supravermian), anterior or lateral to the cerebellar hemispheres, or anterior to the brainstem.

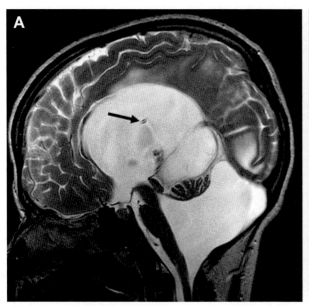
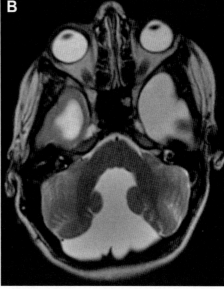

Fig. 2. DWM. (A) Midsagittal and (B) axial T2-weighted images of a child with a DWM show hypoplasia, elevation, and upward rotation of the cerebellar vermis, cystic dilatation of the fourth ventricle extending posteriorly, enlargement of the posterior fossa, mild hypoplasia and anterolateral displacement of the cerebellar hemispheres, and marked ventriculomegaly. A ventriculoperitoneal shunt is noted (arrow). Incidental note is made of a left middle cranial fossa arachnoid cyst.

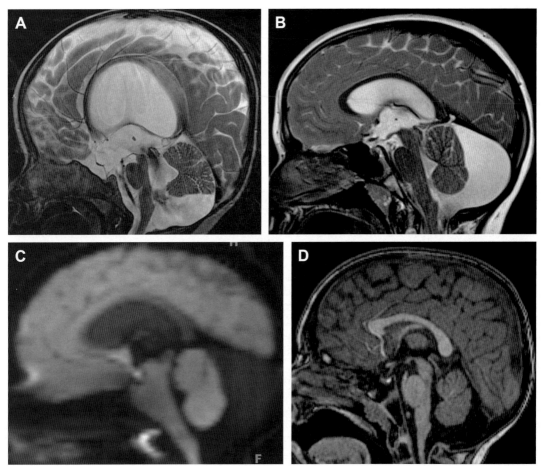

Fig. 3. Cystic malformations of the posterior fossa. (*A*) Midsagittal T2-weighted MR image of a child with a Blake pouch cyst shows enlargement of the fourth ventricle, which communicates with an infravermian cystic compartment corresponding with a Blake pouch cyst, a normal vermis, and tetraventricular hydrocephalus. Cerebrospinal fluid (CSF) flow–related signal void is noted within the region of the sylvian aqueduct and at the level of the widened foramen of Magendie. Significant supratentorial ventriculomegaly is also present. (*B*) Midsagittal T2-weighted MR image and (*C*) midsagittal trace of diffusion maps of a child with a retrovermian arachnoid cyst reveals a CSF isointense cyst with similar diffusion properties to the ventricular system, apparent enlargement of the posterior fossa, scalloping of the occipital bone, mass effect on the dorsal aspect of a normal-appearing vermis, a normal fourth ventricle, and mild supratentorial hydrocephalus. (*D*) Midsagittal T1-weighted MR image of a child with MCM shows a normal vermis, a normal fourth ventricle, a normal posterior fossa, and the absence of hydrocephalus. (*From* [*A*, *B*, *D*] Bosemani T, Orman G, Boltshauser E, et al. Congenital abnormalities of the posterior fossa. Radiographics 2015;35(1):205; with permission.)

Table 1
Key distinguishing neuroimaging findings in DWM and other posterior fossa cystic malformations

Disease	Vermis Size	IV. Ventricle Size	Posterior Fossa Size	Hydrocephalus
DWM	Hypoplastic	Enlarged	Enlarged	Yes (most patients)
BPC	Normal	Enlarged	Normal	Yes
MCM	Normal	Normal	Inconsistently enlarged	No
PFAC	Normal	Normal or reduced	Normal	Possible

Neuroimaging shows a well-circumscribed extra-axial fluid collection, which is isointense to cerebrospinal fluid (CSF) on T2-weighted imaging, may have a slightly higher signal on FLAIR imaging or apparent diffusion coefficient maps because of a higher internal protein content, and does not communicate with the fourth ventricle or subarachnoid space. PFAC may enlarge and produce mass effect on the cerebellum causing hydrocephalus. In addition, remodeling, scalloping, or thinning of the overlying occipital bone may be observed. MCM is an enlarged cisterna magna (≥10-mm diameter on midsagittal images) with an intact vermis and normal fourth ventricle.[16] MCM freely communicates with the fourth ventricle and cervical subarachnoid space, and consequently hydrocephalus is consistently absent. MCM is mostly an incidental finding without clinical relevance.

Rhombencephalosynapsis

Rhombencephalosynapsis is most likely caused by a dorsoventral patterning defect in the rostral dorsal midline regions of rhombomere 1.[4] The genetic basis is still unknown. The sporadic nature of rhombencephalosynapsis contributes to its low recurrence risk.

Most patients are nonsyndromic and present with truncal and/or limb ataxia, abnormal eye movements, head stereotypies, and delayed motor development.[17] In some patients, rhombencephalosynapsis is a key feature of Gómez-López-Hernández syndrome (parietal alopecia, trigeminal anesthesia, and craniofacial dysmorphic signs) or may be seen in VACTERL (Vertebral anomalies, Anal atresia, Cardiac defects, Tracheoesophageal fistula and/or Esophageal atresia, Renal anomalies, and Limb defects) association.[7,18] Long-term cognitive outcome varies from severe impairment to normal cognition. Severe rhombencephalosynapsis, associated holoprosencephaly, or VACTERL features are poor prognostic factors.[7] Systemic involvement is uncommon.

The key neuroimaging findings in rhombencephalosynapsis are agenesis or hypogenesis of the vermis and continuity of the cerebellar hemispheres, dentate nuclei, and often superior cerebellar peduncles (SCP) (Fig. 4). The horizontal folial pattern of the cerebellar hemisphere is best seen on posterior coronal T2-weighted images, whereas axial and sagittal images show the dentate nuclei in the midline (in normal anatomy, the dentate nuclei are separated by the vermis and are consequently off midline). In addition, on midsagittal images the primary fissure is not identified. Rhombencephalosynapsis may be associated with other central nervous system anomalies such as hydrocephalus, mostly because of stenosis of the sylvian aqueduct and forebrain abnormalities, including absent olfactory bulbs, callosal dysgenesis, absent septum pellucidum, and, in rare cases, holoprosencephaly.[7,19]

Cerebellar Dysplasia and Cerebellar Cysts

Cerebellar dysplasia is characterized by abnormal cerebellar foliation and fissuration, white matter arborization, and an abnormal gray-white matter junction.[20] It is a nonspecific feature associated with several different conditions (Table 2) including Chudley-McCullough syndrome,[21] bilateral frontoparietal polymicrogyria caused by GPR56 mutations,[22] Poretti-Boltshauser syndrome caused by LAMA1 mutations,[23,24] and tubulinopathies.[25] In most patients, however, the cause remains unknown. Multiple mechanisms underlie cerebellar

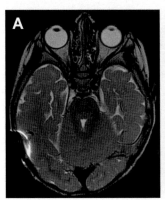
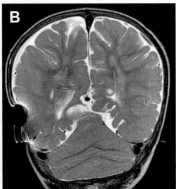
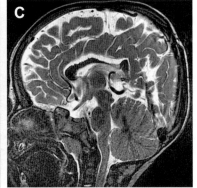

Fig. 4. Rhombencephalosynapsis. (A) Axial, (B) coronal, and (C) midsagittal T2-weighted MR images of a child with rhombencephalosynapsis show continuity of the cerebellar hemispheres, fused dentate nuclei, and SCP without an intervening vermis. Note the keyhole appearance of the fourth ventricle. The cerebellar folia have an abnormal transverse orientation. The dentate nuclei are seen on a midline sagittal image. The ventricles are decompressed after ventriculoperitoneal shunting.

Table 2
Clinical and neuroimaging characteristics of cerebellar dysplasias with known genetic causes

Disease	Genes	Dysplasia Pattern	Distinguishing Features
Chudley-McCullough syndrome	GPSM2	Dysplastic inferior hemispheres	Hearing loss, frontal PMG, heterotopia, partial callosal agenesis
Alpha-dystroglycanopathies	>15 genes	Global cerebellar dysplasia with multiple cysts	Cobblestone brain, brainstem kinking, muscle and eye involvement, increased creatine kinase level
GPR56-related PMG and cerebellar dysplasia	GPR56	Global cerebellar dysplasia with multiple cysts	Bifrontal PMG, T2/FLAIR hyperintense signal of the supratentorial white matter
Poretti-Boltshauser syndrome	LAMA1	Global cerebellar dysplasia with multiple cysts	High myopia, retinal abnormality
Tubulinopathies	TUBA1A, TUBA8, TUBB2B, TUBB3, TUBB5	Diagonal folia across vermis in axial view	Dysmorphic basal ganglia, cortical malformation (PMG to lissencephaly), callosal dysgenesis, asymmetric brainstem
JS	>30 genes	Dysplastic superior vermis and hemispheres	Molar tooth sign

Abbreviation: PMG, polymicrogyria.

dysplasia, including abnormal precursor cell division and neuronal migration. In particular, alpha-dystroglycanopathies, Poretti-Boltshauser syndrome (*LAMA1* mutations), and *GPR56*-associated cerebellar dysplasia are thought to be caused by basement membrane defects that result in abnormal neuronal migration. Chudley-McCullough syndrome is caused by recessive mutations in *GPSM2*, which encodes a GTPase regulator needed for correct orientation of stem-cell division. In some patients, cerebellar dysplasia may be focal and located only in 1 cerebellar hemisphere of reduced volume.[26] A prenatal acquired (disruptive) origin is assumed in view of the focal nature and hemorrhages on fetal MR imaging studies.

The clinical presentation is highly variable and mostly depends on the underlying disease. Isolated cerebellar dysplasia may be an incidental finding or cause severe neurologic impairment.

The key neuroimaging findings of cerebellar dysplasia are abnormal foliation, fissuration (including defective, enlarged, or vertical fissures), white matter arborization, and an obscured gray matter–white matter junction (**Fig. 5**).[3] Cerebellar dysplasia may be associated with a variety of other cerebellar (eg, cerebellar cysts) and supratentorial (eg, polymicrogyria, partial callosal agenesis, and dysmorphic basal ganglia) findings that are usually helpful to differentiate between the causative diseases.

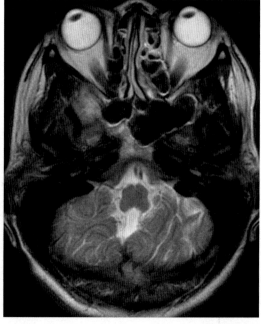

Fig. 5. Cerebellar dysplasia. Axial T2-weighted MR image of a 17-year-old girl reveals abnormal cerebellar foliation and fissuration with loss of the normal white matter architecture in the inferior aspect of the cerebellar hemispheres.

Cerebellar cysts (**Fig. 6**) are uncommon findings in pediatric neuroimaging and may be seen in selected disorders with both malformative and disruptive causes (**Table 3**).[20]

CEREBELLAR AND BRAINSTEM MALFORMATIONS
Pontocerebellar Hypoplasia

The term PCH is often used in a descriptive manner to refer to diseases characterized by reduction in volume of both cerebellum and pons. However, PCH has also been used to refer to a group of autosomal recessive neurodegenerative disorders with prenatal onset as conceptualized by Peter Barth.[27] Accordingly, some PCH types do not represent a malformation (eg, types 1, 2, 4, and 6). To date, 10 subtypes of PCH with different phenotypes and pathogeneses (types 3 and 8 have a nonprogressive course) have been identified (**Table 4**).

Hypoplasia with superimposed atrophy of the cerebellum and absence or significant reduction of the pontine prominence are characteristic findings of PCH (**Fig. 7**).[8] In some cases of PCH (particularly type 2 caused by mutations in *TSEN54*), there is more severe involvement of the cerebellar hemispheres compared with the vermis that is best seen on coronal images (dragonfly appearance created by flattened cerebellar hemispheres and a preserved vermis).[8] The structure of the cerebellar hemispheres seems to be melting and may result in the formation of cavitations (cysts) representing the degenerative nature. Variable cerebral involvement, including atrophy and delayed myelination, may be present.

Mutations in the *CASK*, *RELN*, and *VLDLR* genes may also result in severe cerebellar hypoplasia with pontine hypoplasia. Compared with some of the types of PCH described earlier, PCH caused by mutations in *CASK*, *RELN*, and *VLDLR* represents a malformation. *CASK* encodes a multidomain

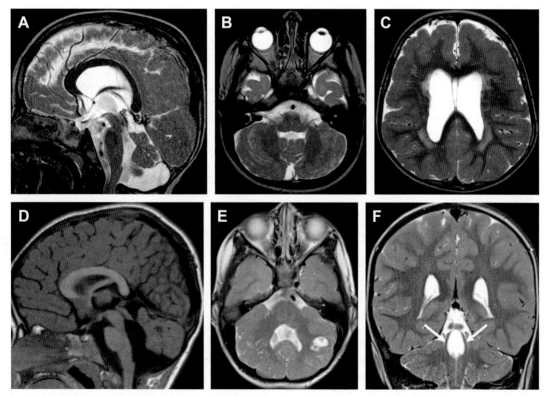

Fig. 6. Cerebellar cysts. (*A*) Midsagittal and (*B, C*) axial T2-weighted MR images of a 3.5-year-old boy with *GPR56* mutations show multiple cysts along the cerebellar fissures and dysplasia of the cerebellar vermis and posterior parts of the cerebellar hemispheres, bilateral migration abnormality, hyperintense signal of the periventricular white matter, and mild ventriculomegaly. (*D*) Midsagittal T1-weighted, (*E*) axial T2-weighted, and (*F*) coronal T2-weighted MR images of a 1.5-year-old girl with *LAMA1* mutations reveal an enlarged, elongated, and square-like formed fourth ventricle, dysplasia, and multiple cortical-subcortical cysts within the cerebellar vermis and both cerebellar hemispheres, and splayed SCP (*arrows*). (*From* [*B, C*] Boltshauser E, Scheer I, Huisman TA, et al. Cerebellar cysts in children: a pattern recognition approach. Cerebellum 2015;14(3):311; with permission.)

Table 3
Differential diagnosis of cerebellar cyst in children

Subgroups		Cause	Comments
Normal structure	Cystic PVS	Mucopolysaccharidosis	Mostly type I + II, rare type III
Isolated cysts		Neuroglial cysts	
Destructive cyst		PCH	Types 1, 2, 6
Malformative		Aicardi syndrome	
		GPR56 related	
		Congenital muscular dystrophies	Mostly alpha-dystroglycanopathy (eg, FKRP, POMT2, LARGE, POMGnT1) Rarely LAMA2 related
		LAMA1 related	
Cerebellar dysplasia		Genetic	Cohen syndrome (rare)
		Unknown pathogenesis (genetic vs acquired)	Diffuse, bilateral dysplasia + cysts
		Disruptive	Focal dysplasia + cysts
Miscellaneous		Leukoencephalopathy with calcifications and cysts Early-onset multiple carboxylase deficiency	

Abbreviation: PVS, perivascular space.

Adapted from Boltshauser E, Scheer I, Huisman TA, et al. Cerebellar cysts in children: a pattern recognition approach. Cerebellum 2015;14(3):309; with permission.

scaffolding protein that regulates expression of genes involved in cortical development, such as RELN.[28] CASK mutations are inherited with an X-linked pattern, occur de novo, and more commonly affect female patients, presumably because they are lethal in male patients. Children with CASK mutations present with ataxia, nystagmus, postnatal microcephaly, severe cognitive impairment, seizures, retinopathy, sensorineural hearing loss, and (inconsistently) cataracts.[29] In patients with CASK mutations, involvement of the cerebellar hemispheres and vermis is usually symmetric, but a dragonfly appearance may also occur (**Fig. 8**).[30] In addition, a simplified gyral pattern involving the

Table 4
PCH subtypes

PCH Subtype	Main Findings	Genotype
PCH1	Anterior horn cells involvement	VRK1, TSEN54, RARS2, EXOSC3
PCH2	Chorea/dystonia, rarely spasticity only	TSEN54 >> TSEN2, TSEN34
PCH3	Optic atrophy; nonprogressive course	PCLO
PCH4	Severe neonatal course with hypertonia and hypoventilation, contractures	TSEN54
PCH5	Lethal course in neonatal period; involvement vermis >> hemispheres	TSEN54
PCH6	Lactic acidemia, high lactate level in CSF (not consistent)	RARS2
PCH7	No palpable gonads with a micropenis	Unknown
PCH8	Proportionate involvement of vermis and hemispheres; nonprogressive course	CHMP1A
PCH9	Dysgenesis of the corpus callosum	AMPD2
PCH10	Dysmorphic features and axonal sensorimotor neuropathy (inconsistent)	CLP1

Adapted from Bosemani T, Orman G, Boltshauser E, et al. Congenital abnormalities of the posterior fossa. Radiographics 2015;35(1):210; with permission.

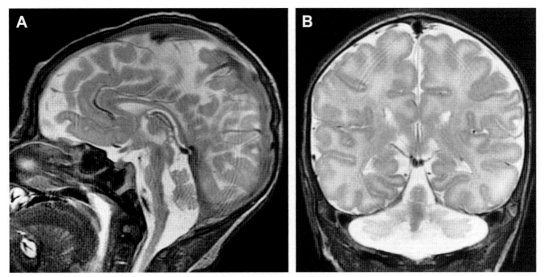

Fig. 7. PCH. (A) Midsagittal and (B) coronal T2-weighted MR images of a child with PCH type 2 and *TSEN54* mutations show hypoplasia of the pons and cerebellum with more severe involvement of the cerebellar hemispheres compared with the vermis (dragonfly appearance). The structure of the cerebellar hemispheres appears to be melting, representing the degenerative nature of the disease. A microcephaly and thin corpus callosum is also noted.

frontal lobes and unmyelinated corpus callosum may be seen in some patients. *RELN* encodes an extracellular matrix–associated glycoprotein (reelin) that is critical for the regulation of neuronal migration during cortical and cerebellar development.[31] Affected children show severe developmental disabilities, microcephaly, seizures, and congenital lymphedema. *VLDLR* encodes the very-low-density lipoprotein receptor, which acts as a coreceptor for the reelin pathway. *VLDLR*-associated PCH is characterized by nonprogressive cerebellar ataxia, moderate to profound intellectual disability, dysarthria, strabismus, and seizures.[32] In patients with *RELN*-related and *VLDLR*-related PCH, mild frontal pachygyria (more severe in patients with *RELN* mutations) and marked cerebellar hypoplasia with more severe involvement of the vermis compared with the

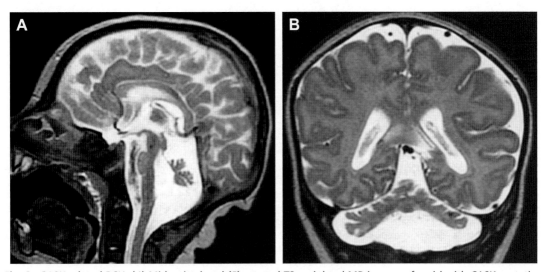

Fig. 8. *CASK*-related PCH. (A) Midsagittal and (B) coronal T2-weighted MR images of a girl with CASK mutation reveal hypoplasia of the pons and cerebellum with proportionate involvement of the cerebellar hemispheres compared with the vermis. The signal intensity of the cerebellar hemispheres is normal (in contrast with PCH 2, as seen in Fig. 7). A microcephaly is also noted.

hemispheres and absent cerebellar folia (more severe in patients with *VLDLR* mutations) are characteristic neuroimaging features.

Congenital Muscular Dystrophies Caused by Defective Alpha-dystroglycan Glycosylation

Alpha-dystroglycanopathies are a group of congenital muscular dystrophies resulting from mutations in more than 15 genes responsible for the O-glycosylation and rarely N-glycosylation of alpha-dystroglycan.[33] Recessive mutations in these genes cause overlapping phenotypes characterized by muscle (weakness, hypotonia, and increased creatine kinase values), brain (intellectual disability, seizures, and tetraspasticity), and eye (microphthalmia, optic nerve hypoplasia, chorioretinal coloboma, cataract, glaucoma, or high myopia) involvement. Based on the severity of the findings, different phenotypes have been described (in order of increasing severity): Fukuyama congenital muscular dystrophy, muscle-eye-brain disease, and Walker-Warburg syndrome.

Infratentorial neuroimaging findings include PCH, cerebellar dysplasia with cysts, dysplastic tectum, ventral pontine cleft, and pontomesencephalic kinking (**Fig. 9**).[34] The cerebellar cysts represent small areas of pia and subarachnoid space herniating inward through gaps in the pial limiting membrane. Supratentorial findings range from mild ventriculomegaly, diffuse periventricular white matter changes, and focal areas of polymicrogyria to severe hydrocephalus, generalized white matter signal changes, and diffuse cortical abnormalities, including cobblestone cortex.[34]

Tubulinopathies

Tubulinopathies are a recently reported group of brain malformations caused by mutations in genes

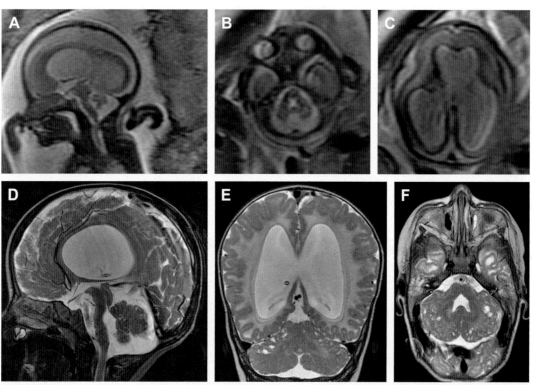

Fig. 9. Alpha-dystroglycanopathy. (*A*) Midsagittal and (*B* and *C*) axial T2-weighted MR images of a 25-week-old fetus with muscle-eye-brain disease and *POMGnT1* mutations show marked enlargement of the lateral ventricles, mild dilatation of the third ventricle, a small fourth ventricle, an abnormal kinking of the brainstem with an elongated and dysplastic midbrain and tectum, as well as thinned pons. (*D*) Midsagittal, (*E*) coronal, and (*F*) axial T2-weighted MR images of the same child at 5 months of age show cerebellar hypoplasia and dysplasia with multiple bilateral subcortical cysts in the cerebellar hemispheres, flattening of the ventral pons, a dysmorphic tectum and midbrain, an abnormal concave posterior border of the brainstem (cleft), an enlarged fourth ventricle, generalized polymicrogyria, abnormal signal intensity of the supratentorial white matter, absence of the septum pellucidum, and supratentorial ventriculomegaly. (*From* [*A–C*] Amir T, Poretti A, Boltshauser E, et al. Differential diagnosis of ventriculomegaly and brainstem kinking on fetal MR images. Brain Dev 2016;38(1):105, with permission; and [*D–F*] Poretti A, Boltshauser E, Doherty D. Cerebellar hypoplasia: differential diagnosis and diagnostic approach. Am J Med Genet 2014;166(2):220, with permission.)

involved in microtubule formation and function (*TUBA1A*, *TUBA8*, *TUBB2B*, *TUBB3*, and *TUBB5*).[35] Most mutations in tubulin genes are de novo, but germline mosaicism and autosomal recessive inheritance have been observed.

The clinical presentation of children with tubulinopathies is wide and includes intellectual disability, tetraspastic cerebral palsy, postnatal microcephaly, and early onset of therapy-resistant seizures.[36] Dysmorphic features are rare and other organs are not affected.

The neuroimaging phenotype is also broad and overlaps between the different genetic causes (**Fig. 10**).[36] Cortical malformations include lissencephaly (usually with an anterior-to-posterior gradient) and polymicrogyria (generalized, asymmetric with left-side preponderance, or only in the perisylvian region). A dysmorphic appearance of the basal ganglia (mostly putamen and caudate) with absence of the anterior limb of the internal capsule is the most characteristic and consistent finding. Ventriculomegaly with abnormal shape of the frontal horns and agenesis/dysgenesis of the corpus callosum and anterior commissure have also been described. Posterior fossa involvement includes different degrees of PCH, cerebellar and tectal dysplasia, and asymmetric midbrain and pons.[35] Cerebellar dysplasia especially involves the superior part of the vermis with diagonal folia (folia crossing the midline at an oblique angle), best visible at the midline on axial images.[25]

In tubulinopathies, DTI and fiber tractography (FT) studies revealed anomalies of several white matter tracts.[37] The anterior commissure is usually missing and fornices may be thin or have a more distant or flattened course. In the posterior fossa, the transverse pontine fibers (TPF) may be markedly thin and have a more slanting course. In addition, the corticospinal tracts (CST) may also be thin and asymmetric in size. All these findings suggest a role of tubulin genes in axonal pathfinding. So far, axonal guidance defects have been associated with mutations in *TUBB3*.[38]

Joubert Syndrome

JS is a midhindbrain malformation with extreme genetic heterogeneity (more than 30 genes have been identified as of April 2016).[39] Mutations in all the genes but OFD1 are autosomal recessively inherited, which results in a recurrence risk of 25%. All genes encode for proteins that localize to primary, nonmotile cilia, which play key roles in the development and functioning of the brain, retina, kidney, liver, and other organs.[40] Primary cilia mediate various signaling processes and brain malformations in JS may result from defects in midline fusion of the developing vermis or defects in sonic hedgehog–mediated granule cell proliferation.[41,42]

Children with JS present with hypotonia, cerebellar ataxia, ocular motor apraxia, neonatal breathing dysregulation, and intellectual disability of variable severity. Systemic involvement may be present and includes kidneys (nephronophthisis), eyes (retinal dystrophy and colobomas), liver (congenital hepatic fibrosis), and skeleton (different forms of polydactyly).[43] Renal and liver involvement may cause high morbidity and mortality and needs appropriate work-up and regular

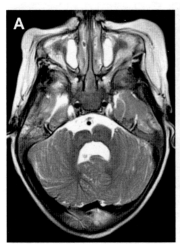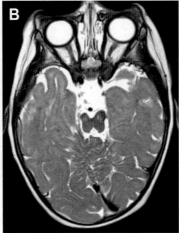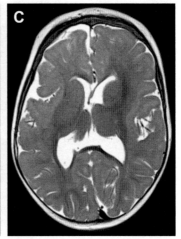

Fig. 10. Tubulinopathy. (*A–C*) Axial T2-weighted MR images of a 15-month-old child with *TUBA1A* mutation reveal marked asymmetry of the brainstem, cerebellar dysplasia involving mostly the superior part of the vermis, a dysmorphic appearance of the bilateral putamen and caudate nucleus with absence of the anterior limb of the internal capsule, and mild ventriculomegaly with abnormal shape of the frontal horns.

follow-up. Based on the systemic involvement, 6 phenotypes have been described.[39] The presence of tongue hamartoma, additional frenula, upper lip notch, mesoaxial polydactyly of 1 or more hands or feet, and/or hypothalamic hamartoma differentiate the oral-facial-digital syndrome type VI (OFDVI) from the other phenotypes.[44] Some degree of genotype-phenotype correlation has been shown. The strongest correlation is between mutations in *TMEM67* and liver involvement.[45]

The molar tooth sign (MTS) is the diagnostic criterion for JS and consists of elongated, thickened, and horizontally oriented SCPs and a deep interpeduncular fossa mimicking a molar tooth on axial imaging (**Fig. 11**). In addition, hypoplasia and dysplasia of the cerebellar vermis is a consistent finding in JS. The spectrum of neuroimaging findings goes beyond MTS and hypodysplasia of the vermis, confirming the heterogeneity of JS.[46] The degree of vermian hypoplasia, shape of the MTS, size of the posterior fossa, and shape and size of the cerebellar hemispheres are variable. Morphologic abnormalities of the brainstem are present in about 30% of patients and include a dysmorphic tectum and midbrain, thickening and elongation of the midbrain, and a small pons. Supratentorial involvement occurs in about 30% of patients and includes callosal dysgenesis, cephaloceles, hippocampal malrotation, migrational disorders, and ventriculomegaly. Neuroimaging is of limited value in classifying patients with JS. Differences in neuroimaging findings were reported in siblings and only a weak neuroimaging-genotype correlation was found.[46] Only the presence of a hypothalamic hamartoma differentiates between OFDVI and the other phenotypes.[44]

In JS, DTI and FT reveal absence of decussation of both the SCP and CST (see **Fig. 11**),[10] as previously shown by neuropathology.[47] JS is now considered an axonal guidance disorder.[48]

PREDOMINANT BRAINSTEM MALFORMATIONS
Pontine Tegmental Cap Dysplasia

PTCD is a rare sporadic brainstem malformation with unknown genotype and no familial recurrence. Children with PTCD present with hearing loss, facial paralysis, trigeminal anesthesia, difficulty in swallowing, and ataxia.[49] Systemic involvement with vertebral segmentation anomalies, rib malformations, and congenital heart defects has been observed. The intellectual prognosis seems to be highly variable, ranging from mild cognitive delay to severe disability.[49]

The conventional neuroimaging findings are pathognomonic and include a flattened ventral pons, vaulted pontine tegmentum (the cap), partial absence of the middle cerebellar peduncles (MCP), absence of the inferior cerebellar peduncles, vermian hypoplasia, a MTS-like aspect of the pontomesencephalic junction, and absent inferior olivary prominence (**Fig. 12**).[11,49] In addition, duplicated internal auditory canals and hypoplastic cranial nerves may be present.[50] The degree of brainstem dysplasia seems to correlate with the developmental disability: mildly affected patients tend to have a rounded bump

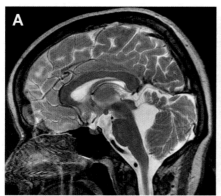
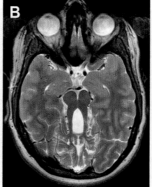
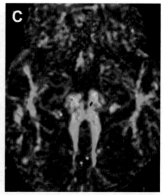

Fig. 11. JS. (*A*) Midsagittal and (*B*) axial T2-weighted MR images of a 5-year-old child with JS show the pathognomonic MTS characterized by elongated, thickened, and horizontally oriented SCP and a deepened interpeduncular fossa, hypoplasia and dysplasia of the vermis, enlargement of the fourth ventricle with upward and posterior displacement of the fastigium, and a narrow pontomesencephalic isthmus. (*C*) Axial color-coded fractional anisotropic (FA) map obtained at the level of the pontomesencephalic junction shows the horizontal orientation of the SCP (green) and the absence of decussation of the SCP (missing midline red dot). (*From* Bosemani T, Orman G, Boltshauser E, et al. Congenital abnormalities of the posterior fossa. Radiographics 2015;35(1):212; with permission.)

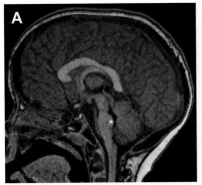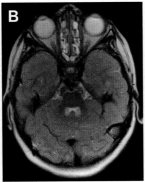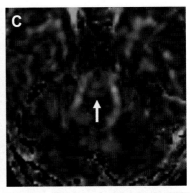

Fig. 12. PTCD. (*A*) Midsagittal T1-weighted and (*B*) axial T2-weighted MR images of a 3-year-old girl with PTCD reveal a flattened ventral pons, a cap covering the dorsal pons (*asterisk*) and protruding into the fourth ventricle, and bilateral hypoplastic MCP. (*C*) Axial color-coded FA map obtained at the level of the pons shows the absence of TPF in the ventral and middle pons, an ectopic band of fibers (horizontal orientation) dorsal to the pons (*arrow*), and small MCP (anteroposterior orientation). (*From* Bosemani T, Orman G, Boltshauser E, et al. Congenital abnormalities of the posterior fossa. Radiographics 2015;35(1):214; with permission.)

(the so-called cap) and those more severely affected tend to have a more angular brainstem protrusion (a so-called beak).[2]

In PTCD, DTI and FT revealed significant additional information regarding the possible pathogenesis. Axial color-coded fractional anisotropy (FA) maps show absence of the TPF and presence of a dorsal transverse axonal band at the level of the cap in the dorsal pons (see **Fig. 12**).[11] Misoriented fibers may be present and connect the basal pons to the cerebellar hemispheres through the MCP (peripontine arcuate fibers), some of which seemed to join the dorsal ectopic band.[51] The SCP decussation is typically missing.[11] The dorsal ectopic axonal band, ectopic peripontine arcuate fibers, and absence of SCP decussation most likely result from abnormal axonal guidance and/or neuronal migration and, to date, PTCD is consequently considered to be an axonal guidance disorder.[48]

Horizontal Gaze Palsy with Progressive Scoliosis

Horizontal gaze palsy with progressive scoliosis (HGPPS) is a rare autosomal recessive disorder caused by mutations in *ROBO3*, which encodes a receptor required for axonal guidance.[52] Children with HGPPS present with congenital absence of horizontal eye movements, preservation of vertical gaze and convergence, and progressive development of scoliosis in childhood.[53] Neurocognitive functions are typically preserved.

Neuroimaging findings are pathognomonic and include a butterfly-shaped medulla caused by the missing prominence of the gracile and cuneate nuclei, and prominent inferior olivary nuclei with respect to the medullary pyramids (**Fig. 13**).[54] In addition, the pons is hypoplastic and has a dorsal midline cleft with absence of the bulging contour of facial colliculi.[54]

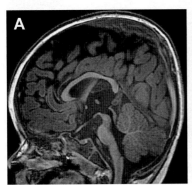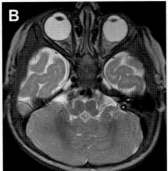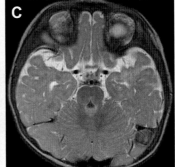

Fig. 13. HGPPS. (*A*) Midsagittal T1-weighted and (*B, C*) axial T2-weighted MR images of a child with HGPPS and *ROBO3* mutations reveal depression of the floor of the fourth ventricle, a butterfly medulla with more prominent inferior olivary nuclei compared with the pyramids, tent-shaped floor of the fourth ventricle with missing prominence of the cuneate and gracile nuclei, and a deep dorsal midline pontine cleft.

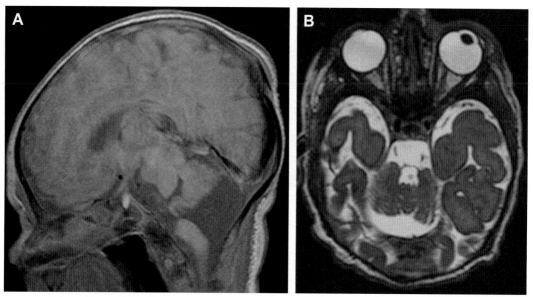

Fig. 14. Brainstem disconnection in a neonate. (*A*) Midsagittal T1-weighted and (*B*) axial T2-weighted MR images show absence of the lower pons with only a thin strand of tissue connecting the upper pons and lower medulla and hypoplasia of the cerebellum. In addition, the basilar artery is not visible. (*From* Poretti A, Boltshauser E, Plecko B. Brainstem disconnection: case report and reveiw of the literature. Neuropediatrics 2007;38(4):211; with permission.)

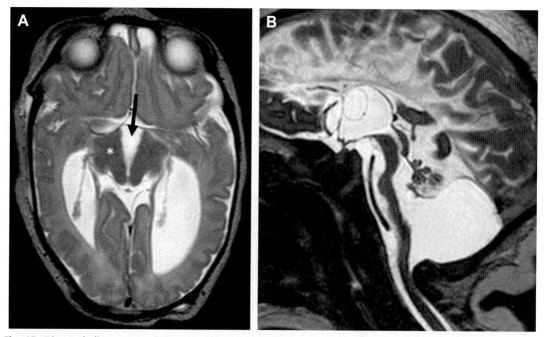

Fig. 15. Diencephalic-mesencephalic junction dysplasia in a newborn. (*A*) Axial T2-weighted MR image reveals reveal fusion of the hypothalamus and midbrain (*asterisk*), an enlargement of the dorsoventral axis of the midbrain, and ventral midbrain clefts (*arrow*) resulting in a butterflylike appearance. (*B*) Midsagittal T2-weighted MR image shows marked brainstem hypoplasia with predominant pontine and cerebellar involvement, elongated midbrain, and kinked bulbomedullary junction. In addition, the corpus callosum and anterior commissure are absent. (*Courtesy of* Drs Mariasavina Severino and Andrea Rossi, Neuroradiology Unit, Istituto Giannina Gaslini, Genova, Italy.)

In HGPPS, DTI and FT show a complete ipsilateral course of the CSTs without decussation at the level of the caudal medulla.[55] The sensorimotor tracts revealed only ipsilateral ascending fibers.[55] The uncrossed ascending course of the sensory tracts may result in lack of bilateral integration of proprioceptive stimuli and is considered to be responsible for the development of scoliosis.

Brainstem disconnection

Brainstem disconnection is a rare congenital anomaly that is defined by the nearly complete absence of a brainstem segment with intact rostral and caudal brainstem portions connected only by a thin cord of tissue (**Fig. 14**).[56] The pathogenesis is unknown. Both malformative and disruptive pathomechanisms have been proposed.

All children are symptomatic at birth, with absent or weak suck and swallowing, central respiratory insufficiency, increased or decreased muscle tone, and reduced or poor visual fixation.[56] Seizures and unstable body temperature may occur.[57] Most children die within the first 2 months after birth and do not achieve any developmental milestones.[57] Extracerebral involvement (congenital cardiac abnormalities, hydronephrosis, and vertebral body anomalies) may occur.[57]

The neuroimaging findings are pathognomonic and are best seen on sagittal images. Brainstem disconnection is consistently associated with cerebellar hypoplasia, whereas supratentorial abnormalities are unusual. The basilar artery is not seen in most patients.

Diencephalic-mesencephalic junction dysplasia

This new malformation is characterized by dysplasia of the diencephalic-mesencephalic junction with a butterflylike contour of the midbrain on axial images.[58,59] Severe cognitive impairment, postnatal progressive microcephaly, axial hypotonia, spastic tetraparesis, and seizures are consistent findings.

Brain MR imaging shows dysplasia of the diencephalic-mesencephalic junction with a characteristic butterflylike contour of the midbrain on axial images (**Fig. 15**). Additional neuroimaging features include variable degrees of supratentorial ventriculomegaly and callosal agenesis or hypoplasia. On axial color-coded FA maps and FT, the CST cannot be identified, suggesting a defect in axonal pathfinding.[58,59]

SUMMARY

Cerebellar and brainstem malformations represent a wide variety of disorders that may involve a single structure within the posterior fossa (eg, the cerebellum alone) or a combination of structures (eg, the pons and cerebellum). Neuroimaging yields detailed anatomic findings and plays a key role in the diagnosis of cerebellar and brainstem malformations. Well-defined neuroimaging-based diagnostic criteria are available for the various disorders and should be used. Accurate classification of cerebellar and brainstem malformations is important for therapy, prognosis, and genetic counseling. In addition, advanced neuroimaging, including DTI and FT, may provide important information about the pathogenesis and may serve as a biomarker for cognitive outcome in selected cerebellar and brainstem malformations.

REFERENCES

1. Barkovich AJ, Millen KJ, Dobyns WB. A developmental and genetic classification for midbrain-hindbrain malformations. Brain 2009;132(Pt 12):3199–230.
2. Doherty D, Millen KJ, Barkovich AJ. Midbrain and hindbrain malformations: advances in clinical diagnosis, imaging, and genetics. Lancet Neurol 2013; 12(4):381–93.
3. Bosemani T, Orman G, Boltshauser E, et al. Congenital abnormalities of the posterior fossa. Radiographics 2015;35(1):200–20.
4. Jissendi-Tchofo P, Severino M, Nguema-Edzang B, et al. Update on neuroimaging phenotypes of midhindbrain malformations. Neuroradiology 2015; 57(2):113–38.
5. Hennekam RC, Biesecker LG, Allanson JE, et al. Elements of morphology: general terms for congenital anomalies. Am J Med Genet A 2013;161A(11): 2726–33.
6. Boddaert N, Klein O, Ferguson N, et al. Intellectual prognosis of the Dandy-Walker malformation in children: the importance of vermian lobulation. Neuroradiology 2003;45(5):320–4.
7. Ishak GE, Dempsey JC, Shaw DW, et al. Rhombencephalosynapsis: a hindbrain malformation associated with incomplete separation of midbrain and forebrain, hydrocephalus and a broad spectrum of severity. Brain 2012;135(Pt 5):1370–86.
8. Namavar Y, Barth PG, Kasher PR, et al. Clinical, neuroradiological and genetic findings in pontocerebellar hypoplasia. Brain 2011;134(Pt 1):143–56.
9. Poretti A, Meoded A, Rossi A, et al. Diffusion tensor imaging and fiber tractography in brain malformations. Pediatr Radiol 2013;43(1):28–54.
10. Poretti A, Boltshauser E, Loenneker T, et al. Diffusion tensor imaging in Joubert syndrome. AJNR Am J Neuroradiol 2007;28(10):1929–33.
11. Jissendi-Tchofo P, Doherty D, McGillivray G, et al. Pontine tegmental cap dysplasia: MR imaging and diffusion tensor imaging features of impaired axonal navigation. AJNR Am J Neuroradiol 2009;30(1): 113–9.

12. Aldinger KA, Lehmann OJ, Hudgins L, et al. FOXC1 is required for normal cerebellar development and is a major contributor to chromosome 6p25.3 Dandy-Walker malformation. Nat Genet 2009;41(9):1037–42.

13. Alexiou GA, Sfakianos G, Prodromou N. Dandy-Walker malformation: analysis of 19 cases. J Child Neurol 2010;25(2):188–91.

14. Correa GG, Amaral LF, Vedolin LM. Neuroimaging of Dandy-Walker malformation: new concepts. Top Magn Reson Imaging 2011;22(6):303–12.

15. Nelson MD Jr, Maher K, Gilles FH. A different approach to cysts of the posterior fossa. Pediatr Radiol 2004;34(9):720–32.

16. Yildiz H, Yazici Z, Hakyemez B, et al. Evaluation of CSF flow patterns of posterior fossa cystic malformations using CSF flow MR imaging. Neuroradiology 2006;48(9):595–605.

17. Poretti A, Alber FD, Burki S, et al. Cognitive outcome in children with rhombencephalosynapsis. Eur J Paediatr Neurol 2009;13(1):28–33.

18. Sukhudyan B, Jaladyan V, Melikyan G, et al. Gómez-López-Hernández syndrome: reappraisal of the diagnostic criteria. Eur J Pediatr 2010;169(12):1523–8.

19. Whitehead MT, Choudhri AF, Grimm J, et al. Rhombencephalosynapsis as a cause of aqueductal stenosis: an under-recognized association in hydrocephalic children. Pediatr Radiol 2014;44(7):849–56.

20. Boltshauser E, Scheer I, Huisman TA, et al. Cerebellar cysts in children: a pattern recognition approach. Cerebellum 2015;14(3):308–16.

21. Doherty D, Chudley AE, Coghlan G, et al. GPSM2 mutations cause the brain malformations and hearing loss in Chudley-McCullough syndrome. Am J Hum Genet 2012;90(6):1088–93.

22. Bahi-Buisson N, Poirier K, Boddaert N, et al. GPR56-related bilateral frontoparietal polymicrogyria: further evidence for an overlap with the cobblestone complex. Brain 2010;133(11):3194–209.

23. Poretti A, Hausler M, von Moers A, et al. Ataxia, intellectual disability, and ocular apraxia with cerebellar cysts: a new disease? Cerebellum 2014;13(1):79–88.

24. Aldinger KA, Mosca SJ, Tetreault M, et al. Mutations in LAMA1 cause cerebellar dysplasia and cysts with and without retinal dystrophy. Am J Hum Genet 2014;95(2):227–34.

25. Oegema R, Cushion TD, Phelps IG, et al. Recognizable cerebellar dysplasia associated with mutations in multiple tubulin genes. Hum Mol Genet 2015;24(18):5313–25.

26. Poretti A, Leventer RJ, Cowan FM, et al. Cerebellar cleft: a form of prenatal cerebellar disruption. Neuropediatrics 2008;39(2):106–12.

27. Namavar Y, Barth PG, Poll-The BT, et al. Classification, diagnosis and potential mechanisms in pontocerebellar hypoplasia. Orphanet J Rare Dis 2011;6:50.

28. Najm J, Horn D, Wimplinger I, et al. Mutations of CASK cause an X-linked brain malformation phenotype with microcephaly and hypoplasia of the brainstem and cerebellum. Nat Genet 2008;40(9):1065–7.

29. Moog U, Kutsche K, Kortum F, et al. Phenotypic spectrum associated with CASK loss-of-function mutations. J Med Genet 2011;48(11):741–51.

30. Burglen L, Chantot-Bastaraud S, Garel C, et al. Spectrum of pontocerebellar hypoplasia in 13 girls and boys with CASK mutations: confirmation of a recognizable phenotype and first description of a male mosaic patient. Orphanet J Rare Dis 2012;7:18.

31. Hong SE, Shugart YY, Huang DT, et al. Autosomal recessive lissencephaly with cerebellar hypoplasia is associated with human RELN mutations. Nat Genet 2000;26(1):93–6.

32. Glass HC, Boycott KM, Adams C, et al. Autosomal recessive cerebellar hypoplasia in the Hutterite population. Dev Med Child Neurol 2005;47(10):691–5.

33. Bonnemann CG, Wang CH, Quijano-Roy S, et al. Diagnostic approach to the congenital muscular dystrophies. Neuromuscul Disord 2014;24(4):289–311.

34. Clement E, Mercuri E, Godfrey C, et al. Brain involvement in muscular dystrophies with defective dystroglycan glycosylation. Ann Neurol 2008;64(5):573–82.

35. Bahi-Buisson N, Poirier K, Fourniol F, et al. The wide spectrum of tubulinopathies: what are the key features for the diagnosis? Brain 2014;137(Pt 6):1676–700.

36. Cushion TD, Dobyns WB, Mullins JG, et al. Overlapping cortical malformations and mutations in TUBB2B and TUBA1A. Brain 2013;136(Pt 2):536–48.

37. Romaniello R, Arrigoni F, Cavallini A, et al. Brain malformations and mutations in alpha- and beta-tubulin genes: a review of the literature and description of two new cases. Dev Med Child Neurol 2014;56(4):354–60.

38. Tischfield MA, Baris HN, Wu C, et al. Human TUBB3 mutations perturb microtubule dynamics, kinesin interactions, and axon guidance. Cell 2010;140(1):74–87.

39. Romani M, Micalizzi A, Valente EM. Joubert syndrome: congenital cerebellar ataxia with the molar tooth. Lancet Neurol 2013;12(9):894–905.

40. Hildebrandt F, Benzing T, Katsanis N. Ciliopathies. N Engl J Med 2011;364(16):1533–43.

41. Lancaster MA, Gopal DJ, Kim J, et al. Defective Wnt-dependent cerebellar midline fusion in a mouse model of Joubert syndrome. Nat Med 2011;17(6):726–31.

42. Aguilar A, Meunier A, Strehl L, et al. Analysis of human samples reveals impaired SHH-dependent cerebellar development in Joubert syndrome/Meckel syndrome. Proc Natl Acad Sci U S A 2012;109(42):16951–6.

43. Bachmann-Gagescu R, Dempsey JC, Phelps IG, et al. Joubert syndrome: a model for untangling recessive disorders with extreme genetic heterogeneity. J Med Genet 2015;52(8):514–22.

44. Poretti A, Vitiello G, Hennekam RC, et al. Delineation and diagnostic criteria of oral-facial-digital syndrome type VI. Orphanet J Rare Dis 2012;7(1):4.

45. Doherty D, Parisi MA, Finn LS, et al. Mutations in 3 genes (MKS3, CC2D2A and RPGRIP1L) cause COACH syndrome (Joubert syndrome with congenital hepatic fibrosis). J Med Genet 2010;47(1):8–21.

46. Poretti A, Huisman TA, Scheer I, et al. Joubert syndrome and related disorders: spectrum of neuroimaging findings in 75 patients. AJNR Am J Neuroradiol 2011;32(8):1459–63.

47. Friede RL, Boltshauser E. Uncommon syndromes of cerebellar vermis aplasia. I: Joubert syndrome. Dev Med Child Neurol 1978;20(6):758–63.

48. Engle EC. Human genetic disorders of axon guidance. Cold Spring Harb Perspect Biol 2010;2(3): a001784.

49. Barth PG, Majoie CB, Caan MW, et al. Pontine tegmental cap dysplasia: a novel brain malformation with a defect in axonal guidance. Brain 2007;130(Pt 9):2258–66.

50. Desai NK, Young L, Miranda MA, et al. Pontine tegmental cap dysplasia: the neurootologic perspective. Otolaryngol Head Neck Surg 2011; 145(6):992–8.

51. Caan MW, Barth PG, Niermeijer JM, et al. Ectopic peripontine arcuate fibres, a novel finding in pontine tegmental cap dysplasia. Eur J Paediatr Neurol 2014;18(3):434–8.

52. Jen JC, Chan WM, Bosley TM, et al. Mutations in a human ROBO gene disrupt hindbrain axon pathway crossing and morphogenesis. Science 2004; 304(5676):1509–13.

53. Bosley TM, Salih MA, Jen JC, et al. Neurologic features of horizontal gaze palsy and progressive scoliosis with mutations in ROBO3. Neurology 2005; 64(7):1196–203.

54. Rossi A, Catala M, Biancheri R, et al. MR imaging of brain-stem hypoplasia in horizontal gaze palsy with progressive scoliosis. AJNR Am J Neuroradiol 2004;25(6):1046–8.

55. Haller S, Wetzel SG, Lutschg J. Functional MRI, DTI and neurophysiology in horizontal gaze palsy with progressive scoliosis. Neuroradiology 2008;50(5): 453–9.

56. Poretti A, Boltshauser E, Plecko B. Brainstem disconnection: case report and review of the literature. Neuropediatrics 2007;38(4):210–2.

57. Poretti A, Denecke J, Miller DC, et al. Brainstem disconnection: two additional patients and expansion of the phenotype. Neuropediatrics 2015;46(2): 139–44.

58. Zaki MS, Saleem SN, Dobyns WB, et al. Diencephalic-mesencephalic junction dysplasia: a novel recessive brain malformation. Brain 2012;135(Pt 8):2416–27.

59. Severino M, Tortora D, Pistorio A, et al. Expanding the spectrum of congenital anomalies of the diencephalic-mesencephalic junction. Neuroradiology 2016;58(1): 33–44.

Prenatal Cerebellar Disruptions
Neuroimaging Spectrum of Findings in Correlation with Likely Mechanisms and Etiologies of Injury

Andrea Poretti, MD[a,b,]*, Eugen Boltshauser, MD[b],
Thierry A.G.M. Huisman, MD, EQNR, FICIS[a]

KEYWORDS

- Cerebellar disruption • Neuroimaging • Prenatal • Hemorrhage • Cerebellar hypoplasia
- Unilateral cerebellar hypoplasia • Cerebellar agenesis • Vanishing cerebellum

KEY POINTS

- The complex and protracted duration of development (from 4 weeks' gestation to 2 years postnatally) results in a high vulnerability of the cerebellum for acquired injury.
- In the last decades, progressing pre- and postnatal anatomic and functional neuroimaging techniques (ultrasound scan and MR imaging) have led to an improved recognition, classification, and understanding of the spectrum of cerebellar disruptions, which include various forms of cerebellar agenesis, unilateral cerebellar hypoplasia, cerebellar cleft, global cerebellar hypoplasia, and vanishing cerebellum associated with Chiari type II malformation.
- Similar disruptive processes may cause a spectrum of cerebellar disruptions as revealed by neuroimaging.
- Timing and chronicity of injury in relation to the stage of cerebellar development impacts the phenotype of cerebellar disruption.
- The recognition of cerebellar disruptions and differentiation from inborn errors of cerebellar development (so-called malformations) is important in terms of diagnosis, prognosis, treatment, and genetic/parental counselling.

INTRODUCTION

The embryogenesis/histogenesis of the cerebellum is a highly complex process that is programmed/determined by a large number of genes and can be summarized in 4 basic steps: (1) characterization of the cerebellar territory in the hindbrain, (2) formation of 2 compartments of cell proliferation giving rise to the Purkinje cells and the granule cells, (3) inward migration of the

Disclosure Statement: The authors have nothing to disclose.
[a] Section of Pediatric Neuroradiology, Division of Pediatric Radiology, Russell H. Morgan Department of Radiology and Radiological Science, Charlotte R. Bloomberg Children's Center, The Johns Hopkins University School of Medicine, Sheikh Zayed Tower, Room 4174, 1800 Orleans Street, Baltimore, MD 21287-0842, USA;
[b] Department of Pediatric Neurology, University Children's Hospital, Steinwiesstrasse 75, Zurich 8032, Switzerland
* Corresponding author. Section of Pediatric Neuroradiology, Division of Pediatric Radiology, The Russell H. Morgan Department of Radiology and Radiological Science, Charlotte R. Bloomberg Children's Center, The Johns Hopkins University School of Medicine, Sheikh Zayed Tower, Room 4174, 1800 Orleans Street, Baltimore, MD 21287-0842.
E-mail address: aporett1@jhmi.edu

Neuroimag Clin N Am 26 (2016) 359–372
http://dx.doi.org/10.1016/j.nic.2016.03.006
1052-5149/16/$ – see front matter © 2016 Elsevier Inc. All rights reserved.

granule cells, and (4) differentiation of cerebellar neurons.[1,2] The cerebellum develops over a long period, extending from the early embryonic period at approximately 4 weeks of gestation into the first postnatal years.[1] The high complexity and long duration of development makes the cerebellum vulnerable for a wide range of pathologic conditions/injuries including inborn errors of development (primary malformations) and acquired/secondary disruptions. Both inborn errors of development (primary malformations) and acquired/secondary disruptions result in morphologic changes (malformed) of the cerebellum and brainstem and are usually named malformations independent on the cause and pathomechanism. The term *malformation*, however, has a more specific significance and implies an alteration of the primary developmental program as pathomechanism of the morphologic anomaly.

Disruptions are defined as nonprogressive, congenital morphologic anomalies caused by the breakdown of a body structure that had a normal developmental potential and was initially normally developing until injured.[3] The timing and nature of the disruptive event/agent may either directly injure or destruct the cerebellum or impair/alter the subsequent sequences of development with resultant perturbation of normal growth and development. There are several possible causes of disruptions, including vascular (eg, hemorrhage and ischemia), infectious, teratogenic, and mechanical.[3] In the prenatal period, the cerebellum is particularly vulnerable to infections and hemorrhages (**Table 1**).[4] In contrast to true malformations (inborn errors of development), disruptions are acquired lesions with low recurrence risk.

Table 1
Cerebellar vulnerability

Category	Cerebellar Vulnerability
Neonatal hypoxic-ischemic injury	+
Postnatal infections	+
Prematurity (<30 wk gestational age)	+
Prenatal infections (particularly CMV)	++
Prenatal hemorrhages	+++
Toxicity/selected drugs	+++
Metabolic disorders	++++

From Poretti A, Prayer D, Boltshauser E. Morphological spectrum of prenatal cerebellar disruptions. Eur J Paediatr Neurol 2009;13(5):405; with permission.

The differentiation between malformations and disruptions is important for genetic counseling and for diagnostic and prognostic purposes. A genetic predisposition for disruptive lesions may, however, be present. For example, dominant mutations in COL4A1 lead to changes in the basal membrane of capillaries resulting in microangiopathy.[5] Within the brain, the microangiopathy increases the risk for hemorrhage or ischemia and subsequent porencephaly or unilateral cerebellar hypoplasia on follow-up.[6,7] Furthermore, homozygous mutations in NED1 are found to cause the fetal brain disruption sequence characterized by severe microcephaly, scalp rugae, and prominent occipital bone.[8]

High-quality anatomic and functional neuroimaging plays a key role in the early and correct diagnosis and differentiation of the many morphologic cerebellar abnormalities that may be seen in the pre-, peri- and postnatal period. In particular, neuroimaging may help differentiate between malformations and disruptions. For example, abnormalities (eg, hypoplasia or dysplasia) involving only 1 cerebellar hemisphere are most likely the sequela of a prenatal disruptive event such as a hemorrhage. High-resolution anatomic MR imaging sequences remain of essential importance for the evaluation/characterization of the normal or abnormal pre- and postnatal posterior fossa contents, which include the cerebellum and brain stem. Advanced, functional neuroimaging techniques such as diffusion tensor imaging (DTI) and susceptibility weighted imaging (SWI) may render additional crucial information to better elucidate certain aspects of the pathogenesis of the encountered cerebellar disruptions. DTI allows exploration of the internal derangement of the fiber architecture. SWI is highly sensitive for blood, blood products, and calcifications and may be of particular help in supporting the notion of a disruptive pathomechanism related to infections or hemorrhages.[9] Additional, less frequently applied techniques include ^{1}H magnetic resonance spectroscopy, and perfusion weighted imaging. Finally, pre- and postnatal ultrasonography with dedicated posterior fossa imaging should not be forgotten as a valuable, widely available, safe, low-cost bedside alternative imaging technique that can be used in critically sick or unstable children. In skilled hands, advanced ultrasound units can give highly diagnostic imaging data, which, because of the ease of serial data collection, allow us to follow and explore the dynamics of cerebellar injury.

This article discusses the morphologic spectrum of prenatal cerebellar disruptions including various forms of cerebellar agenesis, unilateral cerebellar hypoplasia, cerebellar cleft, forms of global cerebellar hypoplasia, and vanishing cerebellum related to Chiari type II malformation. For each cerebellar disruption, the article focuses on the neuroimaging presentation, but the clinical presentation, the presumptive underlying disruptive pathomechanism, and the long-term neurologic outcome are also discussed.

CEREBELLAR AGENESIS

Cerebellar agenesis is a rare finding in pediatric neuroimaging and is defined by the near complete absence of cerebellar tissue (**Fig. 1**).[10,11] The definition of cerebellar agenesis is based on the morphologic pattern/neuroimaging findings and does not suggest the pathogenesis. Cerebellar agenesis may be seen as a primary malformation (eg, mutations in *PTF1A*)[12] or secondary to a disruption. Cerebellar agenesis caused by disruption may be seen in following scenarios: (1) pre- or perinatal hemorrhage, (2) vascular insufficiency/compromise in Chiari II malformation with cerebellar herniation, and (3) as a sequela of prematurity.[4,13] The authors recently reported on a child with normal cerebellar anatomy on prenatal ultrasound scan at 18 and 22 weeks of gestation but isolated cerebellar agenesis at 12 months of age when the patient was referred for an MR imaging examination because of developmental delay.[4] Huissoud and colleagues[14] reported on a fetus with normal anatomy at 12 weeks of gestation but complete absence of cerebellar structures on ultrasound scan at 23 weeks of gestation. After termination of pregnancy at 25 weeks of gestation, neuropathology confirmed a complete and isolated cerebellar agenesis. In 2010, Mohila and colleagues[15] reported on a newborn with cerebellar agenesis in the setting of neonatal alloimmune thrombocytopenia, diffuse body ecchymoses, petechial hemorrhages, and arthrogryposis at birth. She died on day 3 of life because of multisystem organ failure and disseminated intravascular coagulopathy. Neuropathology found complete loss of cerebellar tissue, marked reduction in size of the pons and medulla, acute and chronic germinal matrix hemorrhages, and deposition of blood degradation products and reactive gliosis in the posterior fossa. The neuropathology findings suggest a disruptive pathomechanism of cerebellar agenesis in this neonate. Recently, the authors reported the association of cerebellar agenesis and severe periventricular leukomalacia in a 7-year-old girl who was born at 25 weeks of gestation.[13] The serial ultrasound studies performed at 4.5 and 6 weeks of life showed a normal structure of the cerebellum and brainstem, whereas an ultrasound study at 9 weeks of life found an abnormal hypoechogenic cerebellum. A computed tomography (CT) scan at the age of 12 weeks showed a cerebellar agenesis (**Fig. 2**). In these cases, cerebellar agenesis is secondary to a pre- or perinatal acquired event/complication supporting the possible disruptive etiology of cerebellar agenesis.

All children with cerebellar agenesis are symptomatic. Patients who survive infancy have variable degrees of cerebellar dysfunction (truncal and limb ataxia, dysarthria, and muscular hypotonia) and cognitive impairment including specific

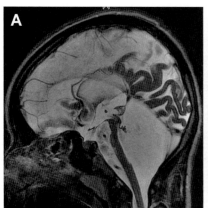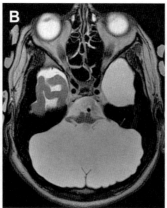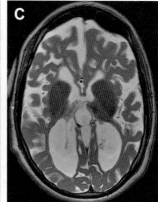

Fig. 1. Cerebellar agenesis. (*A*) Midsagittal and (*B*) Axial T2-weighted MR images of a 15-year-old girl with cerebellar agenesis show near-complete absence of cerebellar structures except for a rudimentary remnant of the anterior vermis, an enlarged posterior fossa, and marked hypoplasia of the pons. (*C*) Axial supratentorial T2-weighted MR image shows severe loss of white matter as seen in severe periventricular leukomalacia that represents a clearly acquired, not hereditary lesion. (*From* Poretti A, Prayer D, Boltshauser E. Morphological spectrum of prenatal cerebellar disruptions. Eur J Paediatr Neurol 2009;13(5):402; with permission.)

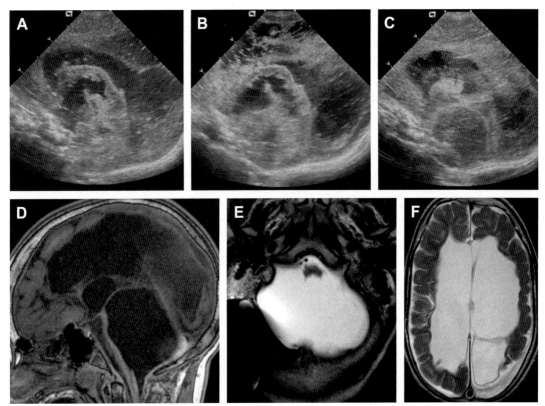

Fig. 2. Cerebellar agenesis. Midline sagittal brain ultrasound images at the age of (A) 4.5 and (B) 6 weeks of life of an extreme preterm neonate born at 25 weeks of gestation show the normal hyperechogenic cerebellar vermis compared with adjacent structures and the present pontine prominence. (C) Midline sagittal brain ultrasound image of the same child at the age of 9 week shows a markedly hypoechogenic cerebellum. (D) Midsagittal T1- and (E) Axial T2-weighted MR images of the same child at the age of 7 years show complete absence of the cerebellum, a shallow pons, and large empty posterior fossa with marked dilatation of the fourth ventricle. (F) Axial supratentorial T2-weighted MR image shows a high-grade volume loss of the hemispheric white matter, including a more focal cortical/subcortical defect in the left parieto-occipital region. Additionally, high-grade ex-vacuo dilatation of the ventricles is seen. A ventriculo-peritoneal shunt catheter is noted in the right posterior, lateral ventricle. (*From* Poretti A, Risen S, Meoded A, et al. Cerebellar agenesis: an extreme form of cerebellar disruption in preterm neonates. J Pediatr Neuroradiol 2013;2:164–5; with permission.)

deficits in planning behavior, visuo-spatial abilities, visual memory, attention, speech com prehension, verbal learning, and declarative memory.[4,10,16]

In cerebellar agenesis, the absence of cerebellar tissue is usually not complete, and remnants of the anterior vermian lobules (particularly vermian lobule III), flocculus, or middle cerebellar peduncles may be present (see Fig. 1).[10,11] A secondary pontine volume loss/hypoplasia and absence of the normal protuberance of the inferior olives are typically seen. The volume of the posterior fossa is variable, mostly of normal or increased size. Cerebrospinal fluid (CSF) pulsations within an "empty skull" may result in the increased size of the posterior fossa as also seen supratentorially in children with hydranencephaly. However, reduced volume has been also reported.[17] Recently, 2 studies

applied DTI and fiber tractography to study 2 patients with cerebellar agenesis. One study applied probabilistic constrained spherical deconvolution tractography in a child with cerebellar agenesis.[18] Findings showed absence of the transverse pontine fibers, which explains the marked pontine hypoplasia and is most likely caused by the absence of cerebellar tissue. In addition, the cerebellothalamic, fronto-cerebellar, and spinocerebellar tracts had aberrant courses. The second article reports on DTI and functional (resting state) MR imaging data in a 48-year-old right-handed man with cerebellar agenesis.[19] Qualitative analysis of DTI data found absence of the transverse pontine fibers, superior cerebellar peduncles and their decussation (most likely secondary to Wallerian degeneration), and the fronto-pontine tracts in the mesial part of the cerebral peduncles. The fronto-pontine tracts are part of the executive control network. Resting-state functional MR imaging confirmed impairment of the executive control network. An empty posterior fossa on ultrasound scan may suggest cerebellar agenesis that needs to be confirmed by MR imaging.

Based on the neuroimaging findings, the diagnosis of cerebellar agenesis is straightforward. The differentiation between a malformative and disruptive nature of cerebellar agenesis may be more challenging but is important for prognosis and genetic counseling of the affected families. Dysmorphic features on the general examination, endocrine disorders (such as diabetes) on metabolic screens, and additional morphologic abnormalities of the central nervous system on neuroimaging may favor a malformative origin. Neonates with cerebellar agenesis should be evaluated for diabetes mellitus, as this association is suggestive of a mutation in *PTF1A*.

GLOBAL CEREBELLAR HYPOPLASIA

Global cerebellar hypoplasia refers to a cerebellum with globally (vermis and cerebellar hemispheres) reduced volume but a normal shape (**Fig. 3**).[20] Global cerebellar hypoplasia is associated with a broad group of etiologies including primary (malformative, genetic) lesions, such as chromosomal aberrations, metabolic disorders, genetic syndromes, and some brain malformations, but may also be secondary to disruptive processes.

Global cerebellar hypoplasia has been reported in children with congenital infections, particularly cytomegalovirus (CMV),[21] and, less commonly, rubella[22] and varicella viruses.[23] The pathomechanism of global cerebellar hypoplasia in congenital CMV infection is still poorly understood. The cerebellum of prenatally infected mice shows global hypoplasia, reduced foliation, and increased thickness of the external granular layer.[24] This pattern of cerebellar abnormalities most likely results from decreased proliferation of granule neurons in the external granular layer, delayed migration of postmitotic neurons from the external granular layer into deeper layers of the cerebellar cortex, and altered morphology of the Purkinje cells.[25] Impaired responsiveness to brain-derived neurotrophins caused by decreased expression of the brain-derived neurotrophic–specific receptor, TrkB, or a strong inflammatory response mediated by several proinflammatory cytokines and chemokines may play key roles. This finding supports an indirect effect of the virus infection rather than a direct virus replication in cerebellar neurons causative of the cerebellar hypoplasia.[25]

Neonates with congenital CMV infection may present with multisystem involvement: lungs (pneumonia), blood (thrombocytopenia and hemolytic anemia), gastrointestinal system (hepatitis and jaundice), eyes (chorioretinitis), and central nervous system (about 50% of children have microcephaly, lethargy, hypotonia, and seizures).[26] Most prenatally infected neonates are asymptomatic at birth, but about 10% may have a variety of central nervous system–related symptoms, including microcephaly, seizures, intellectual disability, tetraspasticity, and sensorineural hearing loss on follow-up.

The spectrum of neuroimaging findings associated with congenital CMV infection is broad and mostly depends on the gestational age time of

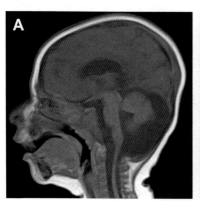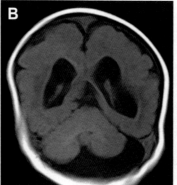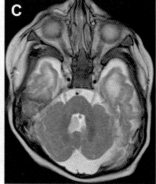

Fig. 3. Global cerebellar hypoplasia. (*A*) Midsagittal T1-, (*B*) Coronal T1-, and (*C*) Axial T2-weighted MR images of a 3-month-old infant with confirmed congenital cytomegalovirus infection show a small, compact cerebellum representing global cerebellar hypoplasia. In addition, a smooth cerebral surface compatible with microlissencephaly and a T2-hyperintense signal of the supratentorial white matter are seen as well-known sequelae of congenital cytomegalovirus infection.

infection. Neuroimaging findings may include multifocal white matter lesions that affect predominantly the temporal/parietal regions, migration abnormalities, ventriculomegaly, white and gray matter calcifications, and subcortical cysts (see **Fig. 3**).[21,27–29] Migration disorders and cerebellar involvement are more severe when infection occurs earlier in pregnancy. Lissencephaly and severe global cerebellar hypoplasia with secondary pontine hypoplasia are found in early infections (before 16–18 weeks of gestation), whereas polymicrogyria and mild global cerebellar hypoplasia are seen in later infections (18–24 weeks of gestation).[30] In third-trimester infections, the cerebellum usually appears normal.[31] Calcifications are located in periventricular regions, basal ganglia, and cerebellar white matter and are best seen on SWI (**Fig. 4**) or ultrasound scan (**Fig. 5**). In congenital CMV infection, head ultrasound scan may also detect ventriculomegaly and severe abnormalities of cortical development.[32]

The entire spectrum of neuroimaging findings and the clinical presentation may suggest the diagnosis. Because postnatal CMV infection is common, diagnostic testing should be performed within the first 3 postnatal weeks. A positive test result thereafter is nonconclusive. If the patient presents beyond the neonatal period, the diagnosis may be confirmed by presence of CMV DNA in dried blood of neonatal screening (Guthrie). This diagnosis is important because of emerging evidence that postnatal antiviral treatment can improve outcomes.[33]

UNILATERAL CEREBELLAR HYPOPLASIA

Unilateral cerebellar hypoplasia is a rare finding with a spectrum of features ranging from complete aplasia to mild asymmetry in the size of the cerebellar hemispheres (**Fig. 6**).[34–36] Increasing experience with prenatal ultrasound scan and fetal MR imaging has found that unilateral cerebellar hypoplasia is of prenatal origin (and thus represents a disruption), with hemorrhage as the leading cause.[35,37] Indeed, an increasing number of cases of prenatal cerebellar hemorrhage between 18 and 24 weeks of gestation has been reported with unilateral cerebellar hypoplasia on follow-up examinations.[38–40]

Cerebellar hemorrhages occur typically early in fetal life, typically between 20 and 24 weeks of gestation and usually not later than 26 weeks of gestation (**Fig. 7**).[37,41] Cerebellar hemorrhages are mostly unilateral, bilateral cases are uncommon.[42,43] Typically, the peripheral and caudal portions of the cerebellar hemispheres are involved.[44]

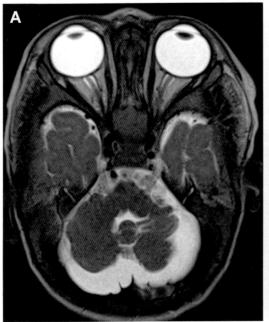 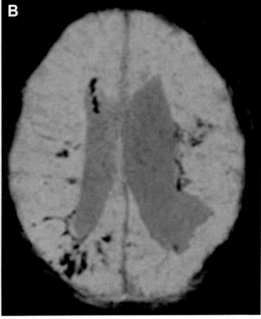

Fig. 4. Global cerebellar hypoplasia. (*A*) Axial T2-weighted MR image of a 2-year-old child with confirmed congenital cytomegalovirus infection shows global cerebellar hypoplasia. (*B*) Axial susceptibility-weighted image of the supratentorial brain shows scattered punctate foci of hypointense signal, suggestive of calcification in the setting of congenital cytomegalovirus infection. (*From* Bosemani T, Orman G, Boltshauser E, et al. Congenital abnormalities of the posterior fossa. Radiographics 2015;35(1):216; with permission.)

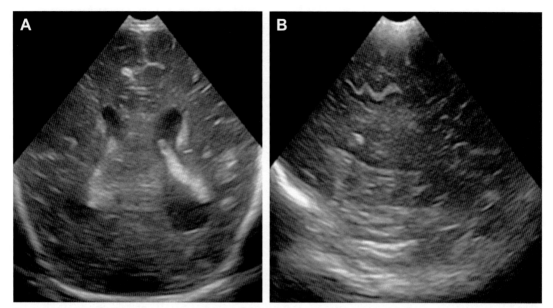

Fig. 5. Congenital cytomegalovirus infection. (*A*) Coronal and (*B*) Sagittal ultrasound scan images of a neonate with confirmed cytomegalovirus infection show multiple hyperechogenic calcifications along the lateral ventricles and within the hemispheric white matter. (*From* Orman G, Benson JE, Kweldam CF, et al. Neonatal head ultrasonography today: a powerful imaging tool! J Neuroimaging 2015;25(1):52; with permission.)

The vermis is reported to be involved in up to half of the fetuses, although vermis involvement may be difficult to determine on prenatal imaging. Cerebellar hemorrhages typically arise from the subependymal germinal matrix of the fourth ventricle or from the external granule layer.[45,46] Neuropathology studies confirm the origin of cerebellar hemorrhages within the deep cerebellar cortex or at the gray-white matter interface near the internal granule layer.[44] The period when cerebellar hemorrhages occur (20–24 weeks of gestation) corresponds to the vulnerable period when the cells from external granular layer start migrating to the internal granular layer.[44,47] The cause of prenatal cerebellar hemorrhage remains unknown in most cases. Reported maternal factors include trauma, sepsis, preeclampsia, seizures, drug abuse (eg, cocaine), and medications altering platelet function.[38,48,49] Fetal etiologies include vascular malformations, congenital infections (eg, cytomegalovirus), congenital tumors, and alloimmune or isoimmune thrombocytopenia.[48–52] Prenatal cerebellar hemorrhages may be caused by maternal and fetal hematologic disorders such as coagulopathies or thrombophilic disorders that cause thrombosis of the placenta or fetal arteries and lead to secondary cerebellar hemorrhagic infarction.[39,53]

The clinical presentation of children with unilateral cerebellar hypoplasia is highly variable. In our experience, minor asymmetry of the cerebellar hemispheres is occasionally seen as an incidental finding without clinical significance, whereas a marked unilateral cerebellar hypoplasia is expected to be of clinical relevance. Cerebellar signs are common and may include truncal and limb ataxia, hypotonia, squint, and head nodding and are usually mild in severity.[35,36] Cognitive outcome is variable, ranging from normal cognitive functions to learning disability of differing severity with IQ scores between 60 and 74.[34,35,54] Abnormalities of the cerebellar vermis is a predictor of poor cognitive functions. Detailed neuropsychological evaluations found selected difficulties in memory and executive functions, graphomotor and arithmetical skills, social perception, and comprehension. In addition, language and speech disorders including dysarthria and expressive language disorder, dysprosody, and limited or lack of expressive language are common in children with unilateral cerebellar hypoplasia. Finally, behavioral disorders including attention deficit hyperactivity disorder, depressive mood, anxiety, and catatonia with obsessive-compulsive disorder may also occur. This pattern of deficits overlaps with the symptom profile of the cerebellar cognitive affective syndrome.[55] In patients with severe unilateral cerebellar hypoplasia, however, this pattern seems to be less specific compared with children with postnatally acquired cerebellar lesions such as cerebellar tumors. Unilateral cerebellar hypoplasia may be also detected by ultrasound scan,

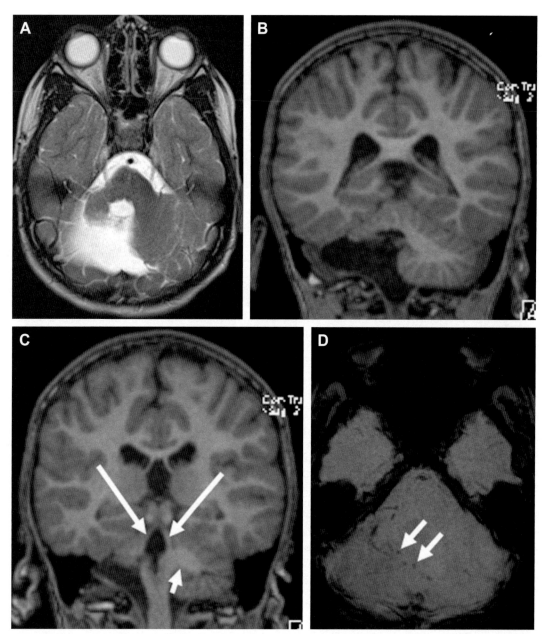

Fig. 6. Unilateral cerebellar hypoplasia. (*A*) Axial T2- and (*B, C*) coronal T1-weighted MR images of a 4-year-old child with unilateral cerebellar hypoplasia show a normal-appearing left cerebellar hemisphere, near-complete absence of the right cerebellar hemisphere and vermis, and an asymmetry of the superior (*long arrows* in *C*) and middle (*arrow* in *C*) cerebellar peduncles with reduction in size of the right cerebellar peduncles. (*D*) Axial susceptibility-weighted image shows scattered punctate foci of hypointense signal (*arrows*), suggestive of previous hemorrhage.

particularly with images through the mastoid fontanel.[56]

In most patients, unilateral cerebellar hypoplasia is an isolated finding. Occasionally, unilateral cerebellar hypoplasia may be an incidental, likely unlinked and consequently unexpected finding in children with complex supratentorial brain malformations such as holoprosencephaly.[4] Unilateral cerebellar has been reported in patients with Moebius syndrome and Goldenhar syndrome in which the cerebellar findings are likely the result of a prenatally vascular compromise with resultant ischemia.[57,58] Unilateral cerebellar hypoplasia may be found as an incidental finding in children

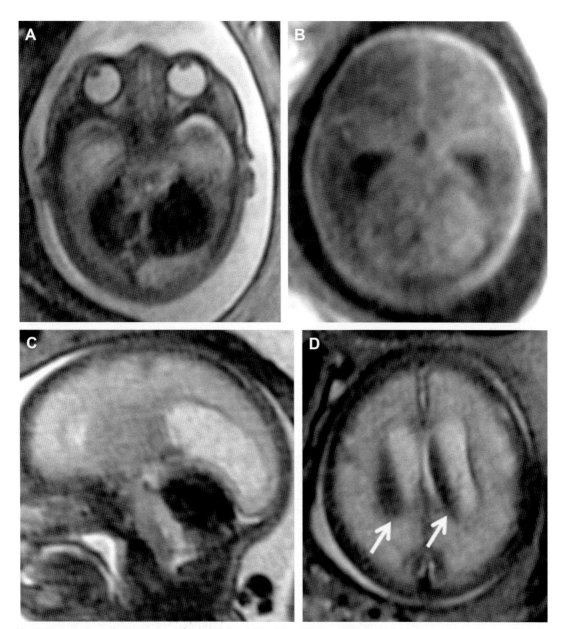

Fig. 7. Prenatal cerebellar hemorrhage. (*A*) Axial T2-, (*B*) axial T1-, and (*C*) sagittal T2-weighted fetal MR images at 27 weeks of gestation show a large T2-hypointense (*A, C*) and T1-hyperintense (*B*) well-marginated lesion located within the entire cerebellum suggestive of a cerebellar hemorrhage. The brain stem appears to be mildly ventrally displaced. (*D*) Supratentorial axial T2-weighted MR image shows a moderate ventriculomegaly with T2-hypointense material within the lateral ventricles (*arrows*) suggestive of extension of the cerebellar hemorrhage into the ventricular system (shifted to the right because of intrauterine fetal position). In addition, the hemispheric white matter appears T2-hyperintense edematous. (*From* Hayashi M, Poretti A, Gorra M, et al. Prenatal cerebellar hemorrhage: fetal and postnatal neuroimaging findings and postnatal outcome. Pediatr Neurol 2015;52(5):530; with permission.)

that are studied for noncerebellar problems, such as headaches or seizures.[4] Unilateral cerebellar hypoplasia has also been reported in children with systemic disorders such as Prader-Willi syndrome or Schimke immunoosseous dysplasia.[59,60]

In these cases, the apparent increased incidence of unilateral cerebellar hypoplasia is likely caused by a selection bias, because children with a syndromic condition are more often investigated with MR imaging.

The characteristic neuroimaging finding of unilateral cerebellar hypoplasia is an asymmetry of the cerebellar hemispheres ranging from aplasia to mild hypoplasia of a cerebellar hemisphere (see **Fig. 6**; **Fig. 8**).[35,36] The vermis is involved in about 50% of the patients (see **Fig. 6**). The volume of the posterior fossa is variable and may be clearly enlarged, normal, or reduced ipsilateral to the hypoplastic hemisphere. In almost all patients, a brainstem asymmetry is present and includes hypoplasia of the ipsilateral middle and superior cerebellar peduncles (see **Fig. 6**) and superior colliculus, a highly asymmetrical pons with absent contralateral olivary body, and contralateral reduction of the red nucleus and the substantia nigra.[35,61] Hemosiderin deposition may be present and is best detected by SWI (see **Fig. 6**) but is not present in most cases. This finding is probably owing to the high prenatal permeability of the blood-brain barrier to hemosiderin-loaded macrophages. Additional intracranial findings may be present and include, for example, supratentorial clastic lesions and ventriculomegaly.

CEREBELLAR CLEFT

Cerebellar clefts are characterized by a CSF-filled tissue defect extending from the surface of the cerebellar hemisphere toward the adjacent white matter or even ventricular system (IV ventricle) (**Fig. 9**).[62,63] Malorientation of the cerebellar foliation and irregular gray/white matter junction confined to the region adjacent to the cleft are additional typical neuroimaging findings. In 2 children with cerebellar clefts, prenatal cerebellar hemorrhages were identified at 24 weeks of gestation.[62,63] In one child with cerebellar cleft, a history of prenatal injury was reported.[64] In addition, cerebellar clefts have been reported in association with supratentorial clastic lesions such as schizencephaly.[7,65,66] These observations suggest a disruptive nature of cerebellar cleft, and prenatal cerebellar hemorrhages are the most likely cause. In addition, cerebellar clefts may occur in preterm neonates with cerebellar hemorrhages. Two patients were born preterm at 24 and 30 weeks of gestation, respectively, after a twin pregnancy with twin-to-twin transfusion in one case.[63] One infant had bilateral intraparenchymal cerebellar hemorrhages at 32 weeks of gestation. A brain MR image at the age of 14 months found bilateral cerebellar clefts. In the other patient, a left cerebellar hemorrhage was detected at 4 months of age (corrected age 40 weeks of gestation). In this child, a brain MR imaging at 1.8 years of age found a left cerebellar cleft.

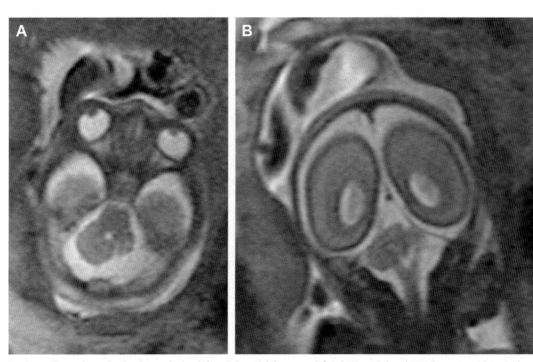

Fig. 8. Unilateral cerebellar hypoplasia. (*A*) Axial and (*B*) coronal fetal T2-weighted MR images at 21 weeks of gestation show severe hypoplasia of the left cerebellar hemisphere. (*From* Poretti A, Limperopoulos C, Roulet-Perez E, et al. Outcome of severe unilateral cerebellar hypoplasia. Dev Med Child Neurol 2010;52(8):720; with permission.)

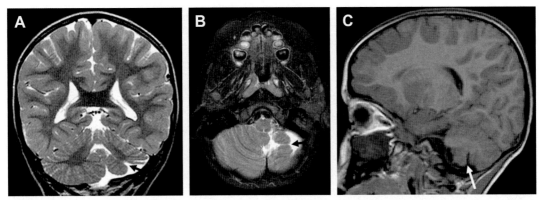

Fig. 9. Unilateral cerebellar cleft. (*A*) Coronal T2-, (*B*) axial T2-, and (*C*) sagittal T1-weighted MR images of a 4-year-old child with unilateral cerebellar cleft show a linear cleft (*arrows*) within the left cerebellar hemisphere running from the surface to the fourth ventricle, along with abnormal cerebellar foliation, fissuration, and white matter arborization around the cleft. In addition, reduction in size of the left cerebellar hemisphere is seen. The appearance and structure of the vermis and right cerebellar hemisphere are normal.

The clinical presentation of children with cerebellar clefts is highly variable and may include cerebellar signs such as truncal ataxia, dysarthria, ocular motor apraxia, intellectual disability, speech impairment, and behavioral changes.[62,63]

Cerebellar clefts may be located within the left or right cerebellar hemispheres, whereas the vermis is consistently spared.[62,63] In rare cases, cerebellar clefts may involve both hemispheres. The cerebellar cortex along the cleft is typically thinned or even interrupted, and the affected cerebellar hemispheres are reduced in volume, resulting in asymmetric sizes of the cerebellar hemispheres. Extension of the cleft into the fourth ventricle may occur. Supratentorial abnormalities are present in some patients and may include schizencephaly, sparse bilateral, asymmetric paratrigonal subependymal heterotopias, mild ventriculomegaly, and atretic occipital encephalocele.[62,63] Cerebellar clefts are difficult to identify on ultrasound scan. Asymmetry of the cerebellar hemispheres and a CSF-filled defect may suggest the cleft and a focal widening of the adjacent subarachnoid space.

VANISHING CEREBELLUM IN CHIARI II MALFORMATION

In non–skin-covered spinal dysraphias, particularly in myelomeningoceles, a small posterior fossa is believed to result from an incomplete or deficient expansion of the rhombo-encephalic vesicle secondary to continuous CSF leakage out of the spinal canal at the level of the spinal dysraphia early in gestation. Because of the too small posterior fossa, the cerebellum herniates through the foramen magnum into the upper cervical spinal canal.

This herniation may result in mild-to-severe parenchymal damage caused by the chronic mechanical compression, altered CSF hemodynamics, and impaired arterial and venous hemodynamics/perfusion of the posterior fossa structures. In a small subgroup of these Chiari II children, the degree of tissue injury is so severe that the cerebellum is nearly completely absent. This infrequent observation was coined as *vanishing cerebellum in Chiari II malformation* by Sener.[67] However, this name does not reflect the remarkable asymmetry of tissue damage that is usually seen and remains unexplained. The damage to the cerebellum typically involves predominantly only 1 cerebellar hemisphere, whereas the vermis is frequently spared or less severely affected (**Fig. 10**). Boltshauser and colleagues[68] reported on 3 patients with this typical pattern of vanishing cerebellum in Chiari II malformation. In one child, the diagnosis was made prenatally at 25 weeks of gestation. In this series, the cerebellar involvement was remarkably asymmetric in all patients. A detailed neurocognitive assessment found a severe cognitive impairment in one child, whereas the other 2 patients could not be adequately tested (one child died early, and the other child was too young for an adequate neurocognitive test). No conclusion can be drawn whether children with Chiari II malformation and vanishing cerebellum have a similar or more severe impairment of cognitive functions compared with children with an uncomplicated Chiari II malformation alone.

SUMMARY

Prenatal cerebellar disruptions are acquired morphologic abnormalities of the cerebellum,

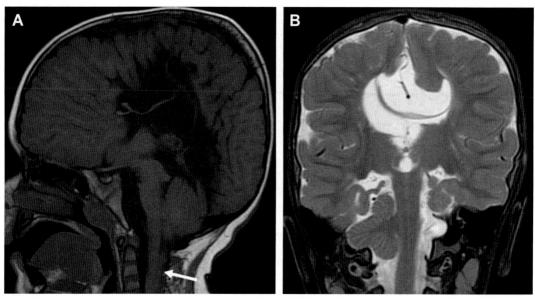

Fig. 10. Vanishing cerebellum in Chiari II malformation. (*A*) Midsagittal T1-weighted MR image of a 2.5-year-old child shows a small posterior fossa, flattening of the ventral pons, herniation of the cerebellar vermis into the spinal canal (*arrow*), an abnormal tectum, a prominent massa intermedia, and dysgenesis of the corpus callosum. (*B*) Coronal T2-weighted MR image of the same child shows absence of the left cerebellar hemisphere, whereas the size of the right cerebellar hemisphere seems to be preserved.

which may be identified intrauterine or in the immediate neonatal period. Various morphologic patterns of cerebellar disruptions have been reported that may be caused by different disruptive agents such as hemorrhages or infections. Neuroimaging is essential for the correct diagnosis of pre- and perinatal cerebellar disruptions. In particular, correct differentiation between acquired/secondary disruptions and inborn errors of development or malformations is essential for estimation of prognosis, choosing treatment options, and parental counseling (**Box 1**).

Box 1
Neuroimaging findings that favor a disruption compared with a malformation

Neuroimaging findings

- Unilateral cerebellar morphologic abnormality with or without involvement of the vermis
- Presence of posterior fossa hemorrhage or blood products as best seen on SWI or ultrasound scan
- Presence of calcifications within the posterior fossa or supratentorial brain as best seen on SWI or ultrasound scan
- Associated supratentorial clastic lesions such as schizencephaly or porencephaly

---

REFERENCES

1. ten Donkelaar HJ, Lammens M, Wesseling P, et al. Development and developmental disorders of the human cerebellum. J Neurol 2003;250(9):1025–36.
2. Butts T, Green MJ, Wingate RJ. Development of the cerebellum: simple steps to make a 'little brain'. Development 2014;141(21):4031–41.
3. Hennekam RC, Biesecker LG, Allanson JE, et al. Elements of morphology: general terms for congenital anomalies. Am J Med Genet A 2013;161A(11):2726–33.
4. Poretti A, Prayer D, Boltshauser E. Morphological spectrum of prenatal cerebellar disruptions. Eur J Paediatr Neurol 2009;13(5):397–407.
5. Gould DB, Phalan FC, Breedveld GJ, et al. Mutations in Col4a1 cause perinatal cerebral hemorrhage and porencephaly. Science 2005;308(5725):1167–71.
6. Vermeulen RJ, Peeters-Scholte C, Van Vugt JJ, et al. Fetal origin of brain damage in 2 infants with a COL4A1 mutation: fetal and neonatal MRI. Neuropediatrics 2011;42(1):1–3.
7. Yoneda Y, Haginoya K, Kato M, et al. Phenotypic spectrum of COL4A1 mutations: porencephaly to schizencephaly. Ann Neurol 2013;73(1):48–57.
8. Paciorkowski AR, Keppler-Noreuil K, Robinson L, et al. Deletion 16p13.11 uncovers NDE1 mutations on the non-deleted homolog and extends the spectrum of severe microcephaly to include fetal

brain disruption. Am J Med Genet A 2013;161A(7): 1523–30.

9. Bosemani T, Poretti A, Huisman TA. Susceptibility-weighted imaging in pediatric neuroimaging. J Magn Reson Imaging 2014;40(3):530–44.

10. Yu F, Jiang QJ, Sun XY, et al. A new case of complete primary cerebellar agenesis: clinical and imaging findings in a living patient. Brain 2015; 138(Pt 6):e353.

11. Poretti A, Boltshauser E. Terminology in morphological anomalies of the cerebellum does matter. Cerebellum Ataxias 2015;2:8.

12. Sellick GS, Barker KT, Stolte-Dijkstra I, et al. Mutations in PTF1A cause pancreatic and cerebellar agenesis. Nat Genet 2004;36(12):1301–5.

13. Poretti A, Risen S, Meoded A, et al. Cerebellar agenesis: an extreme form of cerebellar disruption in preterm neonates. J Pediatr Neuroradiol 2013;2:163–7.

14. Huissoud C, Rudigoz RC, Bisch C, et al. Complete cerebellar agenesis: a very rare abnormality of the posterior fossa. Ultrasound Obstet Gynecol 2009; 33(6):730–1.

15. Mohila CA, Kubicka ZJ, Ornvold KT, et al. Cerebellar loss and brain-stem atrophy associated with neonatal alloimmune thrombocytopenia in a discordant twin. Pediatr Dev Pathol 2010;13(1):55–62.

16. Richter S, Dimitrova A, Hein-Kropp C, et al. Cerebellar agenesis II: motor and language functions. Neurocase 2005;11(2):103–13.

17. Sener RN, Jinkins JR. Subtotal agenesis of the cerebellum in an adult. MRI demonstration. Neuroradiology 1993;35(4):286–7.

18. Mormina E, Briguglio M, Morabito R, et al. A rare case of cerebellar agenesis: a probabilistic constrained spherical deconvolution tractographic study. Brain Imaging Behav 2016;10(1):158–67.

19. Arrigoni F, Romaniello R, Nordio A, et al. Learning to live without the cerebellum. Neuroreport 2015; 26(14):809–13.

20. Poretti A, Boltshauser E, Doherty D. Cerebellar hypoplasia: differential diagnosis and diagnostic approach. Am J Med Genet C Semin Med Genet 2014;166(2):211–26.

21. Oosterom N, Nijman J, Gunkel J, et al. Neuro-imaging findings in infants with congenital cytomegalovirus infection: relation to trimester of infection. Neonatology 2015;107(4):289–96.

22. Cluver C, Meyer R, Odendaal H, et al. Congenital rubella with agenesis of the inferior cerebellar vermis and total anomalous pulmonary venous drainage. Ultrasound Obstet Gynecol 2013;42(2):235–7.

23. Verstraelen H, Vanzieleghem B, Defoort P, et al. Prenatal ultrasound and magnetic resonance imaging in fetal varicella syndrome: correlation with pathology findings. Prenat Diagn 2003;23(9):705–9.

24. Koontz T, Bralic M, Tomac J, et al. Altered development of the brain after focal herpesvirus infection of the central nervous system. J Exp Med 2008;205(2): 423–35.

25. Cekinovic D, Lisnic VJ, Jonjic S. Rodent models of congenital cytomegalovirus infection. Methods Mol Biol 2014;1119:289–310.

26. Noyola DE, Jimenez-Capdeville ME, Demmler-Harrison GJ. Central nervous system disorders in infants with congenital cytomegalovirus infection. Neurol Res 2010;32(3):278–84.

27. Doneda C, Parazzini C, Righini A, et al. Early cerebral lesions in cytomegalovirus infection: prenatal MR imaging. Radiology 2010;255(2):613–21.

28. Fink KR, Thapa MM, Ishak GE, et al. Neuroimaging of pediatric central nervous system cytomegalovirus infection. Radiographics 2010;30(7):1779–96.

29. Manara R, Balao L, Baracchini C, et al. Brain magnetic resonance findings in symptomatic congenital cytomegalovirus infection. Pediatr Radiol 2011; 41(8):962–70.

30. de Vries LS, Gunardi H, Barth PG, et al. The spectrum of cranial ultrasound and magnetic resonance imaging abnormalities in congenital cytomegalovirus infection. Neuropediatrics 2004; 35(2):113–9.

31. Steinlin MI, Nadal D, Eich GF, et al. Late intrauterine cytomegalovirus infection: clinical and neuroimaging findings. Pediatr Neurol 1996;15(3):249–53.

32. Orman G, Benson JE, Kweldam CF, et al. Neonatal head ultrasonography today: a powerful imaging tool! J Neuroimaging 2015;25(1):31–55.

33. Oliver SE, Cloud GA, Sanchez PJ, et al. Neurodevelopmental outcomes following ganciclovir therapy in symptomatic congenital cytomegalovirus infections involving the central nervous system. J Clin Virol 2009;46(Suppl 4):S22–6.

34. Boltshauser E, Steinlin M, Martin E, et al. Unilateral cerebellar aplasia. Neuropediatrics 1996; 27(1):50–3.

35. Poretti A, Limperopoulos C, Roulet-Perez E, et al. Outcome of severe unilateral cerebellar hypoplasia. Dev Med Child Neurol 2010;52(8):718–24.

36. Benbir G, Kara S, Yalcinkaya BC, et al. Unilateral cerebellar hypoplasia with different clinical features. Cerebellum 2011;10(1):49–60.

37. Massoud M, Cagneaux M, Garel C, et al. Prenatal unilateral cerebellar hypoplasia in a series of 26 cases: significance and implications for prenatal diagnosis. Ultrasound Obstet Gynecol 2014;44(4): 447–54.

38. Ranzini AC, Shen-Schwarz S, Guzman ER, et al. Prenatal sonographic appearance of hemorrhagic cerebellar infarction. J Ultrasound Med 1998;17(11): 725–7.

39. Malinger G, Zahalka N, Kidron D, et al. Fatal outcome following foetal cerebellar haemorrhage associated with placental thrombosis. Eur J Paediatr Neurol 2006;10(2):93–6.

40. Malinger G, Lev D, Lerman-Sagie T. The fetal cerebellum. Pitfalls in diagnosis and management. Prenat Diagn 2009;29(4):372–80.

41. Merrill JD, Piecuch RE, Fell SC, et al. A new pattern of cerebellar hemorrhages in preterm infants. Pediatrics 1998;102(6):E62.

42. Limperopoulos C, Benson CB, Bassan H, et al. Cerebellar hemorrhage in the preterm infant: ultrasonographic findings and risk factors. Pediatrics 2005; 116(3):717–24.

43. Hayashi M, Poretti A, Gorra M, et al. Prenatal cerebellar hemorrhage: fetal and postnatal neuroimaging findings and postnatal outcome. Pediatr Neurol 2015;52(5):529–34.

44. Haines KM, Wang W, Pierson CR. Cerebellar hemorrhagic injury in premature infants occurs during a vulnerable developmental period and is associated with wider neuropathology. Acta Neuropathol Commun 2013;1:69.

45. Ecury-Goossen GM, Dudink J, Lequin M, et al. The clinical presentation of preterm cerebellar haemorrhage. Eur J Pediatr 2010;169(10):1249–53.

46. Fumagalli M, Bassi L, Sirgiovanni I, et al. From germinal matrix to cerebellar haemorrhage. J Matern Fetal Neonatal Med 2015;28(Suppl 1): 2280–5.

47. Volpe JJ. Cerebellum of the premature infant: rapidly developing, vulnerable, clinically important. J Child Neurol 2009;24(9):1085–104.

48. Yuksel A, Batukan C. Fetal cerebellar hemorrhage in a severely growth-restricted fetus: natural history and differential diagnosis from Dandy-Walker malformation. Ultrasound Obstet Gynecol 2003;22(2): 178–81.

49. Nomura ML, Barini R, de Andrade KC, et al. Prenatal diagnosis of isolated fetal cerebellar hemorrhage associated with maternal septic shock. Prenat Diagn 2009;29(2):169–71.

50. Sharony R, Kidron D, Aviram R, et al. Prenatal diagnosis of fetal cerebellar lesions: a case report and review of the literature. Prenat Diagn 1999;19(11): 1077–80.

51. Ortiz JU, Ostermayer E, Fischer T, et al. Severe fetal cytomegalovirus infection associated with cerebellar hemorrhage. Ultrasound Obstet Gynecol 2004; 23(4):402–6.

52. Lerner A, Gilboa Y, Gerad L, et al. Sonographic detection of fetal cerebellar cavernous hemangioma with in-utero hemorrhage leading to cerebellar hemi-hypoplasia. Ultrasound Obstet Gynecol 2006;28(7): 968–71.

53. Gorincour G, Rypens F, Lapierre C, et al. Fetal magnetic resonance imaging in the prenatal diagnosis of cerebellar hemorrhage. Ultrasound Obstet Gynecol 2006;27(1):78–80.

54. Gross-Tsur V, Ben-Bashat D, Shalev RS, et al. Evidence of a developmental cerebello-cerebral disorder. Neuropsychologia 2006;44(12):2569–72.

55. Schmahmann JD, Sherman JC. The cerebellar cognitive affective syndrome. Brain 1998;121(Pt 4): 561–79.

56. Robins JB, Mason GC, Watters J, et al. Case report: cerebellar hemi-hypoplasia. Prenat Diagn 1998; 18(2):173–7.

57. Harbord MG, Finn JP, Hall-Craggs MA, et al. Moebius' syndrome with unilateral cerebellar hypoplasia. J Med Genet 1989;26(9):579–82.

58. Martinelli P, Maruotti GM, Agangi A, et al. Prenatal diagnosis of hemifacial microsomia and ipsilateral cerebellar hypoplasia in a fetus with oculoauriculovertebral spectrum. Ultrasound Obstet Gynecol 2004;24:199–201.

59. Dhillon AS, Chapman S, Milford DV. Cerebellar defect associated with Schimke immuno-osseous dysplasia. Eur J Pediatr 2001;160(6):372–4.

60. Titomanlio L, De Brasi D, Romano A, et al. Partial cerebellar hypoplasia in a patient with Prader-Willi syndrome. Acta Paediatr 2006;95(7):861–3.

61. Strong OS. A case of unilateral cerebellar agenesis. J Comp Neurol 1915;25:361–91.

62. Poretti A, Leventer RJ, Cowan FM, et al. Cerebellar cleft: a form of prenatal cerebellar disruption. Neuropediatrics 2008;39(2):106–12.

63. Poretti A, Huisman TA, Cowan FM, et al. Cerebellar cleft: confirmation of the neuroimaging pattern. Neuropediatrics 2009;40(5):228–33.

64. Boddaert N, Desguerre I, Bahi-Buisson N, et al. Posterior fossa imaging in 158 children with ataxia. J Neuroradiol 2010;37(4):220–30.

65. Takano T, Takikita S, Shimada M. Experimental schizencephaly induced by kilham strain of mumps virus: pathogenesis of cleft formation. Neuroreport 1999;10(15):3149–54.

66. Curry CJ, Lammer EJ, Nelson V, et al. Schizencephaly: heterogeneous etiologies in a population of 4 million California births. Am J Med Genet A 2005;137(2):181–9.

67. Sener RN. Cerebellar agenesis versus vanishing cerebellum in Chiari II malformation. Comput Med Imaging Graph 1995;19(6):491–4.

68. Boltshauser E, Schneider J, Kollias S, et al. Vanishing cerebellum in myelomeningocoele. Eur J Paediatr Neurol 2002;6(2):109–13.

The Pediatric Cerebellum in Inherited Neurodegenerative Disorders
A Pattern-recognition Approach

Susan I. Blaser, MD[a],*, Maja Steinlin, MD[b], Almundher Al-Maawali, MD[c], Grace Yoon, MD[d]

KEYWORDS

- Cerebellum • Inborn errors of metabolism • Inherited neurodegenerative disorders

KEY POINTS

- Accurate genetic diagnosis of childhood-onset cerebellar ataxia is complicated by both clinical and genetic heterogeneity.
- Neuroimaging assessment of the cerebellum should include degree of volume loss, gradient of atrophy, signal intensity, magnetic resonance spectroscopy, and change over time.
- Integration of neuroimaging patterns with clinical information is essential to appropriate investigation of childhood-onset cerebellar ataxia.

INTRODUCTION

Inherited neurodegenerative disorders resulting from genetic and inborn biochemical defects can affect the cerebellum at any time, either during development and maturation or later in life. The resultant imaging appearance of the posterior fossa structures can reflect growth arrest (prenatal), growth arrest with superimposed atrophy (prenatal and postnatal), or either stable or progressive cerebellar atrophy (postnatal). Imaging features also include swelling or gliosis, calcification, diffusion restriction, enhancement, cysts, or alterations in magnetic resonance (MR) spectra. Additional features (eg, hyperintensity of the dentate nuclei or cerebellar cortex; specific volume loss patterns of the brainstem, vermis, and cerebellar hemispheres; swelling of the cerebellar white matter; change over time; and involvement of the supratentorial compartment) are crucial in narrowing the differential diagnosis.[1,2] Despite the rapidity with which genetic diagnoses may be made with the decreasing cost and increasing availability of whole-exome sequencing (WES), there are limitations with regard to complete coverage of all coding regions, and difficulties with large genomic rearrangements, trinucleotide repeat sequences, and interpretation of variants.[3] In 2 studies involving pediatric subjects, WES provided genetic diagnoses for 39% and 46% respectively of patients with previously undiagnosed childhood-onset cerebellar ataxia. Diagnosis in the remainder remained occult.[4,5] In another study

Disclosure: The authors have nothing to disclose.
[a] Division of Paediatric Neuroradiology, The Hospital for Sick Children, University of Toronto, 555 University Avenue, Toronto, Ontario M5G 1X8, Canada; [b] Division of Neuropaediatrics, Development and Rehabilitation, University Children's Hospital Inselspital, University of Bern, Freiburgstrasse 4, Bern 3010, Switzerland; [c] Department of Genetics, Sultan Qaboos University Hospital, Al Khoudh, Muscat 123, Oman; [d] Division of Clinical and Metabolic Genetics, The Hospital for Sick Children, University of Toronto, 555 University Avenue, Toronto, Ontario M5G 1X8, Canada
* Corresponding author.
E-mail address: susan.blaser@sickkids.ca

Neuroimag Clin N Am 26 (2016) 373–416
http://dx.doi.org/10.1016/j.nic.2016.03.007

of 126 patients referred for progressive cerebellar ataxia, genetic testing was not always positive.[6] Imaging therefore remains an important tool in the diagnosis, staging, and assessment of therapy for neurodegenerative disorders affecting the cerebellum (**Boxes 1 and 2**).

NEUROIMAGING PATTERN COMPONENTS IN THE CEREBELLUM

Neuroimaging patterns include combinations of: varying degrees of cerebellar volume loss; gradients of volume loss; signal intensity (swelling or gliosis/shrinkage) of the cerebellar cortex or white matter, dentate nuclei, brainstem tracts, and nuclei; diffusion restriction; enhancement; cysts; brain iron or calcifications; specific supratentorial patterns; and MR spectroscopy (MRS) spectra of the supratentorial compartment, cerebellum, or brainstem. The concept of selective vulnerability, caused by the different affinity of noxious insults to different brain structures at differing developmental stages, remains pertinent when discussing the cerebellum. Thus, the appearance at the time of presentation and any change in pattern with further brain development contribute important clues[7–9] (**Box 3**).

BIOMETRY

Multiplanar planimetry, assessing regional length, height, and area of the mesencephalon, pons, medulla, and cerebellar peduncles, adds a degree of specificity in baseline and follow-up assessment in patients with inborn errors of metabolism involving the cerebellum. Although measurements of the

---

Box 1
Imaging and evaluation protocols

- Image in all 3 orthogonal planes (three-dimensional techniques with multiplanar reconstruction may be used)
- Routine T1/T2 with age-appropriate sequence modification; fluid-attenuated inversion recovery (FLAIR)
- Diffusion-weighted imaging (DWI) or diffusion tensor imaging (DTI)
- Sequence sensitive to calcium, hemosiderin, and brain iron: T2*/Multiplanar Gradient-Recalled/Susceptibility Weighted Imaging
- Contrast administration may be helpful if abnormal signal on routine sequences
- MR spectroscopy (MRS)
  - Supratentorial: deep gray/white matter
  - Cerebellum/brainstem

Box 2
Imaging features contributing to patterns of inherited neurodegenerative disorders involving the cerebellum

- Degree of volume loss (or gain)
  - Vermis, cerebellar hemispheres, interfoliate fissures
  - Cerebellar peduncles
  - Brainstem
    - Mesencephalon
    - Pons
    - Medulla
  - Spinal cord
- Gradient of atrophy
  - Superior versus inferior vermis predominant
  - Vermis versus cerebellar hemisphere predominant
  - Cisternal enlargement
- Signal intensity (swelling or gliosis/shrinkage)
  - Cerebellar cortex
  - Cerebellar nuclei (predominantly dentate)
  - Cerebellar white matter
    - Middle cerebellar peduncles
    - Peridentate cerebellar white matter
    - Dentate hilar white matter
  - Brainstem tracts
- Additional imaging clues
  - Diffusion restriction
  - Specific supratentorial white matter patterns
  - Brain iron (dentate, supratentorial gray matter nuclei)
  - Foci of magnetic susceptibility
    - Telangiectasias
    - Hemosiderin
    - Calcifications
    - Brain iron
  - Other: cysts, enhancement
  - Other: chiasmatic enlargement (Krabbe/*GALC*) or atrophy (optic atrophy 1/*OPA1*)
  - Other: change over time
  - MRS: infratentorial, supratentorial

---

mesencephalon are slightly less reproducible because of the variability of slice thickness and partial volume averaging with the interpeduncular cistern, measurements performed on a midsagittal

Box 3
Biometry

- Biometry of cerebellum and vermis
  - Height: vermis
  - Transverse: cerebellum
  - Height of superior and middle cerebellar peduncles
  - Tegmentovermian angle
  - Superior cerebellar peduncle angle
- Biometry of brainstem and cervical spinal cord
  - Anteroposterior: mesencephalon, pons, medulla, clava, spinal cord at C2-C3 disc
  - Height: pons
  - Pontine area on sagittal view

view through the pons, medulla, and clava are robust and reproducible.[10] Craniocaudal vermian height measured between culmen and uvula and measurements of the vermian fissures may also be performed on a midline sagittal view (Fig. 1). Additional measurements performed on axial views include maximum peduncular width, pontine width at the level of the trigeminal nerve origins, and width of the medulla through the medullary waist posterior to the olives. Nomograms have been provided for fetal ultrasonography and for MR imaging studies performed throughout life.[11–13] Volumetric analysis of the cerebellum by automated segmentation allows identification of specific volume loss patterns within lobules of the vermis and cerebellar hemispheres and may be useful in monitoring the course of disease.[14,15] Loss of craniocaudal vermian height and increase in the apparent size of the cisterna magna commonly occur as cerebellar atrophy progresses in the inherited neurodegenerative disorders of childhood, but are not specific findings. Increase in the tegmentovermian angle between the brainstem and vermis on sagittal view also reflects volume loss with compensatory fourth ventricle enlargement.[10] More specific are findings of volume loss of a portion of the vermis (superior vs inferior gradient of atrophy) or regional brainstem atrophy. Spinal MR imaging is not routinely evaluated in most children undergoing MR imaging for inborn errors of metabolism. However, the upper cervical cord is visualized and may be assessed on images obtained for brain imaging at the C2/C3 disc space level or at a level of the top of the odontoid tip.[16] The measurement at the top of the odontoid tip may be difficult to assess in the youngest patients before fusion of ossification centers of the odontoid peg.

DIFFERENTIATING INHERITED AND ACQUIRED DISORDERS WITH CEREBELLAR INVOLVEMENT

Primary malformative and secondary disruptive disorders may also lead to cerebellar volume deficiencies, but are usually readily identified as such. Many of the hindbrain malformative lesions have specific well-described features.[17] Intrauterine destructive lesions, from TORCH (the acronym for toxoplasmosis gondii, other, rubella, cytomegalovirus, herpes simplex virus-2) infections, pseudo-TORCH disorders, maternal trauma or infection, teratogens, and prenatal or perinatal ischemia may cause developmental arrest or focal volume deficiencies.[18,19] As cerebellar development and maturation proceeds during the first year of life, developmental arrest and volume loss also occur in survivors of extreme prematurity, most commonly in association with supratentorial complications, such as hemorrhage and periventricular leukomalacia.[20,21] Specific anterior vermian atrophy in the central region has been shown in cases of profound neonatal hypoxic ischemic insult with thalamic, posterolateral putamina, and Rolandic cortex edema.[22] Postnatal toxin exposures affecting the cerebellum include medically administered medications (anticonvulsant therapy), alcohol, illicit drugs (cocaine, heroin), and environmental exposures (heavy metal, carbon monoxide, manufacturing chemicals, volatile substances, insecticides).[23] These cases are often identified by history or asymmetric findings. Asymmetric cerebellar volume loss only rarely accompanies an inherited disorder for example, with intrauterine or postnatal vasculopathy occurring in COL4A1 mutations[24,25] (Fig. 2).

CEREBELLOVERMIAN VOLUME LOSS: HYPOPLASIA VERSUS ATROPHY

The cerebellar hemispheres and vermis are usually considered together when discussing volume loss. Volumetric cerebellovermian abnormalities, such as hypoplasia and atrophy, are common in the inherited neurodegenerative disorders. Differentiation between hypoplasia and atrophy can be difficult, as shown by the confusion in the literature.[26] However, there are imaging criteria that can be applied in order to reduce some of the confusion. Cerebellar hypoplasia refers to a cerebellum/vermis with a normal or near-normal shape with normal interfoliate fissures and sulci, but reduced volume (Fig. 3). Causes of cerebellar hypoplasia include aneuploidy, genetic syndromes, and teratogen

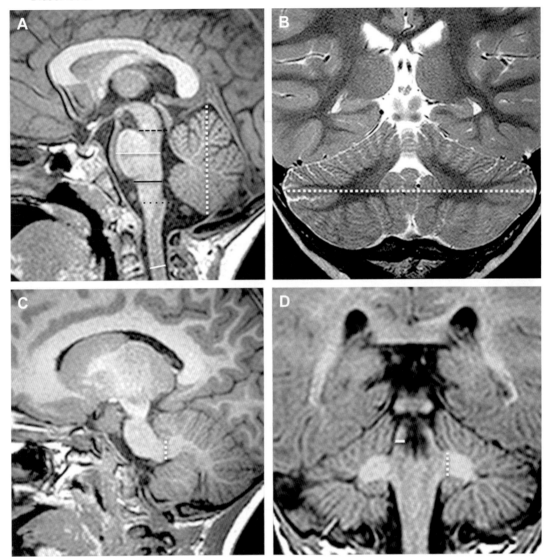

Fig. 1. Biometry. Midline sagittal T1-weighted (T1W) image (*A*) shows normal anteroposterior (AP) measurements of the midbrain AP (*black dashed line*), pons (*white line*), medulla (*black line*), clava (*black dotted line*), and the craniocaudal height of the vermis (*white dotted line*). The AP midbrain and medulla measurements are most reproducible at the pontine junctions. Transverse cerebellar diameter is measured on coronal T2-weighted (T2W) image (*B*). Middle cerebellar peduncle height is shown on parasagittal (*C*) and coronal (*D*) T1W images (*dotted lines*). Superior cerebellar peduncle width (*solid line*) is shown (*D*).

exposure.[27–29] There are many genetic syndromes associated with cerebellovermian hypoplasia. Classic examples include CHARGE syndrome (*CHD7* mutation) and Down syndrome/trisomy 21. CHARGE is the acronym for the constellation of coloboma, heart defect, atresia choanae, retarded growth and development, genital and ear abnormalities. Murine models show that deregulated fibroblast growth factor (FGF) signaling, caused by the effect of *Chd7* gene dosage on *Fgf8* expression, leads to cerebellar hypoplasia in CHARGE (*CHD7*).[30] Similarly, gene dosage effects from triplicated genes in *TsICJe* murine models of Down syndrome show a decrease in granule cell

proliferation in the newborn cerebellum.[31] In cerebellar atrophy, the vermis acquires a skeleton or branchlike configuration with small folia and large interfoliate fissures and sulci.[1] Change or lack of change may be a helpful feature. A useful clue is imaging documenting a previously normal-sized vermis and cerebellum and progressive loss of volume over time. However, early imaging in asymptomatic infants is rarely obtained. In addition, stability of early-onset cerebellovermian atrophy and gliosis has been noted in some disorders, whereas intrauterine growth arrest and postnatal progression of atrophy occurs in the pontocerebellar hypoplasias (PCHs).

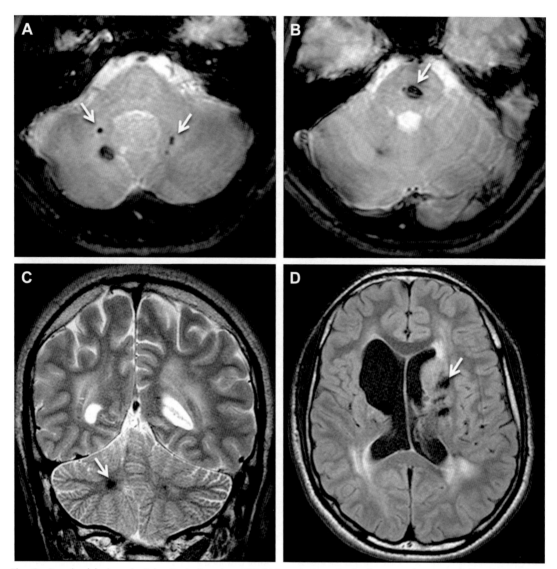

Fig. 2. Acquired lesions in inherited disorder: *COL4A1* mutation. Foci of magnetic susceptibility (*arrows*) are identified in the pons and dentate nuclei on axial T2* sequences (*A, B*), coronal T2W image (*C*), and axial fluid-attenuated inversion recovery (FLAIR) (*D*). The supratentorial, but not the infratentorial, foci were calcium containing on computed tomography. Periventricular hypersignal is present (*C, D*) and there is distortion of the right lateral ventricle caused by porencephaly in this teen with progressive clinical and imaging findings and no history of perinatal distress.

The PCHs are disorders with overlapping features of prenatal growth arrest and subsequent degeneration/atrophy. Head circumference is normal at birth in some patients, but progressive microcephaly develops even when the head circumference is already small. Severe thinning of the brainstem and middle cerebellar peduncles (MCP) occurs both in utero and postnatally. There is specific loss of the basis pons. Severe volume loss of the cerebellar hemispheres leads to enlargement of the fourth ventricle and cisterna magna, which in association with a less shrunken vermis give rise to the dragonfly pattern on coronal images. Eventual supratentorial atrophy occurs with flattening of the caudate nuclei heads (**Fig.** 4). Initially, 2 subtypes were identified, PCH1 and PCH2, classified by the presence or absence of anterior horn cell degeneration. Subsequently, many more causative gene mutations have been identified and PCH subtypes include PCH1 to PCH10. There is mutation-specific variability in the clinical phenotype. Mutations in genes encoding the transfer RNA (tRNA)–splicing endonuclease complex (TSEN) are found in

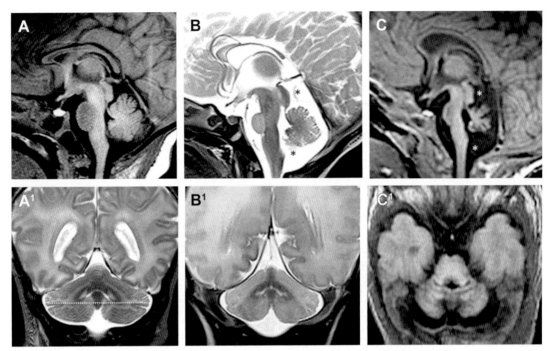

Fig. 3. Comparison of normal, hypoplasia, and atrophy at term. Control: sagittal T1W image (*A*) in a normal 38 weeks' gestational age (GA) infant has normal AP measurements of the midbrain, pons, and medulla; normal cranial-caudal height of the vermis; and normal area (*dotted circle*) of the basis pontis (pontine belly). Coronal T2W image (*A¹*) shows normal transverse diameter obtained at the equator of the cerebellum. Hypoplasia: sagittal T2W image (*B*) in a 37 weeks' GA infant with aneuploidy reveals a small pons and vermian height. The vermian height (*B*) and transverse cerebellar diameter (*B¹*) are small, appropriate for a 31 weeks' GA infant. Cisterns (*asterisks*) are prominent, but interfoliate fissures are normally spaced. Atrophy: sagittal T1W image (*C*) and axial FLAIR (*C¹*) in a term equivalent ex-23 weeks premature infant reveal volume loss of the brainstem, vermis, and cerebellar hemispheres with prominent interfoliate fissures and cisterns (*asterisks*).

infants with PCH2A and PCH4 and a single family described as having PCH5. These subtypes are now thought to be on a spectrum with phenotype reflecting the severity of *TSEN54* mutation. Patients with homozygous *TSEN54* missense mutations typically present with the milder PCH2A phenotype and although they do experience failure to thrive, epilepsy, dystonic attacks, and a reduced lifespan, some make developmental progress. Infants with a common mutation plus either a nonsense mutation or splice site mutation in *TSEN54* present with the severe PCH4 phenotype, formerly called olivopontocerebellar hypoplasia. Compound *TSEN54* heterozygosity was also found in the family formerly classified as PCH5. Newborns with PCH4 and PCH5 are usually ventilator dependent from birth.[32,33] Stunted folial outgrowth with variable loss of Purkinje cells and internal granule cells, cystic cerebellar degeneration, fragmentation of the dentate nuclei, progressive loss of the ventral pontine nuclei and transverse fibers, and segmental loss of neurons of the olives and poor myelin have been shown on autopsy in PCH2. More severe findings in PCH4 include regions of afolial cerebellar hemispheres and folial ghosts carrying remnants of preexistent developed cortex. The folial ghosts and persistent fetal pattern of horseshoe-shaped inferior olivary nuclei reflect arrest of development and the onset of degeneration during fetal life.[34–36]

CEREBELLAR ATROPHY, GENERAL

Atrophy is the most common cerebellar imaging feature found in the inborn errors of metabolism, although it is usually combined with other imaging determinants that help to narrow the differential diagnosis. Mitochondrial disorders, particularly in patients with respiratory chain defects, are the most common of inborn errors of metabolism presenting with cerebellar atrophy. In one large study of 113 children with mitochondrial disease, 26% showed cerebellar volume loss as the predominant imaging pattern.[10] Mutations in *ADCK3*, one of the many genes required for synthesis of coenzyme Q10, are also associated with the cerebellar ataxic phenotype of coenzyme Q10 deficiency.[37]

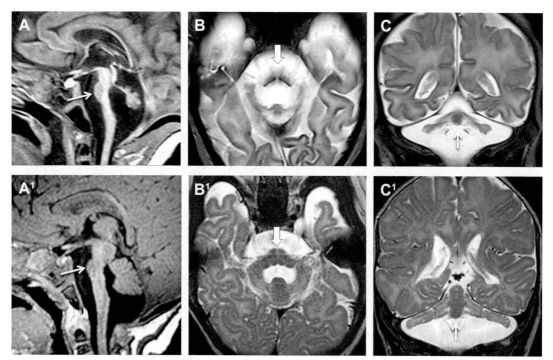

Fig. 4. PCH caused by TSEN4 mutations varies in severity: PCH4 (*top row*) versus PCH2A (*bottom row*). Sagittal images (*A, A¹*) show brainstem thinning and a small vermis in both infants, much more severe in PCH4 (*top row, A*). The pons in each is severely atrophied on sagittal T1W (*A, A¹*) (*arrows*) and axial T2W images (*B, B¹*) (*open arrows*). Although the vermis is small (*arrows*) on coronal T2W images (*C, C¹*), the hemispheres are smaller, giving rise to a dragonfly appearance with crescent-shaped cisterna magna.

Macroscopic patterns of cerebellovermian volume loss are important clues in the evaluation of disorders without a clear diagnosis (**Fig. 5**). Vermian involvement is best evaluated on the sagittal midline view, whereas assessment of the hemispheres and peduncles requires axial and coronal sequences. Predominant corticocerebellar atrophy (CCA) with Purkinje cell loss, spinal cord predominant atrophy with involvement of the Clarke column in the spinal gray matter, and olivopontocerebellar atrophy (OPCA) with loss of ventral pontine nuclei are 3 general patterns based on MR imaging. Progression from the more limited forms to diffuse OPCA may occur over time.

ISOLATED CEREBELLAR ATROPHY

Isolated or pure cerebellar atrophy is a common early, but nonspecific, feature in inborn errors of metabolism. In one study, the most subjects in the category of isolated cerebellar atrophy had no known diagnosis. However, most cases have or develop additional useful imaging features. Persistence of the isolated state is rare, because pure cerebellar atrophy frequently reflects an early stage, before the development of additional disease-specific determinants. The prototype

disorder with isolated and persistent or pure cerebellar atrophy diagnosis is late-onset GM2-gangliosidosis. GM2-gangliosidosis is a lysosomal storage disorder caused by deficiency of beta-hexosaminidase A, combined beta-hexosaminidases A and B, or the much rarer deficiency of the GM2 activator protein. Patients with a late-onset phenotype may present with cerebellar ataxia, dystonia, psychiatric disturbances, or anterior motor neuron disease. Even in late-onset GM2-gangliosidosis, there are 2 neuroradiological subtypes. The most common shows the classic findings of moderately severe, but isolated, cerebellovermian atrophy (**Fig. 6**). Imaging in the less common group also has marked supratentorial atrophy and white matter signal increase. Neuropathologic studies show neuronal GM2 storage throughout the neuroaxis and also show marked loss of granule and Purkinje cells in the cerebellum. The extent of loss is reflected by the decreased *N*-acetylaspartic acid (NAA) level shown on spectroscopy obtained both in the basal ganglia and in the cerebellar hemispheres in both subtypes. In addition, both supratentorial and infratentorial deep nuclear structures lose volume and undergo subtle increased secondary axonal degeneration even

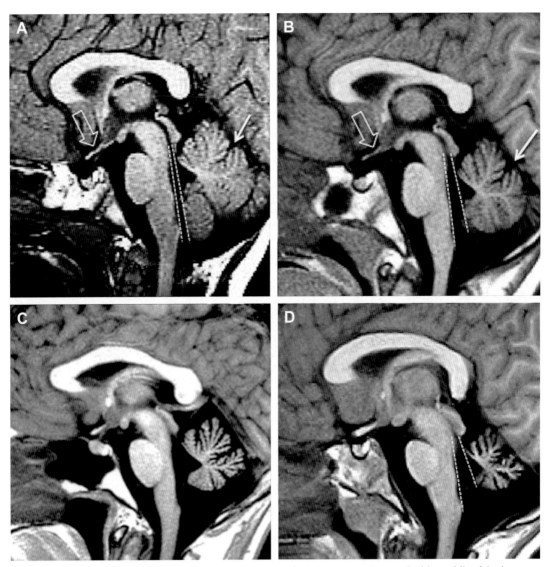

Fig. 5. Grading vermian atrophy. Normal vermis and normal tegmentovermian angle (*dotted lines*) is shown on T1W sagittal image (*A*). Severe optic chiasm atrophy (*open arrow*) preceded development of cerebellar atrophy in a child with optic atrophy 1 (*OPA1*). The primary fissure (*arrow*) and other interfoliate fissures are closed. Mild vermian volume loss and progressive chiasmatic atrophy (*open arrow*) are seen (*B*) on follow-up. The interfoliate fissures of the anterior vermian lobule, above the primary fissure (*arrow*), are open, whereas those below are closed. In mild to moderate vermian atrophy (*C*, late-onset GM2-gangliosidosis) there is progressive prominence of interfoliate fissures above and below the primary fissure. Marked atrophy is present in the final case (*D*) with increased tegmentovermian angle and posterior fossa cisterns.

in the predominantly infratentorial phenotype, resulting in subtle white matter signal of the centrum semiovale and pontine tracts on studies obtained late in the course of disease.[38,39] Similar to late-onset GM2 disorders, cases of neuronal ceroid-lipofuscinosis (NCL) presenting after the neonatal period show hypersignal of the cerebellar cortex late in the disease course. Distinctive imaging features in NCL are low-signal (dark) thalami in T2-weighted (T2W) or fluid-attenuated inversion recovery (FLAIR)

sequences, mild diffuse secondary demyelination of the peritrigonal optic radiations and posterior limb of internal capsule, and rare corticospinal necrosis (**Fig. 7**).[10]

GRADIENTS OF VOLUME LOSS ADD FURTHER SPECIFICITY

Additional inherited neurodegenerative disorders reported to present with isolated cerebellar volume loss or atrophy include ataxia-oculomotor

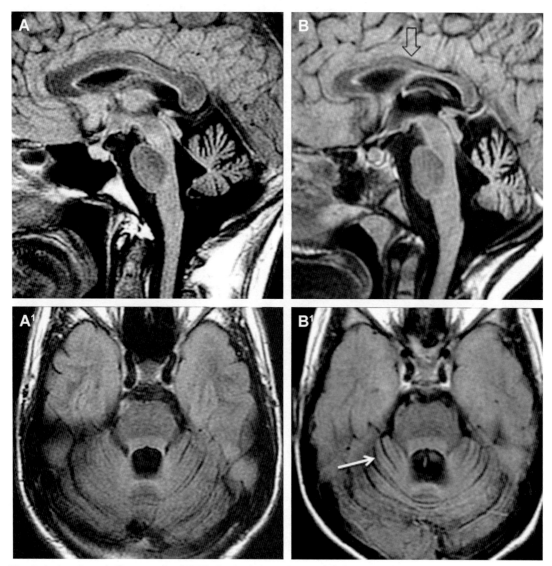

Fig. 6. Isolated cerebellar atrophy (GM2). Sagittal FLAIR image (*A*) shows moderately severe vermian atrophy with widening of the interfoliate fissures above and below the primary fissure (*arrow*). Axial FLAIR image (*A^1*) reveals moderate hemispheric atrophy, but no bright cerebellar cortex. In another teen (*B, B^1*), there is subtle thinning of the corpus callosum (*open arrow*) and mild tram-track hypersignal (*arrow*) of the cerebellar cortex.

apraxia types 1 and 2 and certain of the autosomal dominant and recessive spinocerebellar ataxias (*CACNA1A, TPP1, ANO10, GRM1, ITPR1* mutations).[40] Helpful refining features related to biometry include: gradient of vermian volume loss; anterior versus posterior, discordant involvement of the cerebellar hemispheres and vermis; and involvement of the brainstem and superior, middle, or inferior cerebellar peduncles. For example, cerebellar atrophy in Marinesco-Sjögren syndrome (MSS/*SIL1* mutation) is more pronounced in the vermis than in the hemispheres, whereas patients with SCA15 caused by *ITPR1* mutations show significant vermian atrophy, sparing of the

brainstem, and relative cerebellar hemispheric sparing.[41]

The anterior vermian fissures are normally slightly more prominent than the posterior vermian fissures below primary fissure, a finding that increases with aging in adults. The anterior-predominant gradient of volume loss is also common in inherited neurodegenerative disorders involving the vermis. Inferior vermian–predominant or posterior vermian–predominant atrophy is less common than anterior-predominant vermian atrophy. Inferior vermian–predominant volume loss and high signal of the inferomedial cerebellar cortex may be seen in Christianson syndrome (*SLC9A6*), although

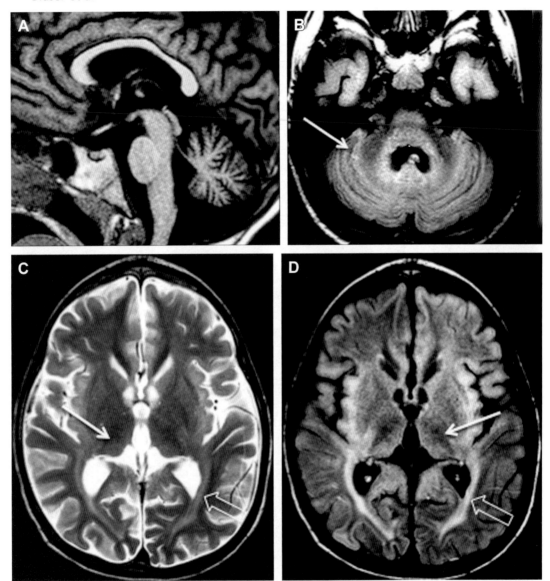

Fig. 7. Neuronal ceroid lipofuscinosis type 2. Sagittal T1W image (A) reveals moderate vermian atrophy and normal brainstem. Axial FLAIR image (B) shows mildly bright cerebellar cortex (arrow) and widened fissures. Axial T2W (C) and FLAIR (D) images show dark thalami (arrow) and high signal of the periventricular white matter and optic radiations (open arrows).

involvement of hemispheres and vermis is often more extensive. In addition to cerebellar hemisphere atrophy, posterior vermian volume loss has been described in patients with autosomal recessive cerebellar ataxia related to mutations in GRM1, which encodes metabotropic glutamate receptor 1 (mGluR1).[42] Congenital disorder of glycosylation, type 1a (CDG1a/PMM2) is only one of the disorders with more pronounced anterior vermian than posterior vermian volume loss. Pronounced anterior vermian atrophy in association with axonal swellings in the posterior lobes suggests progressive degeneration in patients with

CDG1a at 1 month of age.[43] Others include Friedreich Ataxia (FRDA; FRDA/FXN mutation), ataxia telangiectasia (AT/ATM), and autosomal recessive spastic ataxia of Charlevoix-Saguenay (ARSACS/SACS mutation). This anterior gradient may be mild or may be significant, as in ARSACS.

AUTOSOMAL RECESSIVE SPASTIC ATAXIA OF CHARLEVOIX-SAGUENAY; A DISORDER WITH SIGNIFICANT ANTERIOR VERMIAN ATROPHY

Findings in ARSACS, a disorder with ataxia and neuropathy now seen worldwide, include early atrophy of the anterior cerebellar vermis and superior cerebellar peduncles. There is subsequent atrophy of the cerebellar hemispheres and the medulla. The pons and MCP are bulky. The lateral pons and the MCP are also subtly increased in signal intensity. Hypointense linear striations, pontine tigroid hypointensities, are shown on T2 and FLAIR in the base and tegmentum of the pons. Diffusion tensor tractography shows interruption of thin pyramidal tracts by these hyperplastic pontocerebellar fibers at the level of the pons. A rim of T2 hyperintensity around the thalami is a usual feature.[44–48] The cervical spinal cord atrophies late and spinal radiographs show a straight spine.[49] Thickening of the retinal nerve fiber layer is variable, most commonly seen in Quebecois patients and less commonly in cohorts from Europe or the Middle East, can be seen with retinal examination, but is not identifiable on routine imaging (**Fig. 8**).

ABNORMALITIES OF CEREBELLAR PEDUNCLE AND BRAINSTEM VOLUME

MR planimetry of the brainstem and inspection of the cerebellar peduncles are useful in both early-onset and late-onset disorders. The dentate hilum outflow tract, the dentatorubrothalamic tract, traverses the superior cerebellar peduncles to decussate in the midbrain and extends to the red nucleus and thalamus. The inferior cerebellar peduncles are largely composed of the olivocerebellar and spinocerebellar tract fibers, whereas the MCP comprise the pontocerebellar tract arising from the pontine nuclei and extending topographically to the cerebellar cortex. Pontine and MCP enlargement and marked superior cerebellar atrophy are seen in ARSACS (see **Fig. 8**), whereas loss of volume of the MCP and pons is present in PCH2 and PCH4 (**Fig. 9**). MCP and pontine volume loss are also seen in cerebellar ataxia type multiple system atrophy (MSA-C), where loss of the transverse pontine fibers and

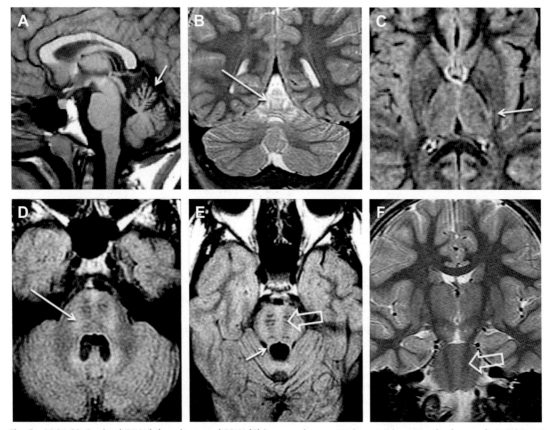

Fig. 8. ARSACS. Sagittal T1W (*A*) and coronal T2W (*B*) images show anterior vermian atrophy (*arrows*). Axial FLAIR (*C*) reveals high-signal rim along the lateral border of the thalamus (*arrow*). Axial FLAIR (*D*) shows high signal of the lateral pons (*arrow*), whereas axial FLAIR (*E*) and coronal T2W images (*F*) show typical thick hypointense pontocerebellar fibers (*open arrows*). There is marked atrophy of the superior cerebellar peduncles (*arrow*) (*E*).

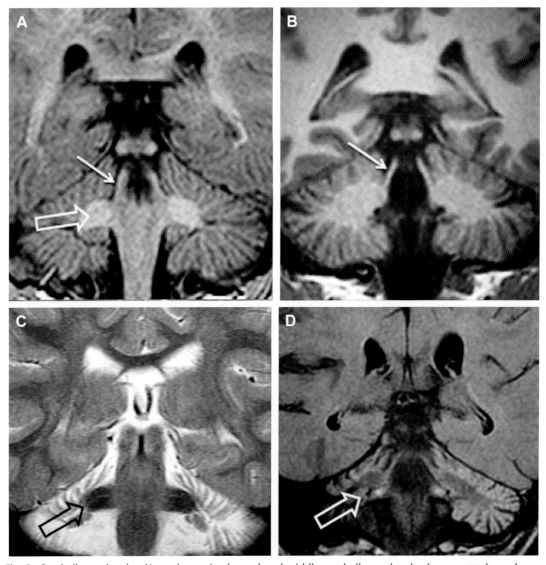

Fig. 9. Cerebellar peduncles. Normal superior (*arrow*) and middle cerebellar peduncles (*open arrow*) are shown on T1W coronal image (*A*), whereas hypoplastic superior cerebellar peduncles (*arrow*) are present in FRDA (*B*). Coronal T2W image (*C*) in CDG1a shows mild atrophy of the middle cerebellar peduncles (MCP) (*open black arrow*) and marked cerebellar cortex atrophy. Coronal FLAIR image (*D*) in another infant with CDG1a shows bright signal and severe atrophy of the MCP (*open arrow*) and cerebellar cortex.

atrophy of the inferior cerebellar peduncles occur. The quarter-note sign, in which an increase in the superior cerebellar peduncle angle obtained at the vertex of the superior cerebellar peduncles on the coronal view reflects degeneration and atrophy of the MCP, is a finding seen with degeneration and atrophy of the basilar portion of the pons.[50] Sparing of the superior cerebellar peduncles in MSA-C helps to differentiate it on imaging from SCA6 (*CACNA1A*), SCA8 (*ATNX8*), CCA, progressive supranuclear palsy (PSP; PSP1/*MAPT*) and striatonigral or parkinsonian type MSA (MSA-P). Atrophy of the superior cerebellar peduncles and midbrain is notable in PSP1,

whereas atrophy of the MCP and pons is more suggestive of MSA-P.[51–53]

FOCAL ABNORMALITIES OF BRAINSTEM BIOMETRY

Diffuse brainstem atrophy, which when associated with cerebellar atrophy is part of the OPCA pattern, is often the end stage of several neurodegenerative disorders, including PCH and CDG1a (*PMM2*). Timely imaging is helpful in identifying specific focal abnormalities. Although midbrain atrophy is common with diffuse brainstem atrophy, severe midbrain atrophy sparing the remainder of the brainstem occurs in early-onset Krabbe (*GALC*). Enlargement of the clava may be the first imaging feature in infantile neuroaxonal dystrophy (INAD; INAD/*PLA2G6*), even before vermian atrophy, whereas a slender medulla and mild posterior vermian atrophy can be seen in spastic paraplegia 35 (*FA2H*), a disorder with mild cerebellar atrophy, T2 hyperintensity of the internal capsules, periatrial white matter and cerebellum, and globus pallidus brain iron (**Fig. 10**). The pons is enlarged in ARSACS (*SACS*), whereas pontine volume loss is seen in Wolfram syndrome types 1 and 2 (*WFS1*/*CISD2*), a neurodegenerative disease characterized with diabetes insipidus, diabetes mellitus (in type 1, not type 2), optic atrophy, and deafness (DIDMOAD), whereas flattening of the pons is seen in patients with congenital disorders of glycosylation CDG1a (*PMM2*) (see **Fig. 8**; **Fig. 11**).

CONGENITAL DISORDER OF GLYCOSYLATION CDG1A (*PMM2*): THE PROTOTYPE FOR DISORDERS WITH PONTINE (AND CEREBELLAR) ATROPHY

Cerebellar and brainstem involvement are the most recognized features of PMM2-CDG (CDG1a), the first described and the most frequent

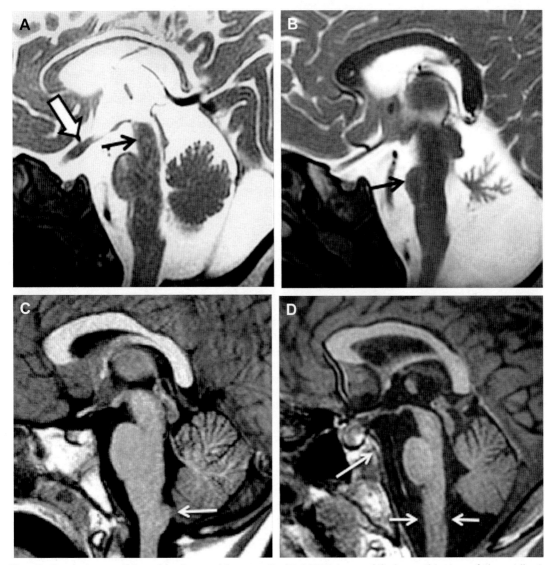

Fig. 10. Focal abnormalities of brainstem biometry. Sagittal T2W image (*A*) shows thinning of the midbrain tegmentum (*black arrow*) and the tectum in Krabbe disease. Note the typical enlarged optic chiasm (*open arrow*). Sagittal T2W image (*B*) in CDG1a reveals decreased pontine area (*arrow*) and severe vermian atrophy. The clava (*arrow*) is enlarged on sagittal T1W image (*C*) in INAD/PLA2G6, whereas the retroclival CSF space (*arrow*) denotes brainstem thinning (*D*) The medulla is thin (*arrows*).

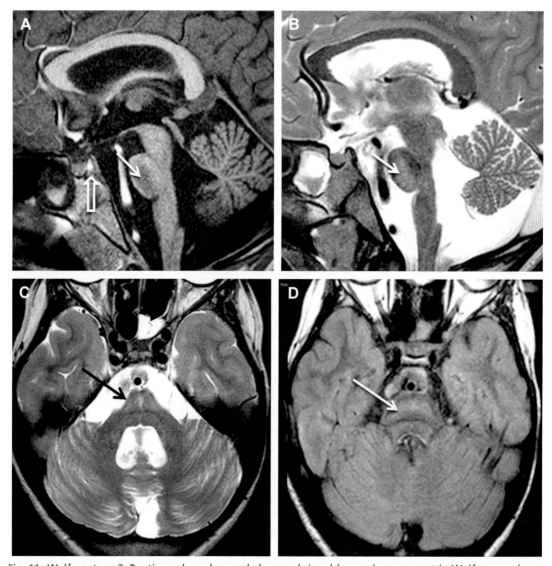

Fig. 11. Wolfram type 2. Pontine volume loss and abnormal signal (*arrows*) are present in Wolfram syndrome in T1W (*A*) and T2W (*B*) sagittal images. The posterior pituitary bright spot (*A, open arrow*) confirms type 2. Cerebellovermian atrophy and increased tegmentovermian angle are present. Axial T2W image (*C*) shows a pyramidal configuration (*black arrow*) of the pons caused by atrophy. Axial FLAIR image (*D*) shows typical high signal of the ventral pontine nuclei (*arrow*) anterior to the hypointense linear transverse trapezoid body fibers.

of the *N*-glycosylation disorders. Classic PMM2-CDG findings have shown progressive cerebellar volume loss and hyperintense cerebellar cortex. Rather than true hypoplasia, early neonatal imaging shows normal biometry of the brainstem and cerebellum before the rapid onset of atrophy. Fetal MR imaging in 1 patient showed a normal cerebellum during the second trimester and normal MR imaging at 6 weeks of age with the development of subsequent cerebellovermian atrophy.[53] Onset of cerebellar and brainstem atrophy have been noted as early as 11 days of life and as late as 9 months of age, but are usual after 3 months

of age. Anterior vermian volume loss, reduction of pontine protuberance, enlarged cerebellar interfoliate fissures and fourth ventricle, and abnormal signal of the olives and cerebellar cortex progress on serial imaging (**Fig. 12**). Although pontine flattening is the first notable brainstem feature, there may be eventual atrophy of the entire brainstem.[54–57] Histopathology shows severe neuronal loss in the pontine nuclei and inferior olives. In keeping with the concept of progressive atrophy, rather than hypoplasia, a fairly intact pons has been shown in an autopsy of a 1-month-old infant with CDG1a (*PMM2-CDG*).[43]

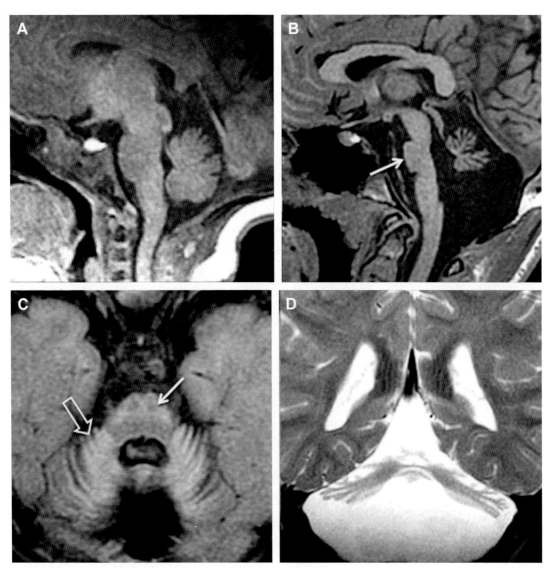

Fig. 12. CDG1a. Sagittal T1W image (*A*) in a newborn with CDG1a shows a normal brainstem and minimal widening of the interfoliate fissures of the anterior vermis. Sagittal T1W image (*B*) in a teen with CDG1a reveals marked pontine flattening (*arrow*) and severe vermian atrophy. Axial FLAIR (*C*) shows hypersignal of the pyramidal-shaped ventral pons (*arrow*) and the cerebellar cortex (*open arrow*). Severe hemispheric atrophy is present on coronal T2W image (*D*).

ATROPHY OF THE SPINAL CORD, GENERAL

Atrophy of the spinal cord and medulla has also been documented as a minor finding on imaging in several disorders. The presence or absence of it in spinocerebellar ataxia may help in differentiating subtypes. For example, the upper cervical spinal cord and medulla show volume loss in SCA3/Machado-Joseph disease (*ATXN3*), a disorder in which anterior horn cells, spinocerebellar tracts, Clarke columns, and dorsal columns are known to be involved, whereas SCA6 (*CACNA1A*), has a cerebellovermian predominance and a relative lack of

spinal cord involvement on imaging.[58] Spinal atrophy on imaging has been reported with increasing age and markedly reduced body weight and severe growth factor deficiency in AT/*ATM*, reflecting anterior horn cell atrophy and demyelination of the spinal cord gracile fascicule.[59,60]

FRIEDREICH ATAXIA IS THE PROTOTYPE FOR NEURODEGENERATIVE DISORDERS WITH PREDOMINANT SPINAL CORD ATROPHY

Assessment of the upper cervical cord is predominantly useful in the evaluation of patients with

Friedreich ataxia (FRDA/*FXN*), in whom cord thinning caused by neuronal loss in the spinal ganglia and Clarke column may be the first imaging clue to the disorder. Increased intramedullary signal reflects gliosis of the fasciculus gracilis and cuneatus (posterior columns) and of the pyramidal tracts (lateral columns).[61] Scoliosis is common. Although thinning of the cervical cord and medulla, and atrophy of the culmen and declive, may be noted visually on assessment of the midline sagittal view, involvement of the cerebellum was initially considered a rare feature in FRDA.

However, volumetric analysis of the cerebellum in FRDA confirms volume loss in the rostral vermis, dorsal medulla, the dentate nuclei, the peridentate white matter, and the associated superior cerebellar peduncle (**Fig. 13**). Increased iron level has been reported, but is neither universal nor reproducible on imaging in the dentate nucleus of patients with FRDA/*FXN*.[62,63] Cerebellar white matter gliosis and loss of dentate nuclei neurons and of the myelinated fibers in the dentate hila are confirmed on pathologic specimens. Mild loss of Purkinje cells of the cerebellar cortex is

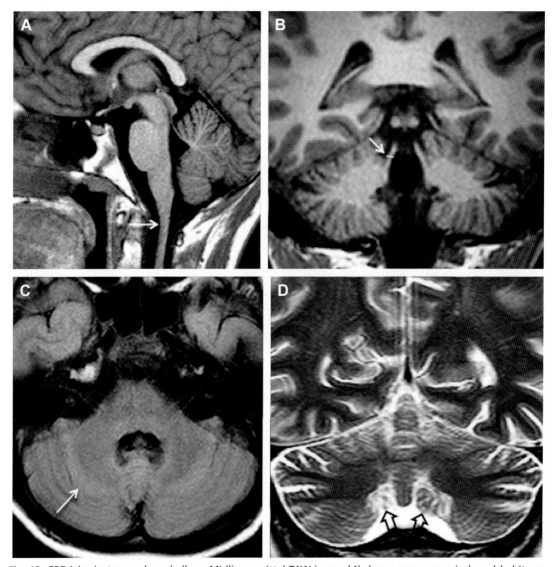

Fig. 13. FRDA brainstem and cerebellum. Midline sagittal T1W image (*A*) shows narrow cervical cord (*white arrow*). The superior cerebellar peduncles (*arrow, white line*) are thin on coronal T1W image (*B*). Subtle increased signal (*arrow*) of the cortex of the cerebellar folia is present on axial FLAIR (*C*). Subtle widening of the lateral interfoliate fissures and the paravermian interfoliate fissures (*open arrows*) on coronal T2W image (*D*) denote mild cerebellar volume loss.

reflected in the mild volume loss of the inferomedial cerebellar lobules.[64,65] Cerebrovascular thrombosis associated with dilated cardiomyopathy in the inherited neuromuscular diseases is considered rare, but does occur.[66] Cardiomyopathy, when present in FRDA, usually consists of a hypertrophic cardiomyopathy, but may progress to a dilated cardiomyopathy (**Fig. 14**). Stroke is reported as a cause of death in 20% of patients with FRDA with dilated cardiomyopathy, caused by atrial fibrillation or mural thrombus.[67]

ADDITIONAL IMAGING FEATURES: FOCI OF MAGNETIC SUSCEPTIBILITY IN ATAXIA TELANGIECTASIA (AND OTHERS)

Cerebellar atrophy is the earliest imaging clue in (AT/*ATM*). Images obtained between 3 and 7 years of age usually show loss of volume of the lateral hemispheres and superior vermis, evolving into diffuse cerebellovermian atrophy later.[68] Subtle increased FLAIR signal of the cerebellar cortex seen after the development of atrophy reflects autopsy findings of Purkinje, and granular and neuronal cell loss. Dentate atrophy also occurs. Telangiectasias only become evident during late childhood and early adult life with the use of T2* techniques and administration of gadolinium.[69,70] Supratentorial white matter hyperintensities correspond with the spongiosis surrounding

telangiectasias on autopsy[60] (**Fig. 15**). Basal ganglia lesions are uncommon, despite the presence of dystonia in some patients.[59] MRS of the cerebellum shows decreased NAA/Cho ratios and increased Cho/creatine (Cr) ratios, typical features of disorders with cerebellar degeneration.[69] Foci of susceptibility caused by small microbleeds can be seen in the brain and cerebellum of children and adults with *COL41A* mutations and also in the cerebellum of infants with methylmalonic acidemia (*MUT^0*) and propionic academia (*PCCA/B*). T2* techniques also detect the presence of calcification in Aicardi-Goutières (*TREX1* and others) and in Coats plus disease (*CTC1*). Aicardi-Goutières is an autoimmune-mediated genetic encephalopathy with imaging findings that resemble congenital TORCH infections. These findings include: variable degrees of white matter atrophy; a range of mild to severe white matter signal abnormalities; temporal lobe cysts; intracranial calcifications involving the white matter, basal ganglia, and dentate nuclei of the cerebellum; and cerebellar and brainstem atrophy. These findings are likely caused in part by a microangiopathy.[71,72] Coats plus syndrome (*CTC1*), a telomere biology disorder with cerebroretinal microangiopathy, shows leukoencephalopathy, calcifications and cysts of the cerebrum and cerebellum, ataxia, and Coats reaction of the retina (retinal telangiectasia) (**Fig. 16**). Progressive intracerebral calcifications

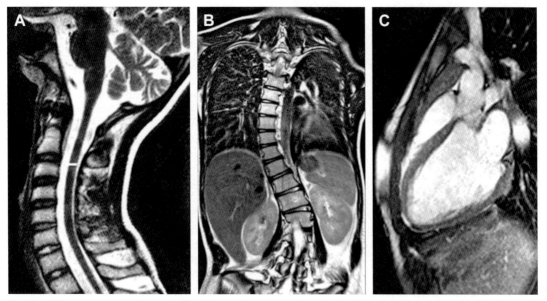

Fig. 14. FRDA spine and cardiomyopathy. The most frequent imaging findings in FRDA do not involve the brain. Sagittal T2W image (*A*) shows mild vermian atrophy and significant cervical spinal cord atrophy (*white line* at C2-C3 disc level). Coronal T2W image (*B*) shows typical scoliosis. Dilated cardiomyopathy is revealed on sagittal T2W image (*C*).

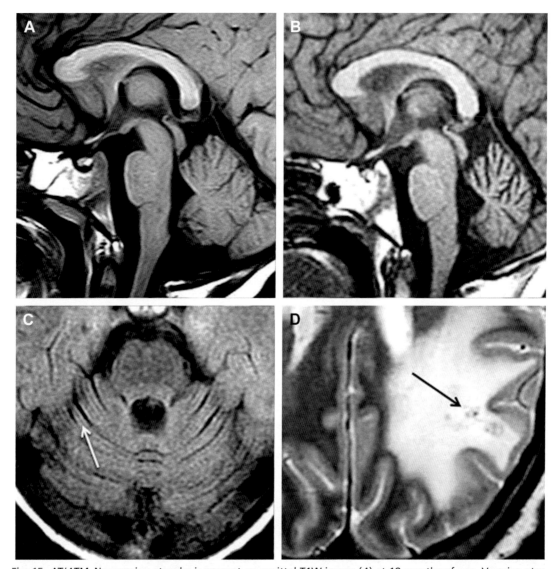

Fig. 15. AT/*ATM*. No vermian atrophy is present on sagittal T1W image (*A*) at 18 months of age. Vermian atrophy is identified on sagittal T1W image (*B*) at 4 years 6 months of age, as has subtle bright tram-tracking (*arrow*) of the cerebellar cortex on FLAIR axial image (*C*) obtained at the same time. Telangiectasias (*arrow*) and surrounding white matter edema are present on T2W axial image (*D*) in another patient with AT at 38 years of age.

of the deep gray nuclei, brainstem, cerebral and cerebellar white matter, dentate nuclei, and diffuse white matter, and cerebral cysts, reflect extensive calcinosis, thickened hyalinized small vessels, obliterative angiopathy, necrosis, cysts and white matter abnormalities.[72,73]

ADDITIONAL IMAGING FINDINGS: CYSTS

Cysts in the cerebellum are an uncommon imaging finding. Large cysts occur in Coats plus syndrome (*CTC1*), whereas small numbers of smaller cerebellar cysts have been described in Aicardi syndrome, PCH type 2, and PCH type 6 (*RARS2*).[34,73–75] Large numbers of very small cysts associated with diffuse cerebellar dysplasia have been shown in dystroglycanopathy (congenital muscular dystrophy with brain and eye anomalies), *GPR56* mutations, cerebellar dysplasias with supratentorial polymicrogyria, and *LAMA1*-related cerebellar dysplasia with ocular motor apraxia with cysts[76–78] (**Fig. 17**). Other disorders with supratentorial cysts, such as megalencephalic leukoencephalopathy with subcortical cysts (*MLC1*) and

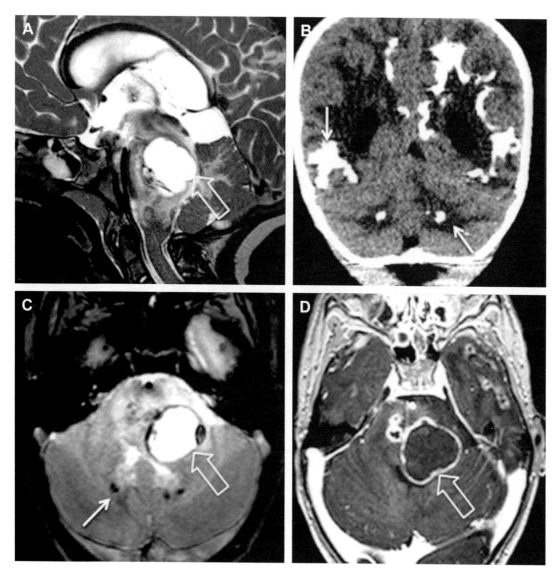

Fig. 16. Coats plus. Sagittal T2W image (*A*) shows swelling of the vermis and brainstem. A large necrotic cyst is present (*open arrow*). Non-enhanced CT (NECT) coronal image (*B*) reveals extensive supratentorial and infratentorial calcification (*arrows*). Axial T2* image (*C*) shows dentate calcifications (*arrow*) and necrotic cyst (*open arrow*). Extensive ring enhancement of multiple small cysts is seen in addition to the larger necrotic cyst (*open arrow*) after gadolinium administration (*D*).

RNASET2-deficient leukoencephalopathy, do not typically show cerebellar cysts.

ADDITIONAL IMAGING FINDINGS: CEREBELLAR ATROPHY WITH INCREASED CEREBELLAR CORTEX SIGNAL ON FLUID-ATTENUATED INVERSION RECOVERY

The cerebellar cortex has 3 layers: the internal granular, the Purkinje layer in the middle, and the outer molecular layer. Two layers, internal granular and molecular, of the cerebellar cortex can be discerned with high-field-strength imaging at 7 T. However, the very thin intervening Purkinje cell layer cannot be resolved, even at 7 T.[79] Intrafoliate white matter lies subjacent to the internal granular layer. High-field 7-T MR imaging is also able to differentiate supratentorial juxtacortical and cortical lesions; however, data regarding evaluation of the layers of the cerebellar cortex in the inherited neurodegenerative disorders involving the cerebellum during childhood are not yet

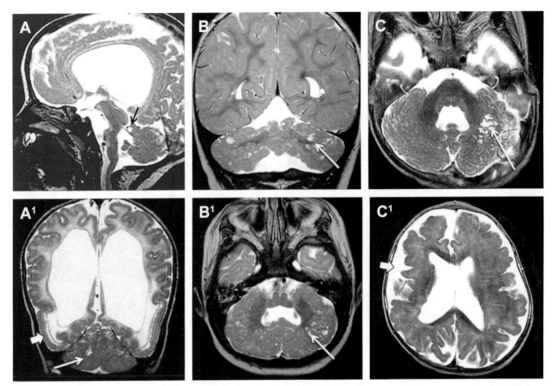

Fig. 17. Cerebellar cysts. Sagittal T2W image in congenital muscular dystrophy (*A*) reveals ventriculomegaly, a Z-shaped brainstem, and dysplastic vermis. Multiple small cerebellovermian cysts (*arrows*) are identified (*A*, *A¹*). Cobblestone lissencephaly (*large arrow*) of the occipital poles is shown on coronal T2W image (*A¹*). Dysplastic cerebellum and multiple small cerebellovermian cysts (*arrows*) are also present in cerebellar dysplasia with ocular motor apraxia (*B*, *B¹*). Extensive small cerebellar cysts (*arrow*) are seen on axial T2W image (*C*) in GPR56 mutation, whereas ventriculomegaly and asymmetric bilateral perisylvian gyral anomalies (*large arrow*) are identified on axial T2W image (*C¹*).

available. Purkinje cell death results in hyperplasia of Bergmann glia, which are located around the Purkinje cell soma, a process called Bergmann gliosis. The fibrillary processes of the Bergmann glia radiate through the molecular layer to the pial surface of the cerebellar cortex. Because the Purkinje cell layer cannot be resolved on routine imaging or even high-field 7-T MR imaging sequences, the cause of the bright cerebellar cortex on FLAIR is assumed to represent reactive gliosis in the cerebellar cortex. The presence of a bright cerebellar cortex on FLAIR or T2-weighted signal adds some specificity on imaging, but the number of disorders in which this sign may occur has expanded. Originally thought to be virtually pathognomonic for congenital disorders of glycosylation (CDG1a [*PMM2*]) and for INAD (*PLA2A6*), it has been documented in patients with Marinesco-Sjögren syndrome (MSS/*SIL1*), Christianson syndrome (*SLC9A6*), and in various mitochondrial disorders, such as coenzyme Q10 deficiency, nonprogressive cerebellar ataxia (*PMPCA*),

mitochondrial myopathy, encephalopathy, lactic acidosis and stroke-like episodes (MELAS), and *POLG1*-related ataxia (**Fig. 18**). Bright cortex signal is thought to reflect the severe cerebellar cortex atrophy with neuronal loss and astrogliosis seen in both MSS and INAD, whereas significant loss of cerebellar cortex Purkinje cells, depletion of granular cells, decreased thickness of the molecular layer, and atrophied cerebellar folia have been shown on pathologic specimens in CDG1a.[43,80] The presence of neuronal cell loss with reactive gliosis and axonal swelling in CDG1a, as well as localization of Purkinje cells within the Purkinje cell layer, is thought to reflect degeneration rather than developmental arrest.[43]

The hyperintense cerebellar cortex on FLAIR is usually symmetric and associated with significant cerebellar atrophy. The bright signal of the cortex on FLAIR may be patchy and asymmetric in some mitochondrial disorders, such as *POLG1*-related ataxia, or diffuse and involve only the inferior cerebellum, as seen in Christianson syndrome.

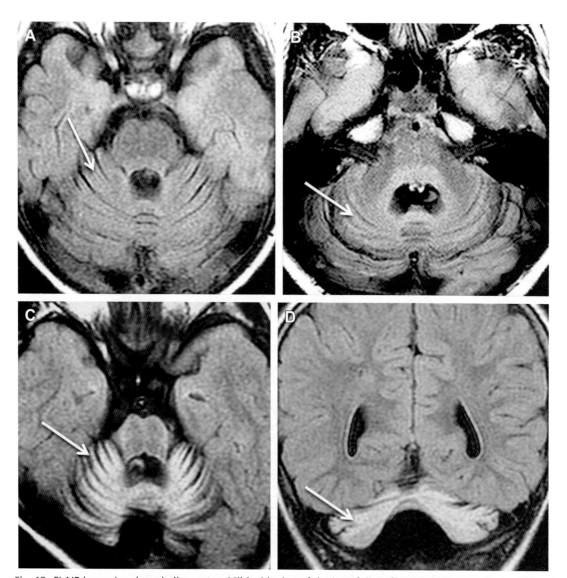

Fig. 18. FLAIR hypersignal cerebellar cortex. Mild widening of the interfoliate fissures and tram-track high signal (*arrow*) of the cerebellar cortex is identified on axial FLAIR image (*A*) in a child with AT. More diffuse cerebellar volume loss and cerebellar cortex signal increase is seen in *POLG1* (*B, arrow*). Markedly increased signal intensity of the cerebellar cortex is present in an infant with CDG1a (*C, arrow*). The pons is also atrophied and increased in signal. In addition, marked high signal of the cerebellar cortex (*arrow*) and prominent subhemispheric cistern is present on coronal FLAIR image (*D*) in an infant with INAD.

DNA-polymerase gamma (*POLG*), responsible for integrity and replication of the mitochondrial genome, is associated with a wide range of encephalopathies with overlapping clusters of clinical and imaging features. It should be noted that classification of POLG-related disorders may be fluid, because other POLG-related manifestations develop over time. The early childhood–onset disorders are currently defined as neonatal-onset mitochondrial DNA depletion (myocerebrohepatopathy spectrum) and infancy/childhood-onset epilepsy with occipital predominance and predilection to sodium-valproate precipitated or accelerated hepatic failure (Alpers-Huttenlocher syndrome). Later-onset disorders are myoclonus, epilepsy, myopathy, sensory ataxia (MEMSA) and the ataxia neuropathy spectrum, which in turn encompasses mitochondrial spinocerebellar ataxia syndrome, mitochondrial recessive ataxic syndrome, sensory ataxic neuropathy with ophthalmoplegia, and spinocerebellar ataxia epilepsy syndrome.[81,82] POLG-encephalopathies share involvement of nervous system and liver, and have episodes of disturbed consciousness, epilepsy, and acute lesions in the posterior parts of the brain. Imaging features include acute predominantly strokelike lesions, which favor the occipital lobes and typically spare the temporal lobes and chronic noncalcifying focal signal abnormalities in the thalami, inferior olivary nuclei, and cerebellum. The supratentorial strokelike lesions are replaced by focal atrophy, retraction, and often persistent increased signal. The thalamic lesions show a particular predilection for the posterior thalamus/pulvinar regions. Dentate atrophy associated with inferior olive lesions is more common in patients with *W748S* (**Fig. 19**). The cerebral cortical, thalamic, and dentate nuclei show evidence of eosinophilic neuronal necrosis, whereas the cerebellum shows Purkinje cell loss and Bergman gliosis. Diffuse white matter hypersignal reflecting spongiosis occurs and is more common

in *A467T* homozygotes. Late atrophy ensues after multiple exacerbations. In addition, dorsal column degeneration has been reported. MELAS differs in acquiring hazy basal ganglia calcifications over time.[81,83]

Male patients with Christianson syndrome, an X-linked neurodevelopmental disorder, present with developmental regression and progressive cerebellar atrophy (**Fig. 20**). Cerebellar atrophy during the second year of life in Christianson syndrome reflects the loss of Purkinje cells within the cerebellar cortex. The dentate nuclei are spared. Cerebellar cortex gliosis is reflected by the hyperintense cortex.[84] The rate of progression of hyperintense cerebellar cortex development is variable. In nonprogressive cerebellar ataxia caused by PMPCA mutations, similar severe vermian atrophy, hyperintense cerebellar cortex, and brainstem sparing were seen in individuals as young as 21 months of age and as old as 40 years

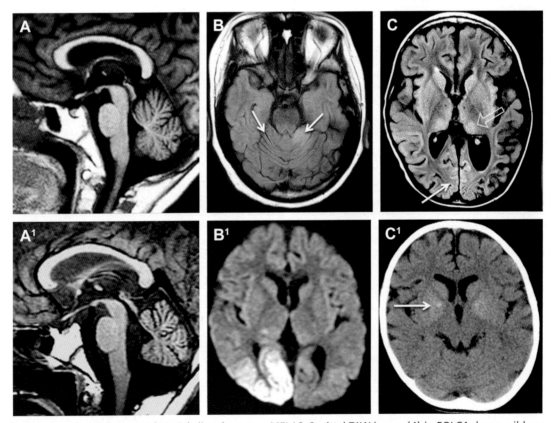

Fig. 19. Polymerase gamma 1 (*POLG1*) disorder versus MELAS. Sagittal T1W image (*A*) in POLG1 shows mild vermian atrophy. There is subtle tram-track high signal on FLAIR (*B*) and asymmetric swelling on the left (*arrows*). Bilateral occipital pole atrophy and high signal of the cortex and juxtacortical white matter are present (*arrow*) and bilateral typical posterior thalamic (*open arrow*) high signal is present on axial FLAIR (*C*). Sagittal T1W image in MELAS (*A¹*) also reveals mild vermian atrophy. Axial DWI (*B¹*) shows diffusion restriction of the right occipital pole, whereas NECT (*C¹*) reveals hazy calcification of the globus pallidus (*arrow*).

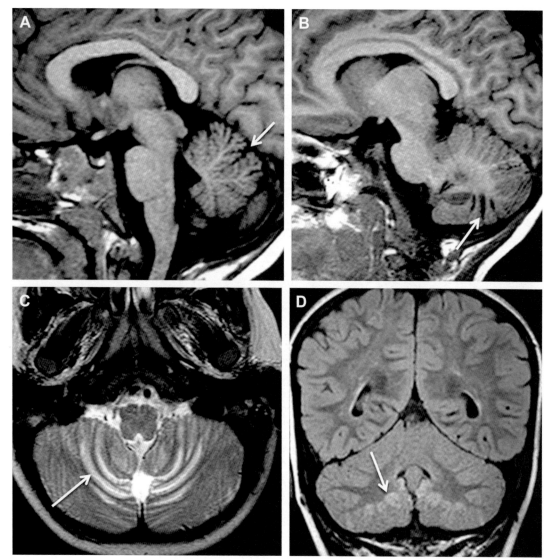

Fig. 20. Christianson syndrome. Sagittal T1W image (*A*) shows mild enlargement of the cerebellar folia (*arrow*), whereas focal atrophy at the depth of the folia is seen in the hemispheres (*arrow*) on (*B*). Axial T2W image (*C*) and FLAIR coronal image (*D*) reveal hypersignal at the depth of the inferomedial cerebellar folia (*arrow*).

of age.[85] In contradistinction, late-onset GM2 gangliosidosis, usually classified with disorders showing isolated or pure cerebellar atrophy, may develop a bright cerebellar cortex very late in the course of disease.[10,80,86]

DENTATE NUCLEI

The dentate nucleus is the largest and most recognizable of the deep cerebellar nuclei. It has a predictable imaging appearance reflecting the stage of myelin maturation in the dentate hilum and the cerebellar white matter surrounding the dentate nucleus during the first year of life. At term, the dentate nucleus is T1 hypointense and T2 hyperintense with a dark serrated rim. By 6 months of age, myelin maturation within the dentate renders the nucleus difficult to distinguish from the surrounding white matter on T1-weighted (T1W) images, whereas the central nucleus remains marginally brighter on T2W images and the dark serrated rim blends with the surrounding mature myelin. Noticeably increased signal on T2W or FLAIR sequences after that time is abnormal. Diffusion restriction at any age is abnormal[87] (**Fig. 21**).

Disorders with defective mitochondrial DNA commonly affect the posterior fossa structures leading to variable neuronal loss of the Purkinje

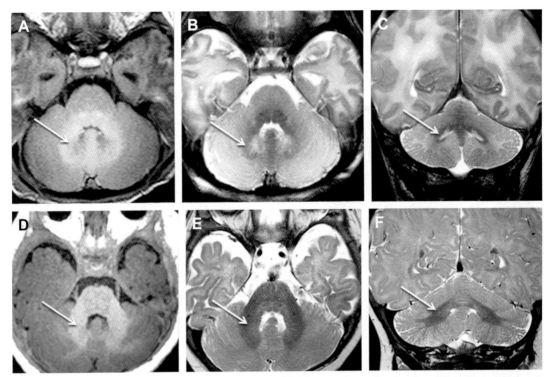

Fig. 21. Normal dentate nucleus maturation. (*Top row*) At 39 weeks the dentate nucleus (*arrow*) is subtly low in signal compared with adjacent white matter on T1W axial image (*A*), whereas the central hilus of the dentate nucleus is low. The dentate nucleus appears as a crenellated low-signal-intensity ribbon (*arrows*) on axial (*B*) and coronal T2W (*C*) images, and the central hilar white matter maintains an increased signal. (*Bottom row*) At 6 months, with myelin maturation of the adjacent cerebellar white matter in the brachium pontis and the central hilus, the dentate nucleus (*arrows*) is barely discernable on T1W (*D*) and T2W (*E, F*) images.

cells, the olivary and dentate nuclei, and the granule cells.[88] *SURF1* is an assembly factor of the oxidative phosphorylation complexes. Although cerebellar atrophy is very rarely the first abnormal MR feature in patients with *SURF1* mutations, and although there may be associated leukodystrophy or demyelinating neuropathy, a Leigh syndrome pattern involving the brainstem and cerebellum should raise the consideration of *SURF1*-related cytochrome-c oxidase deficiency.[83,89] Symmetric T2/FLAIR signal increase, reflecting capillary proliferation, necrosis, astrogliosis, or demyelination, occurs in the medulla, inferior cerebellar peduncles, dentate nuclei, central tegmental tracts, substantia nigra, and subthalamic nuclei. Supratentorial involvement of the thalami and basal ganglia is considerably less common.[89–91] Hypertrophic olivary degeneration (HOD) can be seen in both *SURF1* mutations and mutations in the DNA-POLG gene (**Fig. 22**). Typical dentate and brainstem abnormalities have been shown in patients with *SURF1* with HOD, whereas, in *POLG1* mutations with cerebellar involvement, HOD can be accompanied by cerebellar atrophy, and cerebellar white matter and supratentorial putaminal abnormalities.[92,93]

DENTATE NUCLEI AND CEREBELLAR WHITE MATTER

Involvement of the dentate, hilum, and surrounding white matter by inherited neurodegenerative disorders can be partial or complete. The differential diagnosis can include mitochondrial encephalopathies, organic acidurias, and amino acidopathies. Acute phase swelling during the acute metabolic stage with volume loss and less prominent signal during the atrophic-necrotic stage are common.[2] Specific attention to the pattern of involvement of the specific layers may be helpful. Involvement of the white matter of the hilum with involvement of the dentate nucleus, but sparing of the white matter peripheral to the dentate nucleus, can give a cockle-shell appearance. This appearance has been shown in children with L2OH glutaric aciduria (*L2HGDH*), who are known to have involvement of supratentorial subcortical white matter, the globus pallidus, caudate nucleus, and putamina.[94,95] The

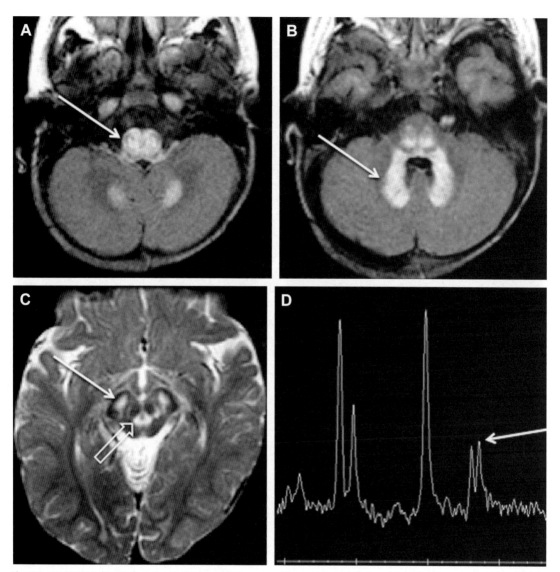

Fig. 22. SURFEIT 1 (SURF1). Axial FLAIR images show swelling of the medulla with HOD (*A, arrow*) and cerebellar white matter (*B, arrow*). Increased signal intensity is present in the subthalamic nuclei (*arrow*) and periaqueductal gray matter (*open arrow*) on axial T2W image (*C*). Single-voxel TE 288 MRS (*D*) placed over the brainstem and cerebellar white matter reveals a large lactate doublet (*arrow*).

dentate nucleus and hilar outflow tracts are involved, but there is sparing of the cerebellar white matter (Fig. 23). There may be very slow progressive atrophy of the dentate and hila by adulthood.[95] A spared dentate nucleus sandwiched between hyperintense cerebellar white matter and hilar outflow tracts leads to a 3-layered pattern that can be present in infantile-onset Krabbe (*GALC*), a lysosomal leukodystrophy caused by galactocerebrosidase β-galactosidase deficiency. Early-onset cases also present with hypersignal on T2W sequences of the periventricular and centrum semiovale white matter; hypertrophy of

the optic chiasm; the hummingbird configuration of midbrain atrophy; faint calcifications or computed tomography hyperdensity of the thalami, cerebellum, caudate, and involved white matter; and eventual corticospinal tract necrosis.[96,97] Involvement of the cerebellum is a poor prognostic indicator, whereas lack of cerebellar involvement on the first MR scan is reported in long-term survivors.[98] It is also seen in the early-onset peroxisomal disorders, in which it starts in the outflow tracts of the dentate nucleus, the hilum, and superior cerebellar peduncles, with eventual involvement of the cerebellar white matter, the

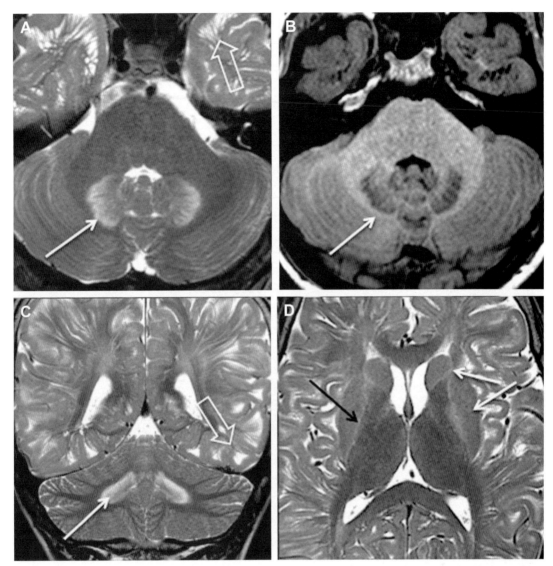

Fig. 23. Abnormal bright dentate signal. L2OH glutaric aciduria: T2W and T1W axial images (*A, B*) show abnormally increased signal of the dentate nucleus (*arrow*) and hilar white matter in an infant with L2OH glutaric aciduria. The surrounding cerebellar white matter is normal in signal. Juxtacortical white matter rarefaction and increased signal (*open arrows*) are present on T2W images (*A, C, D*). There is typical periventricular white matter sparing. Abnormally increased signal of the caudate nuclei, putamina, and globi pallidi (*arrows*) is present on T2W axial image (*D*). There is a typical white rim (*black arrow*) on the lateral aspects of the globi pallidi, putamina, and caudate nuclei. White matter of the corpus callosum, forceps minor, and internal capsule is normal.

pyramidal tracts, medial lemniscus, the remainder of the cerebellar peduncles and the splenium, forceps major, and posterior limb of internal capsule.[99,100] Cerebrotendinous xanthomatosis (*CYP27A1*) may show this pattern in association with hyperintense spinal cord, substantia nigra, posterior limbs of the internal capsule, and periventricular supratentorial white matter (**Fig. 24**).[101]

CEREBELLAR WHITE MATTER, INCLUDING THE BRIGHT MIDDLE CEREBELLAR PEDUNCLE SIGN

The paired MCP, the largest of the cerebellar peduncles, consist of afferent fibers extending from the pons to the cerebellum.[102] MCP white matter normally shows mildly increased FLAIR hyperintensity.[103] Symmetric ovoid or diffuse

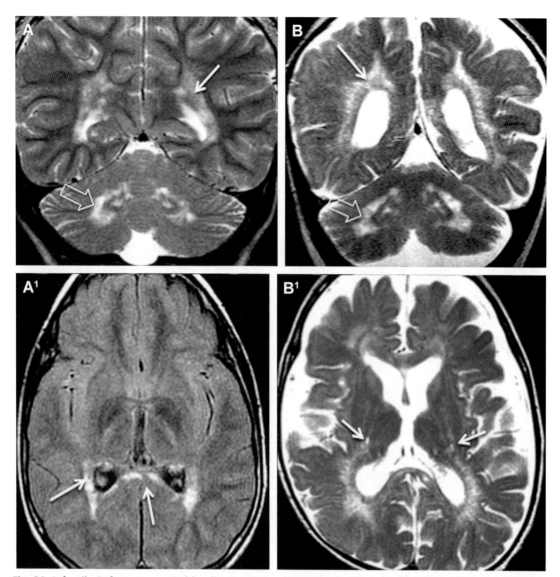

Fig. 24. Infantile Refsum versus Krabbe disease. Coronal T2W images (*A*, infantile Refsum) and (*B*, Krabbe disease) show similar location of high signal periventricular white matter (*arrows*), although striations are present in Krabbe. Both show a 3-layered (*open arrows*) of high-signal peridentate and hilar white matter and spared intervening dentate nucleus. Axial FLAIR (*A¹*) in infantile Refsum, an early-onset peroxisomal disorder, shows high-signal splenium and forceps major (*arrows*), whereas axial T2W image (*B¹*) in Krabbe disease, a lysosomal leukodystrophy, reveals focal necrosis of the corticospinal tracts (*arrows*).

high T2 signal intensity of the MCP can be seen in various acquired and inherited neurodegenerative disorders, including wallerian degeneration of the pontocerebellar tracts following pontine injury. The hyperintense MCP sign has been widely reported in neurodegenerative disorders with late onset, including late-onset adrenoleukodystrophy (ALD), some of the adult-onset autosomal dominant spinocerebellar ataxias/atrophies, and the alpha-synucleinopathies, such as the sporadic

OPCAs and multisystem atrophies (MSA/*COQ2*). Other disorders that may exhibit the bright cerebellar peduncle sign include Wilson disease (*ATB7P* mutation), spinocerebellar ataxia (SCA2/*ATXN2* and SCA6/*CACNA1A*), progressive supranuclear palsy (PSP1/*MAPT* mutation), dentatorubral-pallidoluysian atrophy (DRPLA/*ATN1* mutation), and fragile X syndrome (*FMR1* mutation). MCP involvement may also present in mitochondrial oxidative phosphorylation disorders, with or without diffusion restriction (**Fig. 25**). Additional pediatric disorders involving the cerebellar white matter and MCP include the late phase of infantile GM2 gangliosidoses and the hypomyelinating disorders with failure of myelin maturation.[104–106]

In Pelizaeus-Merzbacher (*PLP1*), the prototype for hypomyelinating disorders, there is diffuse failure of cerebellar white matter maturation, although the early myelinated structures are better myelinated than other structures. Eventual cerebellar atrophy occurs. In contrast, in hypomyelination of early myelinating structures or HEMS (*PLP1*), there is mild T2 hyperintensity of the medulla, pons, hilus of dentate, and the peridentate white matter.[107] Although there is no significant cerebellar atrophy in Pelizaeus-Merzbacher–like disease, white matter abnormalities in the pyramidal tracts or entire pons may occur and there is abnormal signal of the dentate hila[108] (**Fig. 26**). A few additional hereditary white matter disorders with cerebellar involvement are megalencephalic leukoencephalopathy with subcortical cysts (*MLC1*), hypomyelination with atrophy of the basal ganglia and cerebellum

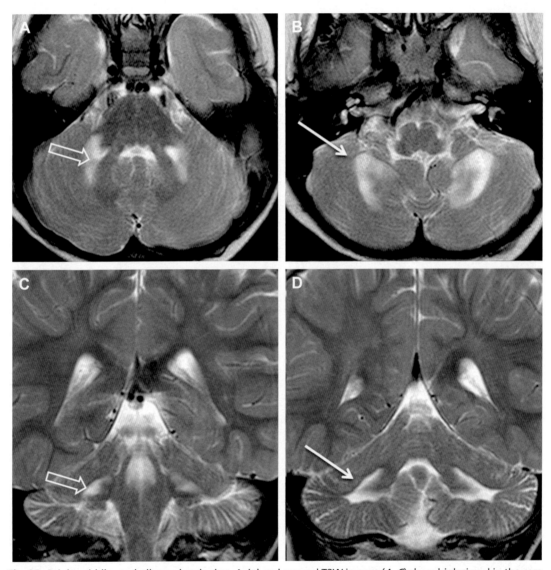

Fig. 25. Bright middle cerebellar peduncle sign. Axial and coronal T2W images (*A, C*) show high signal in the cerebellar peduncle (*open arrows*), whereas axial and coronal T2W images (*B, D*) show hypersignal of the cerebellar hemispheric white matter (*arrows*). There is sparing of the dentate nuclei and of the hilar white matter in this child with Leigh syndrome caused by cytochrome c oxidase (*COX15*) deficiency.

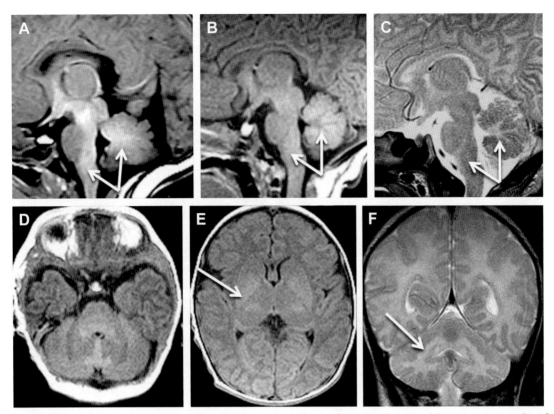

Fig. 26. Hypomyelinating disorders, Pelizaeus-Merzbacher Disease (PMD/*PLP1*). Normal hyperintense myelin of the brainstem and vermian white matter (*arrows*) is seen on T1W sagittal image (*A*). Compare with lack of normal hyperintense myelin signal (*arrows*) on sagittal T1W (*B*) and normal hyposignal (*arrows*) of myelin on T2W sagittal (*C*) and coronal (*F*) images in a newborn boy with Pelizaeus-Merzbacher. There is a lack of normal hyperintense myelin signal of the cerebellar white matter on axial T1W image (*D*). The posterior limb of the internal capsule (*arrow*) on axial T1W image (*E*) also lacks normal myelin signal in this full-term infant.

(HABC/*TUBB4A*), and 4H leukodystrophy (*POLR3A/POLR3B*). In MLC1, diffuse abnormal signal of the cerebellar white matter is present in association with anterotemporal and parietal cysts. Hypomyelination with atrophy of the basal ganglia and cerebellum (HABC/*TUBB4A*) shows abnormal myelin signal of the cerebellum, increased signal of the MCP and pyramidal tracts, progressive cerebellar atrophy, and typical supratentorial hypomyelination and basal ganglia atrophy[109,110] (Fig. 27). In hypomyelination, hypodontia, hypogonadotropic hypogonadism, or 4H leukodystrophy (*POLR3A*, *POLR3B*), cerebellovermian atrophy and abnormally increased signal intensity of the MCP are present, although patients with *POLR3A* show less cerebellar atrophy and patients with *POLR3B* show milder degrees of hypomyelination.[111,112]

CEREBELLAR WHITE MATTER IN SELECTED MITOCHONDRIAL DISORDERS

Imaging patterns of involvement can include the presence of lactate on MRS, predominant cerebellar atrophy, cerebellar white matter abnormalities, brainstem and dentate signal change, HOD, and spinal cord signal increase. Kearns-Sayre syndrome (KSS), Leigh syndrome with *SURF1* mutations, *POLG1*-related disorders, and 2 disorders caused by mutations in genes encoding mitochondrial tRNA synthetases, leukoencephalopathy with brainstem and spinal cord involvement and high lactate (LBSL/*DARS2*) and hypomyelination with brainstem and spinal cord involvement and leg spasticity (HBSL/*DARS*), are a few of the mitochondrial-related disorders with fairly specific cerebellar involvement. Myelinopathy is the prominent feature in KSS, in which imaging reflects splitting of myelin lamellae in the juxtacortical/subcortical white matter thalamus, brainstem, and cerebellum, and oligodendrocyte dysfunction.[113] Preferential loss of myelin-associated glycoprotein (MAG), a sign of distal dying-back oligodendrogliopathy, is considered a primary event in KSS. MAG loss is not evident in other mitochondrial encephalopathies, such as Leber hereditary optic neuropathy, MELAS,

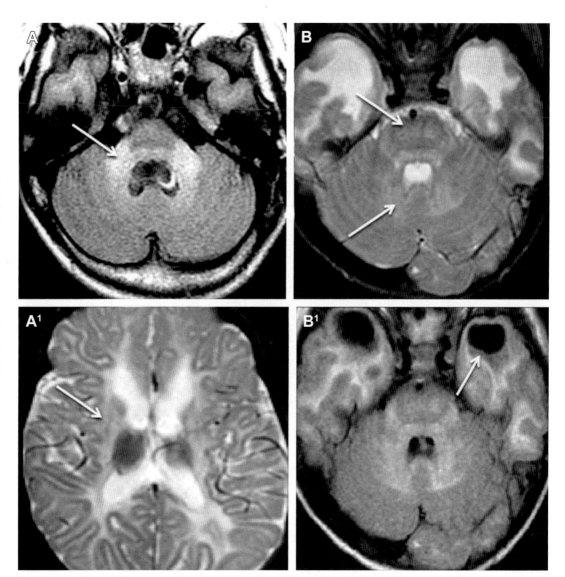

Fig. 27. Hereditary white matter disorders. HABC: the white matter of the MCP (*arrow*) is diffusely increased in signal on FLAIR axial image (*A*) in this child with HABC. There is hypomyelination of the cerebellum and supra-tentorial brain. Thalami are diffusely low in signal and the caudates, putamina, and globi pallidi are severely atro-phied (*A¹, arrow*). MLC1: hazy increased signal of the pontine tracts (*arrow*) and cerebellar white matter (*arrows*) on axial T2W image (*B*). Diffuse white matter swelling of the temporal lobes is present, but the cerebellum is not swollen. Anterior-temporal cysts (*arrow*) are shown within the swollen temporal lobe white matter on FLAIR axial image (*B¹*) in this infant with *MLC1*.

myoclonic epilepsy associated with ragged-red fi-bers, mitochondrial neurogastrointestinal enceph-alopathy/*TYMP*, or POLG-related disorders, in which myelin protein loss correlates with the de-gree of neuroaxonal degeneration[88] (**Fig. 28**).

DARS and *DARS2* are disease-associated paralogues encoding mitochondrial tRNA synthe-tases. Leukoencephalopathy with brain stem and spinal cord involvement and increased lactate level (LBSL) caused by mutations in the *DARS2* gene was first described more than a decade ago. In LBSL, selective tract involvement provides a unique pattern. There is involvement of the intra-parenchymal trajectories of the trigeminal nerve, mesencephalic trigeminal tracts, and the medial lemniscus. The pyramidal tracts are involved through the posterior limbs of the internal capsule into the lateral corticospinal tracts. In addition,

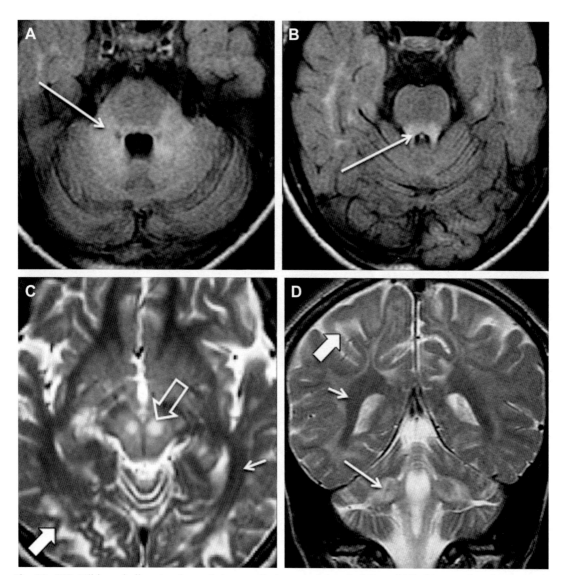

Fig. 28. KSS. Mild cerebellar atrophy and abnormally increased signal of the middle (*A, arrow*) and superior (*B, arrow*) cerebellar peduncles is present on FLAIR images. Hypersignal of the juxtacortical white matter (*large white arrows*) is present on axial (*C*) and coronal T2W images (*D*). The immediate periventricular white matter is spared (*small arrows*). There is high signal of the red nuclei (*open arrow*) on axial T2W image (*C*). Coronal T2W image (*D*) reveals increased signal of the superior cerebellar peduncles (*arrow*).

there is involvement of the posterior corpus callosum and extensive signal changes are present in periventricular and deep temporal white matter, with relative sparing of the U fibers. Cerebellar connections are also involved. There is early involvement of the superior and inferior cerebellar peduncles and late involvement of the brachium pontis or MCP. The cerebellar white matter, first subcortical and then diffuse, is involved with late development of cerebellar atrophy. Hypomyelination with brainstem and spinal cord involvement and leg spasticity shows similar involvement of

the superior and inferior cerebellar peduncles, the medial lemniscus, and pyramidal tracts in the brain stem and the dorsal columns, and the lateral corticospinal tracts in the spinal cord in addition to hypomyelination[114,115] (**Fig. 29**).

ADDITIONAL IMAGING FEATURES: DIFFUSION RESTRICTION

Diffusion restriction is common in the mitochondrial disorders involving the cerebellum, particularly those with *SURF1* mutations. More extensive

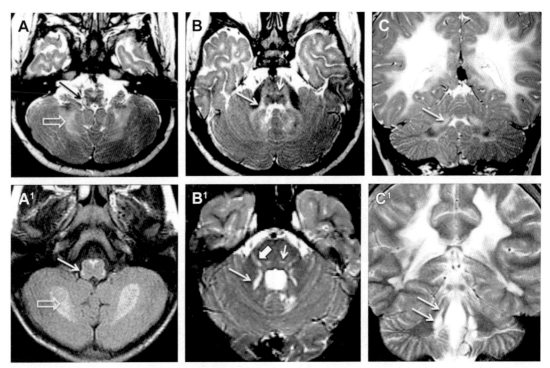

Fig. 29. HBSL (*DARS*), top row, versus LBSL (*DARS2*), bottom row. Axial T2W image (*A*) in HBSL and FLAIR image (*A¹*) in LBSL show high signal of the cerebellar white matter (*open arrows*), whereas black (*A*) and white arrows (*A¹*) show high signal of the inferior cerebellar peduncles. On axial T2W image (*B*) in HBSL and on axial T2W image (*B¹*) in LBSL, increased signal of the superior cerebellar peduncle (*white arrows*) and medial lemniscus (*short arrows*) is seen. There is characteristic high signal of the trajectory of the fifth cranial nerve (*B¹, thick white arrow*). Abnormal signal of the cerebellar peduncles is again identified on coronal T2W (*C*) image in HBSL and in LBSL (*C¹*). There is diffuse hyperintensity of the white matter (*C*) in HBSL. In LBSL, there is sparing of the juxtacortical/subcortical white matter (*C¹*).

infratentorial and supratentorial swelling with T2 hyperintensity and diffusion restriction involving gray and white matter is seen with thiamine transporter deficiency (*SLC19A3*) presenting in the first month of life. Cystic degeneration and atrophy follow, with Leigh-like brain lesions present on autopsy[116] (**Fig. 30**). Other disorders that present acutely with the neonatal disorders are maple syrup urine disease (MSUD/*BCKDHA/B*), methylmalonic academia (*MUT⁰*) and nonketotic hyperglycinemia (*AMT/GLDC/GCSH*). MSUD (*BCKDHA/B*) presents in the first days to weeks of life with acute metabolic decompensation (**Fig. 31**). Early myelinated structures of the cerebellum and brainstem tract acutely restrict on diffusion-weighted imaging (DWI) because of vacuolating myelinopathy. Follow-up imaging after the child is no longer in crisis shows resolution of diffusion restriction and a change in the imaging pattern. There is subsequent loss of normal myelin signal in the cerebellum and brainstem and

prominent abnormally increased signal in the globus pallidus. MRS obtained during MSUD crisis often reveals lactate in addition to a peak at 0.9 parts per million (ppm) caused by methyl resonance peak.[94,117,118] Specific findings on DWI in acutely decompensating newborns with nonketotic hyperglycinemia (NKH) include symmetric linear diffusion restriction in the cerebellar cortex, MCP, dorsal brain stem, cerebral peduncles, and posterior limbs of the internal capsules (**Fig. 32**). Spectroscopy is particularly useful and shows a peak at 3.55 ppm.[118,119] Methylmalonic academia (MMA/*MUT*) is a disorder of methylmalonate and cobalamin metabolism and is genetically heterogeneous. Children typically present with diffusion restriction and high signal of the globi pallidi. Additional posterior fossa features in children presenting past the newborn stage are hemorrhagic foci of the white matter, delay in supratentorial and infratentorial myelin maturation, and hyperintense pontine cerebellar tracts. However, infants

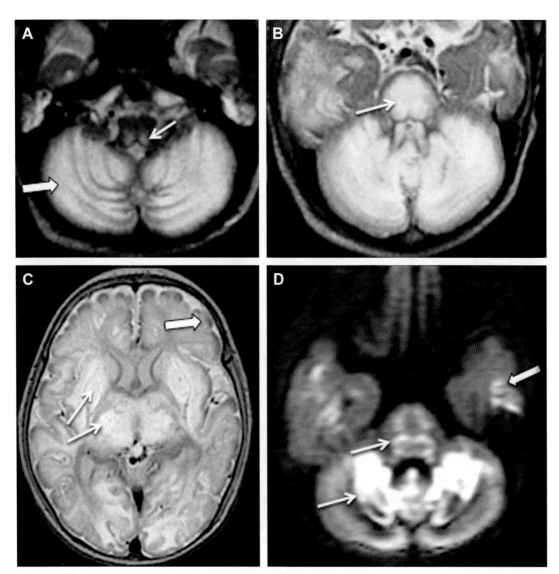

Fig. 30. Diffusion restriction in thiamine transporter dysfunction syndrome 2 (*SLC19A3*). Involvement of the cerebellar cortex (*large arrow*), cerebellar white matter, and the dorsal medulla (*arrow*) is seen on axial T2W image (*A*). Diffuse hypersignal and swelling of the pons (*arrow*) is present on axial T2W image (*B*). The basal ganglia and thalami are swollen, high in signal, and show early internal necrosis (*arrows*) on axial T2W image (*C*). The domes of the gyri (*large arrow*) are spared. Diffusion restriction of the inferior temporal cortex (*large white arrow*), the dentate nuclei, cerebellar white matter (*arrow*), pontine tracts, and medial lemnisci (*arrow*) is present on axial DWI (*D*).

with complete (*MUT⁰*) enzyme deficiency may present in the newborn period with imaging showing diffusion restriction in the cerebellar and brainstem white matter and subsequent cerebellar volume loss[120] (**Fig. 33**).

ADDITIONAL IMAGING FEATURES: ENHANCEMENT FOLLOWING CONTRAST ADMINISTRATION

Imaging in juvenile Alexander disease (*GFAP*) differs from infantile-onset Alexander disease in the gradient of involvement of abnormal signal and enhancement. The frontal-predominant pattern present in infantile-onset Alexander disease shifts to a posterior-predominant pattern in the later-onset cases (**Fig. 34**). There are medulla and spinal cord abnormalities with focal enhancement and the presence of garlands along the lateral ventricle walls.[121]

X-linked ALD, a peroxisomal disease caused by *ABCD1* mutations, has several phenotypes including childhood ALD, adolescent-onset or adult-onset ALD, adrenomyeloneuropathy (AMN),

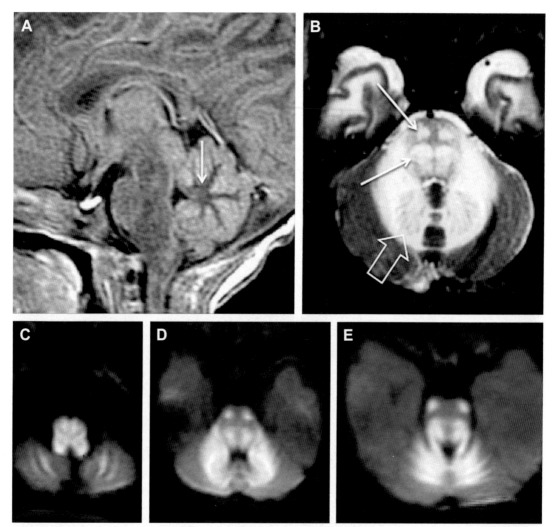

Fig. 31. Diffusion restriction in MSUD. Sagittal T1W image (*A*) shows marked swelling of the pons, brainstem, and cerebellar white matter (*arrow*). Axial T2W image (*B*) shows hypersignal of the pyramidal and tegmental tracts (*arrows*) with sparing of the dentate nucleus (*open arrow*). Diffusion-weighted images (*C–E*) reveal extensive diffusion restriction of the medulla, pyramidal, and tegmental tracts; cerebellar peduncles; and cerebellar white matter.

spinocerebellar ALD, and hypoadrenalism or primary hypogonadism. The cerebral form is usually associated with a rapidly progressive inflammatory demyelination, whereas AMN is predominantly a noninflammatory axonopathy of the long tracts of the spinal cord. In AMN, autopsy shows loss of axons and secondary demyelination of the dorsal fascicles and pyramidal tracts in the cord with a dying-back myelopathy. The usual childhood-onset parieto-occipital pattern shows confluent symmetric caudorostral progression starting in the splenium of the corpus callosum and spreading outwards into the forceps major and parietooccipital white matter. Three layers of involvement have been described. The peripheral outer zone is the leading edge of active demyelination and the intermediate zone is composed of active inflammation and breakdown of the blood-brain barrier. The degree of enhancement predicts aggressive progression. The inner, largely destroyed zone shows irreversible gliosis scarring and punctate calcification. The cortex and gray matter nuclei are typically spared. Eventually, the posterior limbs of the internal capsules, optic pathways, and pyramidal tracts in brainstem and spinal cord are involved. Specific

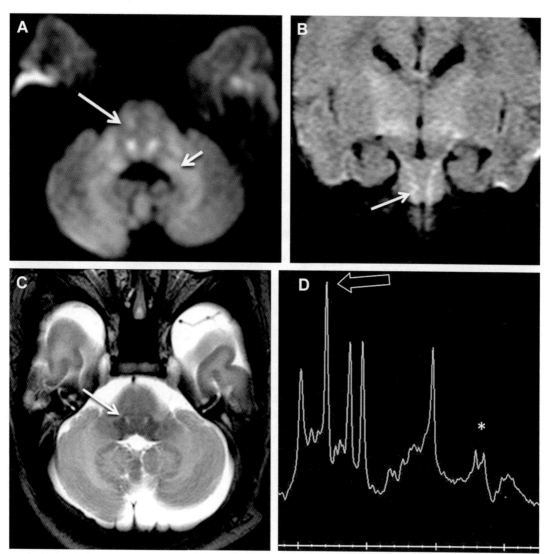

Fig. 32. Diffusion restriction in NKH. Axial DWI (*A*) shows diffusion restriction of the pyramidal (*arrow*) and tegmental white matter tracts and the MCP (*short arrow*). Coronal DWI (*B*) confirms extension along the pyramidal tracts (*arrow*). Axial T2W image (*C*) shows focal increased signal in the tegmental white matter tracts (*arrow*). MRS (*D*) confirms glycine peak at 3.6 ppm (*arrow*). Lactate doublet is present at 1.33 ppm (*asterisks*).

areas of demyelination include the primary visual and auditory pathways, the pyramidal tracts, internal and external capsules, lateral lemnisci, and frontopontine and pontocerebellar tracts. Although the white matter of the cerebellum is less extensively involved than supratentorial white matter, involvement occurs in aggressive cases or in cases of the rare spinocerebellar variant (**Fig. 35**). As with supratentorial involvement, the cerebellar cortex and dentate nuclei are typically spared.[122–124]

MAGNETIC RESONANCE SPECTROSCOPY

Feasibility studies have shown the reproducibility of single-voxel 1H-MRS of the structures of the posterior fossa. Voxels placed in the mesencephalon, pons, medulla, upper vermis, and cerebellar hemisphere centered on the dentate nucleus in normal patients documented regional variations of NAA/Cr, choline (Cho)/Cr, and NAA/Cho ratios. For example, the pons has the highest NAA/Cr and Cho/Cr ratios, whereas these ratios are lowest

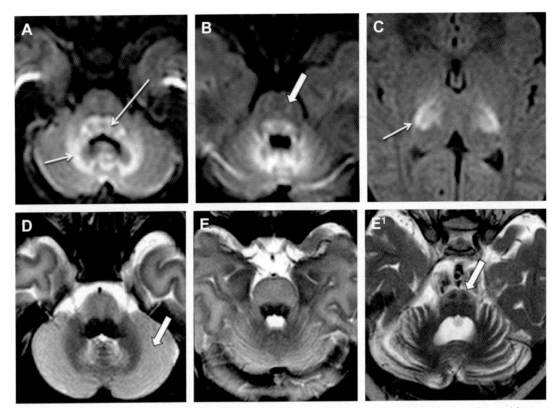

Fig. 33. Diffusion restriction in neonatal MMA. Axial diffusion (*A*) shows abnormal signal in the peridentate white matter (*arrow*), the MCP, and the pontine tegmentum (*long arrow*). The pyramidal tracts (*B, large white arrow*) are not restricting, unlike MSUD. The posterior limbs of internal capsule (*arrow*) and adjacent internal medullary lamina of the thalami are restricting (*C*). The cerebellar cortex is bright (*large white arrow*) on T2 axial image (*D*), but was not shown to be restricting on DWI (*A*). There is no cerebellar atrophy on axial T2W images (*D, E*) obtained during the first week of life. On follow-up T2W axial image (*E¹*) obtained at 3 years of age, there is atrophy of the cerebellar pons, white matter, and cortex. The pyramidal tracts (*large arrow*) are spared.

in the dentate and vermis. Regional variations likely represent the variable proportions of gray and white matter in the voxel. The proximity of skull base, adjacent cerebrospinal fluid, and blood vessels may cause challenges with field inhomogeneity and shimming; however, these problems may be ameliorated with increased field strength and resultant increased signal/noise ratio allowing a smaller voxel size.[125] Comparison of supratentorial with infratentorial 1H-MRS voxel sampling also shows regional variability in metabolite concentration. The N-acetylaspartic acid (NAA peak) peak of infratentorial structures is lower than is found in supratentorial structures, but remains higher than the choline (Cho) and creatine (Cr) peaks in the same voxel at 1.5, 3, and 7 T.[126,127] Decrease in posterior fossa structure NAA levels or NAA/Cr ratio is a common finding in the neurodegenerative

disorders involving the brainstem and cerebellum, rendering MRS nonspecific (**Fig. 36**). However, abnormal levels and ratios of these metabolites can show dysfunction of the brainstem or cerebellum even before atrophy of those structures is fully developed.[128] Using multiple voxel placements and assessing more than the usual NAA, Cr, and Cho peaks may increase specificity and aid in differentiation between different neurodegenerative disorders.[129,130] For example, the combination of low NAA and glutamate levels (both neuronal markers) and increased myoinositol (a glial marker) and Cr levels has been noted in the pons and cerebellum of patients with SCA1, SCA2, SCA3, and SCA7.[131] Decreased NAA and increased myoinositol levels have been shown on cerebellar MRS in Marinesco-Sjögren syndrome and late-onset GM2.[80,132] Marked increase of

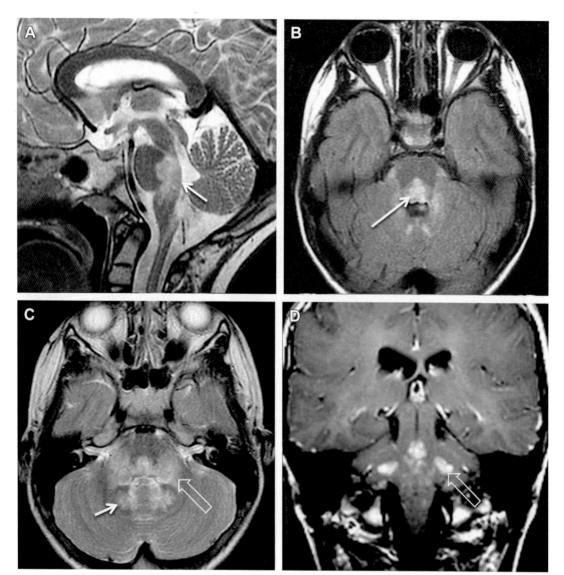

Fig. 34. Abnormal enhancement in juvenile Alexander disease (*GFAP*). Sagittal T2W (*A*) and axial FLAIR (*B*) images show swelling and signal increase of the dorsal pons (*arrows*). T2W (*C*) axial images show hypersignal of the dentate hila (*arrow*) and MCP (*open arrow*). Enhancement of the involved areas (*open arrow*) is present after gadolinium on T1 C+ (*D*).

vermian and pontine myoinositol levels distinguished cerebellar multisystem atrophy from the spinocerebellar ataxias in one study, reflecting the involvement of glial cells in the disorder.[133] Reduction of glutathione level in the cerebellum has been reported with cellular damage from oxidative stress in FRDA/*FXN*, autosomal dominant ataxia type 14 (SCA14), and other neurodegenerative disorders.[134]

Additional more specific markers have been reported. Although the presence of lactate in no way confirms the diagnosis of a mitochondrial disorder, 1H-MRS voxels placed in the dentate nucleus of the cerebellum may reveal increased brain lactate levels in patients with respiratory chain deficiency presenting with cerebellar atrophy or signal change, even when no putaminal lactate is detected (see **Fig. 22**).[135] Similarly, lactate is often absent in unaffected areas of the brain in POLG-related disorders.[81] Although Cr levels are often maintained or increased in patients with SCA, total Cr levels in the cerebellar hemispheres have been shown to be decreased in patients with *CACNA1A* compared with controls.[136] Glycine has been

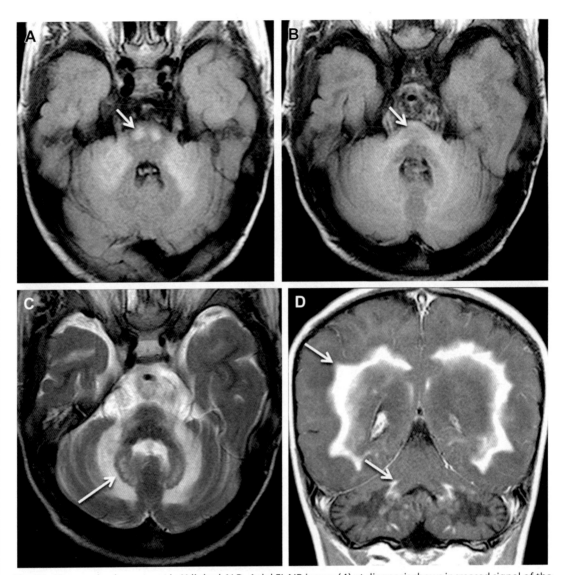

Fig. 35. Abnormal enhancement in X-linked ALD. Axial FLAIR image (*A*) at diagnosis shows increased signal of the pyramidal tract (*arrow*) and MCP extending into the cerebellar white matter. Axial FLAIR image (*B*) on follow-up reveals progression of signal abnormalities (*arrow*). Abnormal white matter signal extends into the peridentate white matter on axial T2W image (*C*). The dentate nucleus (*arrow*) is spared. Extensive enhancement is present in supratentorial and infratentorial white matter (*arrows*) T1W coronal image (*D*).

documented at higher levels in the involved early myelinated structures, such as the cerebellar white matter in neonates with NKH, than in the less severely involved (and incompletely myelinated) supratentorial compartment.[118,119] Focusing MRS sampling on affected areas can be extremely useful in showing metabolic aberrations. For example, an MRS voxel placed supratentorially in normal-appearing brain in a patient with CDG1a showed normal spectral peaks, whereas posterior fossa voxel in the atrophied cerebellum revealed low NAA and increased myoinositol levels.[137] However, posterior fossa sampling of many of the inborn errors of metabolism by spectroscopy has not yet been documented, despite pathologic and imaging confirmation of cerebellar involvement. In those cases, supratentorial confirmation of abnormal metabolites remains a useful adjunct.[138]

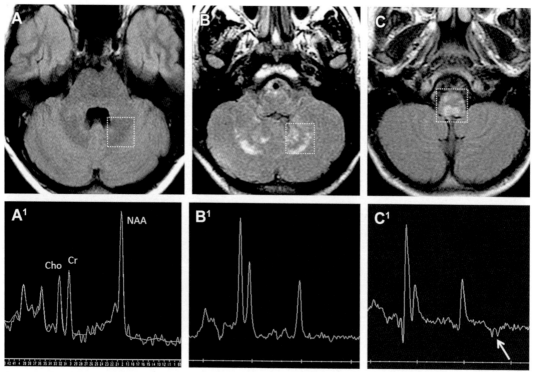

Fig. 36. MRS of the cerebellum. Axial FLAIR image (*A*) shows voxel placement in a normal control. MRS spectrum (*A¹*) reveals normal Cho, Cr, and NAA peaks. Axial FLAIR image (*B*) in infantile Refsum shows voxel placement in the dentate nucleus and peridentate white matter. MRS spectrum (*B¹*) shows increased Cho and decreased NAA peaks. Axial FLAIR image (*C*) in juvenile Alexander shows voxel placement in the brainstem. Spectra (*C¹*) reveals increased Cho and decreased Cr and NAA peaks and a small lactate doublet (*arrow*).

REFERENCES

1. Steinlin M, Blaser S, Boltshauser E. Cerebellar involvement in metabolic disorders: a pattern-recognition approach. Neuroradiology 1998;40(6): 347–54.

2. Patay Z. The cerebellum in amino and organic acidurias. Neuroradiol J 2007;20:439–48.

3. Pyle A, Smertenko T, Bargiela D, et al. Exome sequencing in undiagnosed and inherited and sporadic ataxias. Brain 2015;138:276–83.

4. Obha C, Osaka H, Iai M, et al. Diagnostic utility of whole exome sequencing in patients showing cerebellar and/or vermis atrophy in childhood. Neurogenetics 2013;14:225–32.

5. Sawyer SL, Schwartzentruber J, Beaulieu CL, et al. Exome sequencing as a diagnostic tool for pediatric-onset ataxia. Hum Mutat 2014;35:45–9.

6. Bargiela D, Shanmugarajah P, Lo C, et al. Mitochondrial pathology in progressive cerebellar ataxia. Cerebellum Ataxias 2015;2:16.

7. van der Knaap MS, Valk J, de Neeling N, et al. Pattern recognition in magnetic resonance imaging of white matter disorders in children and young adults. Neuroradiology 1991;33(6):478–93.

8. Schiffman R, van der Knaap MS. Invited article: an MRI-based approach to the diagnosis of white matter disorders. Neurology 2009;72:750–9.

9. Poretti A, Wolf NI, Boltshauser E. Differential diagnosis of cerebellar atrophy in childhood: an update. Neuropediatrics 2015;46:359–70.

10. Al-Maawali A, Blaser S, Yoon G. Diagnostic approach to childhood-onset cerebellar atrophy: a 10-year retrospective study of 300 patients. J Child Neurol 2012;27(9):1121–32.

11. Leibovitz Z, Shkolnic C, Krajden Haratz K, et al. Assessment of fetal midbrain and hindbrain in mid-sagittal cranial plane by three-dimensional multiplanar sonography. Part 1: comparison of new and established nomograms. Ultrasound Obstet Gynecol 2014;44:575–80.

12. Koehler PR, Haughton VM, Daniels DL, et al. MR measurement of normal and pathologic brainstem diameters. AJNR Am J Neuroradiol 1985;6(3): 425–7.

13. Raininko R, Autti T, Vanhanen SL, et al. The normal brainstem from infancy to old age. A morphometric MRI study. Neuroradiology 1994;36:364–8.

14. Park MTM, Pipitone J, Baer LH, et al. Derivation of high-resolution MRI atlases of the human cerebellum

at 3T and segmentation using multiple automatically generated templates. Neuroimage 2014;95:217–31.

15. Yang Z, Ye C, Bogovic JA, et al. Automated cerebellar lobule segmentation with application to cerebellar structural analysis in cerebellar disease. Neuroimage 2016;127:435–44.

16. Liu Z, Yaldizli O, Pardini M, et al. Cervical cord area measurement using volumetric brain magnetic resonance imaging in multiple sclerosis. Mult Scler Relat Disord 2015;4(1):52–7.

17. Doherty D, Millen KJ, Barkovich AJ. Midbrain and hindbrain malformations: advances in clinical diagnosis, imaging, and genetics. Lancet Neurol 2013; 12(4):381–93.

18. Merlini L, Fluss J, Dhouib A, et al. Mid-hindbrain malformations due to drugs taken during pregnancy. J Child Neurol 2014;29(4):538–44.

19. Zhao J, Chen Y, Xu Y, et al. Effect of intrauterine infection on brain development and injury. Int J Dev Neurosci 2013;31:543–9.

20. Limperopoulos C, Soul JS, Gauvreau K, et al. Late gestation cerebellar growth is rapid and impeded by premature birth. Pediatrics 2005; 115(3):688–95.

21. Srinivasan L, Allsop J, Coundsell SJ, et al. Smaller cerebellar volumes in very preterm infants at term-equivalent age are associated with the presence of supratentorial lesions. AJNR Am J Neuroradiol 2006;27(3):573–9.

22. Sargent MA, Poskitt KJ, Roland EG, et al. Cerebellar vermian atrophy after neonatal hypoxic-ischemic encephalopathy. AJNR Am J Neuroradiol 2004;25(6):1008–15.

23. Alekseeva N, McGee J, Kelley RE, et al. Toxic-metabolic, nutritional, and medicinal induced disorders of cerebellum. Neurol Clin 2014;32:901–11.

24. Vermeulen RJ, Peeters-Scholte C, van Vugt JJMG, et al. Fetal origin of brain damage in 2 infants with a COL4A1 mutation: fetal and neonatal MRI. Neuropediatrics 2011;42(1):1–3.

25. Yoneda Y, Haginoya K, Kato M, et al. Phenotypic spectrum of COL4A1 mutations: porencephaly to schizencephaly. Ann Neurol 2013;73(1):48–57.

26. Poretti A, Boltshauser E. Terminology in morphological anomalies of the cerebellum does matter. Cerebellum Ataxias 2015;2:8.

27. Boltshauser E. Cerebellum—small brain but large confusion: a review of selected cerebellar malformations and disruptions. Am J Med Genet A 2004;126:376–85.

28. Basson MA, Wingate RJ. Congenital hypoplasia of the cerebellum: developmental causes and behavioral consequences. Front Neuroanat 2013;7:29.

29. Poretti A, Boltshauser E, Doherty D. Cerebellar hypoplasia: differential diagnosis and diagnostic approach. Am J Med Genet C Semin Med Genet 2014;166C:211–26.

30. Basson MA. Epistatic interactions between Chd7 and Fgf8 during cerebellar development: implications for CHARGE syndrome. Rare Dis 2014;2: e28688.

31. Laffaire J, Rivals I, Dauphinot L, et al. Gene expression signature of cerebellar hypoplasia in a mouse model of Down syndrome during postnatal development. BMC Genomics 2009;10:138.

32. Namavar Y, Barth PG, Kasher PR, et al. Clinical, neuroradiological and genetic findings in pontocerebellar hypoplasia. Brain 2011;134:143–56.

33. Sánchez-Albisua I, Frolich S, Barth PG, et al. Natural course of pontocerebellar hypoplasia type 2A. Orphanet J Rare Dis 2014;9:70.

34. Barth PG, Aronica E, de Vries L, et al. Pontocerebellar hypoplasia type 2: a neuropathological update. Acta Neuropathol 2007;114(4):376–8.

35. Cassandrini D, Biancheri R, Tessa A, et al. Pontocerebellar hypoplasia: clinical, pathologic, and genetic studies. Neurology 2010;75:1459–64.

36. Rudnik-Schöneborn S, Barth PG, Zerres K. Am J Med Genet C Semin Med Genet 2014;166C: 173–83.

37. Doimo M, Desbats MA, Cerqua C, et al. Genetics of coenzyme Q10 deficiency. Mol Syndromol 2014;5: 156–62.

38. Maegawa GHB, Banwell BL, Blaser S, et al. Substrate reduction therapy in juvenile GM2 gangliosidosis. Mol Genet Metab 2009;98:215–24.

39. Inglese M, Nusbaum AO, Pastores G, et al. MR imaging and proton spectroscopy of neuronal injury in late-onset GM2 gangliosidosis. AJNR Am J Neuroradiol 2005;26(8):2037–42.

40. Wolf NI, Koenig M. Progressive cerebellar atrophy: hereditary ataxias and disorders with spinocerebellar degeneration. Handb Clin Neurol 2013;113: 1869–78.

41. Marelli C, van de Leemput J, Johnson JO, et al. SCA15 due to large ITPR1 deletions in a cohort of 333 white families with dominant ataxia. Arch Neurol 2011;68(5):637–43.

42. Guergueltcheva V, Azmanov DN, Angelicheva D, et al. Autosomal-recessive congenital cerebellar ataxia Is caused by mutations in metabotropic glutamate receptor 1. Am J Hum Genet 2012; 91(3):553–64.

43. Aronica E, van Kempen AA, van der Heide M, et al. Congenital disorder of glycosylation type Ia: a clinicopathological report of a newborn infant with cerebellar pathology. Acta Neuropathol 2005; 109(4):433–42.

44. Martin M-H, Bouchard J-P, Sylvain M, et al. Autosomal recessive spastic ataxia of Charlevoix-Saguenay: a report of MR imaging in 5 patients. AJNR Am J Neuroradiol 2007;28:1606–8.

45. Prodi E, Grisoli M, Panzeri M, et al. Supratentorial and pontine MRI abnormalities characterize

recessive spastic ataxia of Charlevoix-Saguenay. A comprehensive study of an Italian series. Eur Neurol 2013;20:138–46.

46. Shimazaki H, Takiyama Y, Honda J, et al. Middle cerebellar peduncles and pontine T2 hypointensities in ARSACS. J Neuroimaging 2013;23(1):82–5.

47. Synofzik M, Soehn AS, Gburek-Augustat J, et al. Autosomal recessive spastic ataxia of Charlevoix Saguenay (ARSACS): expanding the genetic, clinical and imaging spectrum. Orphanet J Rare Dis 2013;8:41.

48. Parkinson MH, Bremner F, Giunti P. Autosomal recessive spastic ataxia of Charlevoix-Saguenay. ACNR 2014;V13(7):12–6.

49. Gazulla J, Benavente I, Vela AC, et al. New findings in the ataxia of Charlevoix-Saguenay. J Neurol 2012;259:869–78.

50. Ochi T, Taoka T, Miyasaka T, et al. "Cerebellar peduncle quarter notes" formed by the superior and middle cerebellar peduncles: comparison with a diffusion tensor study of spinocerebellar degeneration. Jpn J Radiol 2015;33:210–5.

51. Qualltrone A, Nicoletti G, Messina D, et al. MR imaging index for differentiation of progressive supranuclear palsy from Parkinson disease and the Parkinson variant of multiple system atrophy. Radiology 2008;246(1):214–21.

52. Hussl A, Mahlknecht P, Scherfler C, et al. Diagnostic accuracy of the magnetic resonance Parkinsonism index and the midbrain-to-pontine area ratio to differentiate progressive supranuclear palsy from Parkinson's disease and the Parkinson variant of multiple system atrophy. Mov Disord 2010;25(14):2444–9.

53. Kakeda S, Korogi Y, Yoneda T, et al. A novel tract imaging technique of the brainstem using phase difference enhanced imaging: normal anatomy and initial experience in multiple system atrophy. Eur Radiol 2011;21:2202–10.

54. Drouin-Garraud V, Belgrand M, Grünewald S, et al. Neurological presentation of a congenital disorder of glycosylation CDG-Ia: implications for diagnosis and genetic counseling. Am J Med Genet 2001; 101(1):46–9.

55. Mader I, Döbler-Neumann M, Küker W, et al. Congenital disorder of glycosylation type Ia: benign clinical course in a new genetic variant. Childs Nerv Syst 2002;18(1–2):77–80.

56. Al-Maawali AA, Miller E, Schulze A, et al. Subcutaneous fat pads on body MRI - an early sign of congenital disorder of glycosylation PMM2-CDG (CDG1a). Pediatr Radiol 2014;44:222–5.

57. Barone R, Fiumara A, Jaeken J. Congenital disorders of glycosylation with emphasis on cerebellar involvement. Semin Neurol 2014;34:357–66.

58. Eichler L, Bellenberg B, Hahn HK, et al. Quantitative assessment of brain stem and cerebellar atrophy in spinocerebellar ataxia types 3 and 6: impact on clinical status. AJNR Am J Neuroradiol 2011;32:890–7.

59. Kieslich M, Hoche F, Reichenbach J, et al. Extracerebellar MRI-lesions in ataxia telangiectasia go along with deficiency of the GH/IGF-1 axis, markedly reduced body weight, high ataxia scores and advanced age. Cerebellum 2010;9:190–7.

60. Kamiya M, Yamanouchi H, Yoshida T, et al. Ataxia telangiectasia with vascular abnormalities in the brain parenchyma: report of an autopsy case and literature review. Pathol Int 2001;51(4):271–6.

61. Mascalchi M, Salvi F, Piacentini S, et al. Friedreich's ataxia: MR findings involving the cervical portion of the spinal cord. AJR Am J Roentgenol 1994;163: 163–91.

62. Solbach K, Kraff O, Minnerop M, et al. Cerebellar pathology in Friedreich's ataxia: atrophied dentate nuclei with normal iron content. Neuroimage Clin 2014;6:93–9.

63. Waldvogel D, van Gelderen P, Hallett M. Increased iron in the dentate nucleus of patients with Friedreich's Ataxia. Ann Neurol 1999;46:123–5.

64. Della Nave R, Ginestroni A, Giannelli M, et al. Brain structural damage in Friedreich's ataxia. J Neurol Neurosurg Psychiatry 2008;79:82–5.

65. Bhidayasiri R, Perlman SL, Pulst S-M, et al. Late-onset Friedreich ataxia: phenotypic analysis, magnetic resonance imaging findings and review of the literature. Arch Neurol 2005;6(12):1865–9.

66. Biller J, Ionasescu V, Zellweger H, et al. Frequency of cerebral infarction in patients with inherited neuromuscular diseases. Stroke 1987;18(4):805–7.

67. Tsou AY, Paulsen EK, Lagedrost SJ, et al. Mortality in Friedreich ataxia. J Neurol Sci 2011;307:46–9.

68. Tavani R, Zimmerman RA, Berry GT, et al. Ataxia-telangiectasia: the pattern of cerebellar atrophy on MRI. Neuroradiology 2003;45:315–9.

69. Wallis LI, Griffiths PD, Ritchie SJ, et al. Proton spectroscopy and imaging at 3T in ataxia-telangiectasia. AJNR Am J Neuroradiol 2007;28(1):79–83.

70. Lin DDM, Barker PB, Lederman HM, et al. Cerebral abnormalities in adults with ataxia-telangiectasia. AJNR Am J Neuroradiol 2014;35:119–23.

71. Ramantani G, Niggemann P, Bast T, et al. Reconciling neuroimaging and clinical findings in Aicardi-Goutières syndrome: an autoimmune-mediated encephalopathy. AJNR Am J Neuroradiol 2010;31(7):E62–3.

72. Vanderver A, Prust M, Kadom N, et al. Early-onset Aicardi-Goutières syndrome: magnetic resonance imaging (MRI) pattern recognition. J Child Neurol 2015;30(10):1343–8.

73. Linnankivi T, Valanne L, Paetau A, et al. Cerebroretinal microangiopathy with calcifications and cysts. Neurology 2006;67(8):1437–43.

74. Hopkins B, Sutton VR, Lewis RA, et al. Neuroimaging aspects of Aicardi syndrome. neuroimaging

aspects of Aicardi syndrome. Am J Med Genet A 2008;146A(22):2871–8.

75. Glamuzina E, Brown R, Hogarth K, et al. Further delineation of pontocerebellar hypoplasia type 6 due to mutations in the gene encoding mitochondrial arginyl-tRNA synthetase RARS2. J Inherit Metab Dis 2012;35:459–67.

76. Demaerel P, Lagae L, Casaer P, et al. MR of cerebellar cortical dysplasia. AJNR Am J Neuroradiol 1998;19:984–6.

77. Poretti A, Häusler M, von Moers A, et al. Ataxia, intellectual disability and ocular apraxia with cerebellar cysts: a new disease. Cerebellum 2014;13: 79–88.

78. Aldinger KA, Mosca SJ, Tetreault M, et al. Mutations in LAMA1 cause cerebellar dysplasia and cysts with and without retinal dystrophy. Am J Hum Genet 2014;95:227–34.

79. Marques JP, van der Zwaag W, Granziera C. Cerebellar cortical layers: in vivo visualization with structural high-field-strength MR imaging. Radiology 2010;254(3):942–8.

80. Harting I, Blaschek A, Wolf NI, et al. T2-hyperintense cerebellar cortex in Marinesco-Sjögren syndrome. Neurology 2004;63(12):2448–9.

81. Tzoulis C, Neckelmann G, Mørk SJ, et al. Localized cerebral energy failure in DNA polymerase gamma-associated encephalopathy syndromes. Brain 2010;133(Pt 5):1428–37.

82. Cohen BH, Chinnery PF, Copeland WC. POLG-related disorders. In: Pagon RA, Adam MP, Ardinger HH, et al, editors. GeneReviews [Internet]. Seattle (WA): University of Washington, Seattle; 2014. p. 1993–2016.

83. Bindu PS, Arvinda H, Taly AB, et al. Magnetic resonance imaging correlates of genetically characterized patients with mitochondrial disorders: a study from South India. Mitochondrion 2015;25:6–16.

84. Bosemani T, Zanni G, Hartman A, et al. Christianson syndrome: spectrum of neuroimaging findings. Neuropediatrics 2014;45(4):247–51.

85. Jobling RK, Assoum M, Gakh O, et al. PMPCA mutations cause abnormal mitochondrial protein processing in patients with non-progressive cerebellar ataxia. Brain 2015;138(Pt 6):1505–17.

86. Feraco P, Mirabelli-Badenier M, Severino M, et al. The shrunken, bright cerebellum: a characteristic MRI finding in congenital disorders of glycosylation type 1a. AJNR Am J Neuroradiol 2012;33:2062–7.

87. McErlean A, Abdalla K, Donaghue V, et al. The dentate nucleus in children: normal development and patterns of disease. Pediatr Radiol 2010;40:326–39.

88. Lax NZ, Campbell GR, Reeve AK, et al. Loss of myelin-associated glycoprotein in Kearns-Sayre syndrome. Arch Neurol 2012;69(4):490–9.

89. Xie S, Xiao JX, Qi ZY, et al. Heterogeneity of magnetic resonance imaging in Leigh syndrome with SURF1 gene 604G>C mutation. Clin Imaging 2009;33(1):1–6.

90. Farina L, Chiapparini L, Uziel G, et al. MR findings in Leigh syndrome with COX deficiency and SURF-1 mutations. AJNR Am J Neuroradiol 2002;23:1095–100.

91. Rossi A, Biancheri R, Bruno C, et al. Leigh syndrome with COX deficiency and SURF1 gene mutations: MR imaging findings. AJNR Am J Neuroradiol 2003;24:1188–91.

92. Kinghorn K, Kaliakatsos M, Blakely E, et al. Hypertrophic olivary degeneration on magnetic resonance imaging in mitochondrial syndromes associated with POLG and SURF1 mutations. J Neurol 2012; 260:3–9.

93. Bindu PS, Taly AB, Sonam K, et al. Bilateral hypertrophic olivary nucleus degeneration on magnetic resonance imaging in children with Leigh and Leigh-Like syndrome. Br J Radiol 2014;87:20130478.

94. Patay Z. Diffusion-weighted MR imaging in leukodystrophies. Eur Radiol 2005;15:2284–303.

95. Steenweg ME, Salomons GS, Yapici Z, et al. L-2-hydroxyglutaric aciduria: pattern of MR imaging abnormalities in 56 patients. Radiology 2009; 251(3):856–65.

96. Finelli DA, Tarr RW, Sawyer RN, et al. Deceptively normal MR in early infantile Krabbe disease. AJNR Am J Neuroradiol 1994;15:167–71.

97. Zuccoli G, Narayanan S, Panigrahy A, et al. Midbrain morphology reflects extent of brain damage in Krabbe disease. Neuroradiology 2015;57:739–45.

98. Abdelhalim AN, Alberico RA, Barczykowski AL, et al. Patterns of magnetic resonance imaging abnormalities in symptomatic patients with Krabbe disease correspond to phenotype. Pediatr Neurol 2014;50:127–34.

99. van der Knaap MS, Wassmer E, Wolf NI, et al. MRI as diagnostic tool in early-onset peroxisomal disorders. Neurology 2012;78:1304–8.

100. Poll-The BT, Gartner J. Clinical diagnosis, biochemical findings and RMI spectrum of peroxisomal disorders. Biochim Biophys Acta 1822;2012:1421–9.

101. Pudhiavan A, Agrawal A, Chaudhari S, et al. Cerebrotendinous xanthomatosis - The spectrum of imaging findings. J Radiol Case Rep 2013;7(4):1–9.

102. Terajima K, Matsuzawa H, Shimohata T, et al. Tract-by-tract morphometric and diffusivity analyses in vivo of spinocerebellar degeneration. J Neuroimaging 2009;19(3):220–6.

103. Ngai S, Tang YM, Du L, et al. Hyperintensity of the middle cerebellar peduncles on fluid-attenuated inversion recovery imaging: variation with age and implications for the diagnosis of multiple system atrophy. AJNR Am J Neuroradiol 2006;27: 2146–8.

104. Morales H, Tomsick T. Middle cerebellar peduncles: magnetic resonance imaging and pathophysiologic correlate. World J Radiol 2015;7(12):438–47.

105. Okamoto K, Tokiguchi S, Furusawa T, et al. MR features of diseases involving bilateral middle cerebellar peduncles. AJNR Am J Neuroradiol 2003; 24:1946–54.

106. Uchino A, Sawada A, Takase Y, et al. Symmetrical lesions of the middle cerebellar peduncle: MR imaging and differential diagnosis. Magn Reson Med Sci 2004;3(3):133–40.

107. Kevelam SH, Taube JR, van Spaendonk RML, et al. Altered PLP1 splicing causes hypomyelination of early myelinated structures. Ann Clin Transl Neurol 2015;2(6):648–61.

108. Steenweg ME, Vanderver A, Blaser S, et al. Magnetic resonance imaging pattern recognition in hypomyelinating disorders. Brain 2010;133(10):2971–82.

109. van der Knaap MS, Barth PG, Stroink H. Leukoencephalopathy with swelling and a discrepantly mild clinical course in eight children. Ann Neurol 1995; 37:324–34.

110. Simons C, Wolf NI, McNeil N, et al. A de novo mutation in the β-tubulin gene TUBB4A results in the leukoencephalopathy hypomyelination with atrophy of the basal ganglia and cerebellum. Am J Hum Genet 2013;92(5):767–73.

111. Wolf NL, Vanderver A, van Spaendonk RM, et al. Clinical spectrum of 4H leukodystrophy caused by POLR3A and POLR3B mutations. Neurology 2014;83(21):1898–905.

112. Takanashi J-I, Osaka H, Saitsu H, et al. Different patterns of cerebellar abnormality and hypomyelination between POLR3A and POLR3B mutations. Brain Dev 2014;36(3):259–63.

113. Kevelam SH, Bugiani M, Salomons GS, et al. Exome sequencing reveals mutated SLC19A3 in patients with an early-infantile, lethal encephalopathy. Brain 2013;136:1–10.

114. Wong L-JC. Mitochondrial syndromes with leukoencephalopathies. Semin Neurol 2012;32:55–61.

115. van der Knaap M, van der Voorn P, Barkhof F, et al. A new leukoencephalopathy with brainstem and spinal cord involvement and high lactate. Ann Neurol 2003;53:252–8.

116. Taft RJ, Vanderver A, Leventer RJ, et al. Mutations in DARS cause hypomyelination with brain stem and spinal cord involvement and leg spasticity. Am J Hum Genet 2013;92(5):774–80.

117. Ben-Omran TI, Blaser S, Phillips S, et al. Atypical phenotype in a boy with a maple syrup urine disease. J Inherit Metab Dis 2006;29:195–200.

118. Poretti A, Blaser SI, Lequin M, et al. Neonatal neuroimaging findings in inborn errors of metabolism. J Magn Reson Imaging 2013;37:294–312.

119. Huisman TA, Thiel T, Steinmann B, et al. Proton magnetic resonance spectroscopy of the brain of a neonate with nonketotic hyperglycinemia; in vivo-in vitro (ex vivo) correlation. Eur Radiol 2002;12(4):858–61.

120. Harting I, Seitz A, Geb S, et al. Looking beyond the basal ganglia: the spectrum of MRI changes in methylmalonic acidaemia. J Inherit Metab Dis 2008;31:368–78.

121. van der Knaap MS, Schiffmann RV, Blaser S, et al. Alexander disease: ventricular garlands and abnormalities of the medulla and spinal cord. Neurology 2006;66(4):494–8.

122. Jung S, Chung JW, Yun JY, et al. A case of adrenoleukodystrophy presenting as progressive cerebellar dysfunction. J Mov Disord 2009;2(2): 91–4.

123. Ogaki K, Koga S, Aoki N, et al. Adult-onset cerebello-brainstem dominant form of X-linked adrenoleukodystrophy presenting as multiple system atrophy: case report and literature review. Neuropathology 2016;36(1):64–76.

124. de Munter S, Verheijden S, Regal L, et al. Peroxisomal disorders: a review on cerebellar pathologies. Brain Pathol 2015;25(6):663–78.

125. Mascalchi M, Brugnoli R, Guerrine L, et al. Single-voxel long TE 1H-MR spectroscopy of the normal brainstem and cerebellum. J Magn Reson Imaging 2002;16:532–7.

126. Costa MOR, Lacerda MTC, Otuday MCG, et al. Proton magnetic resonance spectroscopy: normal findings in the cerebellar hemisphere in childhood. Pediatr Radiol 2002;32:787–92.

127. Terpstra M, Cheong I, Lyu T, et al. Test-retest reproducibility of neurochemical profiles with short-echo, single-voxel MR spectroscopy at 3T and 7T. Magn Reson Med 2015. http://dx.doi.org/10.1002/mrm.26022.

128. Mascalchi M, Cosottini M, Lolli F, et al. Proton MR spectroscopy of the cerebellum and pons in patients with degenerative ataxia. Radiology 2002; 223:371–8.

129. Viau M, Boulanger Y. Characterization of ataxias with magnetic resonance imaging and spectroscopy. Parkinsonism Relat Disord 2004;10:335–51.

130. Viau M, Marchand L, Bard C, et al. (1)H magnetic resonance spectroscopy of autosomal ataxias. Brain Res 2005;1049:191–202.

131. Adanyeguh IM, Henry PG, Nguyen TM, et al. In vivo neurometabolic profiling in patients with spinocerebellar ataxia types 1, 2, 3, and 7. Mov Disord 2015;30:662–70.

132. Jamrozik Z, Logowska A, Golebioski M, et al. Late onset GM2 gangliosidosis mimicking spinal muscular atrophy. Gene 2013;527(2):679–82.

133. Öz G, Iltis I, Hutter D, et al. Distinct neurochemical profiles of spinocerebellar ataxias 1, 2, 6 and cerebellar multiple system atrophy. Cerebellum 2011; 10(2):208–17.

134. Doss S, Rinnenthal JL, Schmitz-Hubsch TS, et al. Cerebellar neurochemical alterations in spinocerebellar

ataxia type 14 appear to include glutathione deficiency. J Neurol 2015;262(8):1927–35.

135. Boddaert N, Romano S, Funalot B, et al. 1H MRS spectroscopy evidence of cerebellar high lactate in mitochondrial respiratory chain deficiency. Mol Genet Metab 2008;93:85–8.

136. Harno H, Heikkinen S, Kaunisto MA, et al. Decreased cerebellar total creatine in episodic ataxia type 2: a 1H MRS study. Neurology 2005; 64:542–4.

137. Takeuchi M, Harada M, Hisaoka S, et al. Magnetic resonance imaging and proton MR spectroscopy of the brain in a patient with carbohydrate-deficient glycoprotein syndrome type 1. J Magn Reson Imaging 2003;17:722–5.

138. Cecil KM, Lindquist DM. Chapter 11, Metabolic disorders. In: Blüml S, Panigrahy A, editors. MR spectroscopy of pediatric brain disorders. New York: Springer Science+Business Media, LLC, Springer; 2013. p. 123–48. http://dx.doi.org/10.1007/978-1-4419-5864-8_11.

Pediatric Neurocutaneous Syndromes with Cerebellar Involvement

 CrossMark

Thangamadhan Bosemani, MD*,
Thierry A.G.M. Huisman, MD, EQNR, FICIS, Andrea Poretti, MD

KEYWORDS

- Neurocutaneous syndromes • Cerebellum • Intracranial • Children • MR imaging

KEY POINTS

- Neurocutaneous syndromes are associated with widespread cerebellar involvement.
- Cerebellar involvement in certain types of neurocutaneous syndromes may cause neurocognitive deficits, in particular with regard to language and visuospatial abilities in children.
- Accurate characterization of cerebellar involvement may help in the diagnosis and influences long-term neurocognitive prognosis of children with neurocutaneous syndromes.
- In neurocutaneous disorder, cerebellar tumors such as medulloblastoma in basal cell nevus syndrome have a significantly different management regime compared with sporadic medulloblastoma.

INTRODUCTION

Neurocutaneous syndromes (NCS) are a group of congenital disorders of histogenesis in which the overall brain structure may be normal but anomalous cells persist and continue to differentiate. NCS primarily involves structures derived from the neuroectoderm and, consequently, typically affect the skin and central and/or peripheral nervous system. Most textbooks and reviews focus on the description of the typical supratentorial findings in NCS, with few focusing on the coexisting infratentorial lesions. Neuroimaging has proven to play a key role in the characterization, definition, and diagnosis of NCS. The cerebellum is, however, involved in various types of NCS and its careful evaluation should be part of every neuroimaging study in children with NCS. Cerebellar involvement may (1) be helpful or needed

for the diagnosis of certain types of NCS and (2) explain the cognitive and behavioral phenotype (eg, impaired visuospatial ability, impaired language, or abnormal social behavior) of children with some NCS.

This article describes various types of NCS with cerebellar involvement. For each disease or syndrome, clinical features, genetic, neuroimaging findings, and the potential role of the cerebellar involvement is discussed.

NEUROFIBROMATOSIS TYPE 1

Neurofibromatosis type 1 (NF1; Online Mendelian Inheritance in Man [OMIM] entry 162200) is the most common NCS with a prevalence of 1 in 2500 to 3000 individuals.[1] It is an autosomal dominant disorder caused by heterozygous mutation in the neurofibromin gene on chromosome 17q11.2.

Disclosure: The author reports no conflicts of interest.
Section of Pediatric Neuroradiology, Division of Pediatric Radiology, Russell H. Morgan Department of Radiology and Radiological Science, The Johns Hopkins University School of Medicine, Baltimore, MD, USA
* Corresponding author. Section of Pediatric Neuroradiology, Division of Pediatric Radiology, Russell H. Morgan Department of Radiology and Radiological Science, Charlotte R. Bloomberg Children's Center, The Johns Hopkins University School of Medicine, Sheikh Zayed Tower, Room 4174, 1800 Orleans Street, Baltimore, MD 21287-0842.
E-mail address: tbosema1@jhmi.edu

Neurofibromin is widely expressed with high levels in the nervous system and acts as a tumor suppressor. Neurofibromin reduces cell growth and proliferation by negative regulation of the cellular proto-oncogene p21RAS and by control of the serine threonine kinase mammalian target of rapamycin (mTOR).[2] Impaired neurofibromin function predisposes to benign and malignant tumor formation.

The principal clinical manifestations of NF1 involve the skin and the nervous system, but the complications are variable and may involve most of the body systems.[3]

Neuroimaging abnormalities in NF1 include intracranial neoplasms, parenchymal T2-hyperintense lesions, cerebral vasculopathy, and sphenoid wing dysplasia. Intracranial neoplasms include glioma, cranial nerve schwannoma, and plexiform neurofibroma.[4] Gliomas generally develop in the optic pathways, brainstem, and, rarely, cerebellum. Optic pathway gliomas are the most

frequent neoplasms seen in about 15% of children with NF1 and are typically low-grade pilocytic astrocytomas. Parenchymal T2-hyperintense lesions, also referred to as unidentified bright objects, can be seen in up to 75% of pediatric patients with NF1 and tend to decrease in prevalence with advancing age (**Fig. 1**A).[4] These lesions are not space occupying, do not or very rarely show contrast enhancement, and are typically located in the basal ganglia, internal capsule, brainstem, and cerebellum. Increased apparent diffusion coefficient (ADC) values in unidentified bright objects match the histopathological finding of myelin vacuolation and spongiotic changes attributed to increased water accumulation.[5]

Primary cerebellar tumors are a rare presentation in NF1. In a series of 600 NF1 subjects, only 2 children had low-grade astrocytomas arising primarily from the cerebellar hemisphere (**Fig. 1**B).[6] Vinchon and colleagues[7] showed an overall better outcome for cerebellar gliomas

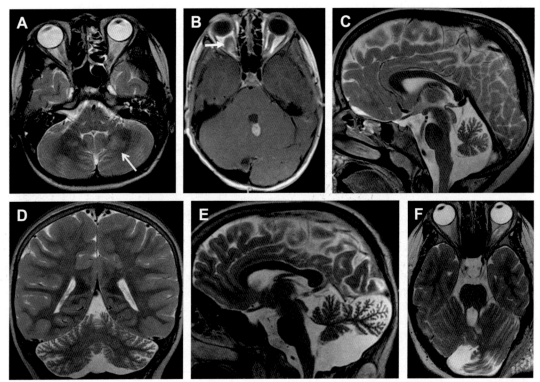

Fig. 1. Neurofibromatosis type 1. (*A*) Axial T2-weighted image showing cerebellar parenchymal T2-hyperintense lesions (*arrow*), also referred to as unidentified bright objects. (*B*) Axial T1 postcontrast image demonstrating an enhancing glioma in the rostral and medial aspect of the cerebellar vermis and optic glioma on the left (*arrow*). (*C*) Sagittal and (*D*) coronal T2-weighted images showing normal size of the cerebellar vermis and hemispheres with stable enlargement of the interfoliar spaces consistent with cerebellar hypoplasia. (*E*) Sagittal and (*F*) axial T2-weighted images showing enlargement of the left cerebellar hemisphere. The posteromedial part of the left cerebellar hemisphere is bulky, crosses the midline, and its interfoliar spaces are enlarged, consistent with cerebellar dysmorphia. (*From* Toelle SP, Poretti A, Weber P, et al. Cerebellar hypoplasia and dysmorphia in neurofibromatosis type 1. Cerebellum 2015;14(6):642–9; with permission.)

associated with NF1 compared with sporadic cerebellar gliomas. Cerebellar parenchymal T2-hyperintense lesions can be distinguished from neoplasms based on absence of mass effect and lack of enhancement. Children with cerebellar parenchymal T2-hyperintense lesions showed a lower intelligence quotient and an altered cognitive profile compared with children without the lesions, particularly with regard to language and visuospatial abilities.[8] Malformative cerebellar abnormalities, including cerebellar hypoplasia and dysmorphia (defined as enlargement of a cerebellar hemisphere with widening of the interfoliar spaces of its posterior part, which is bulky and crosses the midline), are a rare but most likely an underestimated cerebellar manifestation of NF1 (Fig. 1C–F).[9]

TUBEROUS SCLEROSIS COMPLEX

Tuberous sclerosis complex (TSC) is caused by either *TSC1* (OMIM 191100) or *TSC2* (OMIM 613254). It is an autosomal dominant NCS characterized by hamartomas in several organs, including the skin, brain, heart, eyes, kidney, lung, and liver.[10] TSC is due to an inactivating mutation in 1 of the 2 genes, *TSC1* (on chromosome 9q34) encoding hamartin or *TSC2* (on chromosome 16p13.3) encoding tuberin.[10] Hamartin and tuberin work together to inhibit the mTOR pathway that stimulates protein translation, cell growth, and proliferation. Mutations of hamartin or tuberin in TSC cause hyperactivation of the downstream mTOR pathway, which leads to disorganized cellular overgrowth, abnormal differentiation, increased protein translation, and the formation of tumors. Estimated prevalence of TSC is 1 in 6000 to 7000 newborns.

The identification of either a *TSC1* or *TSC2* pathogenic mutation in DNA from normal tissue is sufficient to make a definite diagnosis of TSC.[11] Between 10% and 25% of TSC patients have no mutation identified by conventional genetic testing and a normal result does not exclude TSC or have any effect on the use of clinical diagnostic criteria to diagnose TSC.[11]

Clinical features of TSC most commonly involve the brain (seizures, including infantile spasms, intellectual disability, autism, and self-injurious or aggressive behavior), skin (hypomelanotic macules, angiofibromas, ungula fibromas, shagreen patch, and confetti skin lesions), kidneys (angiomyolipomas and multiple renal cysts), heart (cardiac rhabdomyomas), eyes (multiple retinal hamartomas), and lungs (lymphangioleiomyomatosis in female patients). The 2012 International TSC Consensus Conference updated diagnostic clinical criteria now include 11 major features and 6 minor features. The 2012 consensus is based on definite (2 major features or 1 major feature with ≥2 minor features) or possible (either 1 major feature or ≥2 minor features) diagnosis.[11] Interestingly, some neurologic symptoms such as seizures and intellectual disability are not part of the diagnostic criteria. Three major diagnostic criteria are based on neuroimaging studies (cortical dysplasias, including tubers and cerebral white matter radial migration lines [RMLs], subependymal nodules, and subependymal giant cell astrocytoma). This means that the diagnosis can be made by brain MR imaging alone.

The neuroimaging manifestations of TSC include cortical tubers, subependymal nodules, subependymal giant cell astrocytomas, and white matter RMLs.[4] White matter RMLs are the most frequent neuroimaging finding and are strongly associated with age of seizure onset, intelligence outcomes, and level of autistic features.[12] RMLs represent residual or altered heterotopic glial cells and neurons along the course of glial neuronal migration. Cortical tubers observed in approximately 90% of TSC patients are a type of focal cortical dysplasia and may occur in the cerebellum. The pathologic and clinical overlap between cortical tuber as a major feature and RML as a minor feature in the 1998 diagnostic criteria were replaced with a single major feature, cortical dysplasia, in the new 2012 classification.[11]

Cerebellar tubers are present in 24% to 36% of TSC patients and have a different imaging pattern compared with cerebral tubers.[13,14] Cerebellar cortical tubers differ from the supratentorial tubers in their imaging features. They are triangular with a broad base towards the cerebellar cortex. The shape results from the differing neuronal migration within the cerebellum compared with the cerebrum. Cerebellar tubers are T1-hypointense, and T2-hyperintense (Fig. 2A). Contrast enhancement with a striated or zebra-like pattern (Fig. 2B) and calcification (Fig. 2C) may be seen.[13,15] Cerebellar tubers were demonstrated to increase in size, enhancement, or calcification, within the first 8 years of life (Fig. 2D).[13] Elevated ADC values in cerebellar tubers have been attributed to gliosis and hypomyelination.[13,15] An increasing number of cerebellar tubers on MR imaging has been correlated with the severity of autistic spectrum disorder.[16] In addition, reduced cerebellar volume has been observed in TSC patients, particularly patients with *TSC2* mutations and a more severe phenotype.[17] Evidence of the role of cerebellar involvement in cognition and behavior in TSC was provided by animal studies. In a *Tsc1* mouse model, Tsai and colleagues[18] showed a decrease

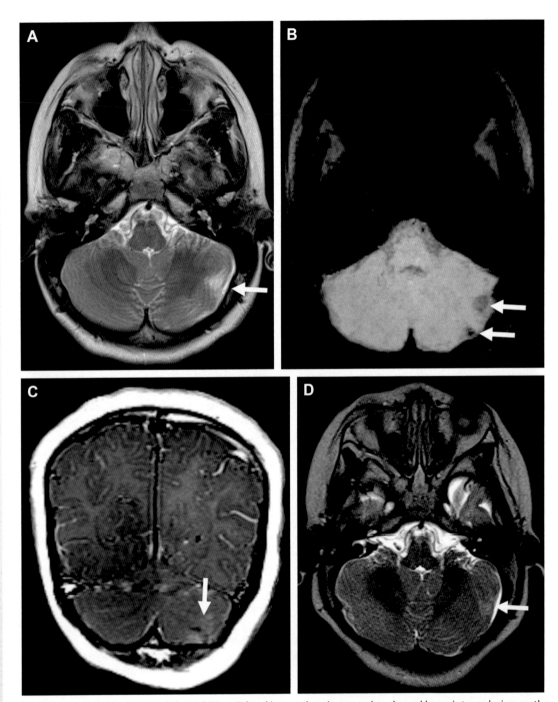

Fig. 2. 5-year-old girl with TSC. (*A*) Axial T2-weighted image showing a wedge-shaped hyperintense lesion on the left consistent with a cerebellar tuber (*arrow*). (*B*) Axial susceptibility-weighted image (SWI) demonstrates hypo-intensity within the tuber (*arrows*), suggesting calcification. (*C*) Coronal T1 postcontrast image showing striated or zebra-like pattern of enhancement (*arrow*). (*D*) Axial T2-weighted image at 10-months of age shows a subtle T2 bright cerebellar tuber on the left (*arrow*) with interval significant increase in dimension at 5-years of age.

in the number of Purkinje cells compared with control. This is the most likely explanation for smaller cerebellar volume in TSC patients. In addition, mutated mice showed an autistic-like behavior as seen in TSC patients.

STURGE-WEBER SYNDROME

Sturge-Weber syndrome (SWS; OMIM 185300) is a sporadic NCS characterized by a facial cuta-neous capillary malformation (port-wine stain) in the ophthalmic distribution of the trigeminal nerve, ipsilateral vascular glaucoma, vascular malformation of the choroid, and a concomitant vascular malformation of the brain and meninges (leptomeningeal angioma).[19] The estimated prevalence of SWS ranges between 1 in 20,000 to 50,000 live births. Specific somatic mosaic activating mutation in GNAQ is associated with both SWS and nonsyndromic port-wine stains.[20] It is hypothesized that GNAQ mutation causes dysregulation of vascular endothelin that may result in malformed, progressively dilated, and abnormally innervated blood vessels.[20] Pathophysiological mechanism in SWS can be explained by venous dysplasia producing focal venous hypertension and resultant tissue hypertrophy.[21] The absence of a mature venous system is initially compensated by the persistence and enlargement of the primitive primordial cerebral venous system. This primitive venous system becomes progressively insufficient with the rapid brain development resulting in intraparenchymal venous hypertension, venous ischemia, tissue injury, and atrophy. Compensatory collateral venous circulatory pathways (eg, dilated intramedullary veins) draining into the deep venous system partially compensate for the venous insufficiency.[22] The clinical course of SWS is variable but typically includes seizures, hemiparesis, headache, stroke-like episodes, developmental delay, and visual field defects.[23]

Typical neuroimaging findings in SWS include a prominent leptomeningeal angiomatosis (especially well seen on contrast-enhanced T1-weighted and FLAIR images),[24] dilated medullary veins, enlargement of the ipsilateral choroid plexus, and underlying slowly progressive cortical or subcortical atrophy. The occipital lobes are primarily affected; in severe cases the central zone, as well as frontal lobes, may also be involved. Rare cases of bilateral involvement have been recorded. Susceptibility-weighted imaging (SWI) is an advanced MR imaging technique that can detect deoxygenated blood in small veins without contrast administration. SWI can detect dilation of transmedullary veins secondary to venous hypertension.[25] In addition, progressive cortical calcifications secondary to long-standing venous hypertension or ischemia is easily identified by the T2* blooming artifacts on SWI.

Cerebellar involvement in SWS is rare and includes leptomeningeal enhancement (Fig. 3A), atrophy, and developmental venous anomaly (Fig. 3B–D). ADC-values of the cerebellar white matter remote from the location of the leptomeningeal angioma may be increased.[26]

PHACE SYNDROME

PHACE syndrome (OMIM 606519) is an NCS characterized by posterior fossa malformation, infantile hemangioma (IH), arterial anomalies, coarctation of the aorta, eye abnormalities, and ventral developmental defects, specifically sternal defects, and/or supraumbilical raphe. The cause and pathogenesis of PHACE is unknown and its diagnosis is based on the presence of a characteristic hemangioma and other major or minor clinical or imaging criteria.[27]

Isolated IH are subtle or absent at birth, usually becoming more evident within the first days to weeks of life. IH associated with PHACE tend to be large (>5 cm in diameter), telangiectatic in appearance, and typically segmental in distribution in the face.[27] Most patients have a normal neurologic examination in infancy but may develop focal seizures, developmental delay, and recurrent headaches.[27] Early neurologic findings are typically related to structural brain anomalies.

The presence of a segmental cervicofacial IH should prompt neuroimaging to evaluate for the presence of intracranial abnormalities that may be related to PHACE. Hence, neuroimaging plays a key role in establishing the diagnosis. Intracranial anomalies (cerebrovascular and posterior fossa) are the most common extracutaneous feature of PHACE and are typically ipsilateral to the IH.[28,29] Intracranial and cervical arteriopathy diagnosed by MR angiography can be categorized as dysgenesis, narrowing, nonvisualization, persistent embryonic carotid-vertebrobasilar arterial connections, and abnormalities in arterial course and/or origin.[28] Arterial dysgenesis is the most common vascular manifestation and is characterized by eccentric outpouching, fusiform enlargement, or aneurysm formation.[28] Arteriopathy is more common in the anterior circulation (internal carotid artery) than in the posterior circulation. Perinatal arterial ischemic stroke may be seen. Supratentorial brain abnormalities associated with PHACE include callosal dysgenesis, hemispheric hypoplasia, subependymal heterotopia, polymicrogyria, and extra-axial hemangiomas.[30] Posterior fossa anomalies are the most commonly reported brain anomalies in PHACE.[27,28,30] The typical posterior fossa anomaly is unilateral cerebellar hypoplasia (Fig. 4) with or without involvement of the vermis; whereas a Dandy-Walker malformation (DWM) is less common.[28]

VON HIPPEL-LINDAU DISEASE

von Hippel-Lindau (VHL) disease (OMIM 193300) is an autosomal dominant NCS characterized by

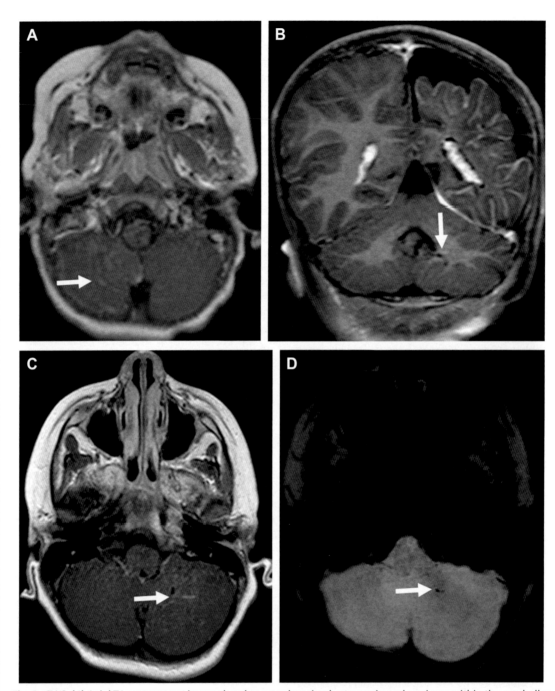

Fig. 3. SWS. (*A*) Axial T1 postcontrast image showing an enhancing leptomeningeal angioma within the cerebellar fissures on the right (*arrow*). (*B*) Coronal (*arrow*) and (*C*) axial T1 postcontrast image showing developmental venous anomaly (DVA) in the left cerebellar hemisphere (*arrow*) and atrophy in the left cerebrum. (*D*) Axial SWI image showing hypointense signal in the left cerebellar hemisphere DVA (*arrow*). (*From* [A] Arulrajah S, Ertan G, M Comi A, et al. MR imaging with diffusion-weighted imaging in children and young adults with simultaneous supra- and infratentorial manifestations of Sturge-Weber syndrome. J Neuroradiol 2010;37:51–9; with permission.)

various benign and malignant tumors of the central nervous system (CNS), kidneys, adrenal glands, inner ear, and reproductive adnexal organs such as retinal, cerebellar, and spinal hemangioblastoma and endolymphatic sac tumor. VHL results from a germline mutation in the *VHL* tumor suppressor gene on chromosome 3p25.3, which inactivates a *VHL* allele, with the carriers

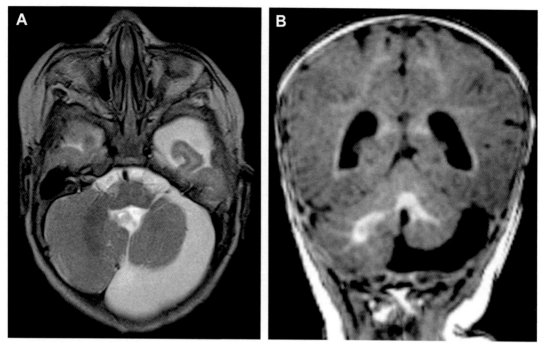

Fig. 4. 4-month-old girl with PHACE syndrome. (*A*) Axial T2 and (*B*) coronal T1-weighted images showing unilateral cerebellar hypoplasia with volume loss in the left cerebellar hemisphere and vermis with a normal sized posterior fossa and a prominent extra-axial CSF space subjacent to it.

of this mutation being subject to a second inactivating event (2-hit hypothesis).[31] This mutation results in complete functional loss of the tumor suppressor and, therefore, overexpression of proteins that mediate angiogenesis. The estimated incidence of VHL is about 1 in 36,000 live births.[4] Outside the CNS, multisystem visceral involvement includes renal cysts, renal cell carcinomas, pancreatic cysts, and pheochromocytomas. CNS hemangioblastoma is observed in 65% of patients with VHL and is a defining feature in VHL.[32]

The cerebellum is the most common location (about 65%) for CNS hemangioblastomas. They are highly vascular benign World Health Organization (WHO) grade 1 tumors that show solid enhancement, appear pial-based, and are, therefore, peripherally located in the cerebellum (**Fig. 5**). When the tumors enlarge, they appear cystic with an enhancing mural nodule and the natural history of progression shows a faster rate of cystic expansion than growth of the causative solid tumor, eventually resulting in pressure effect and clinical symptoms.[33] Hemangioblastomas are T1-isointense and T2-hyperintense. Heterogeneous T2 signal may be seen in the presence of intralesional hemorrhage. Mural nodules are well demarcated and show homogenous enhancement. If present, flow voids appear T2 hypointense

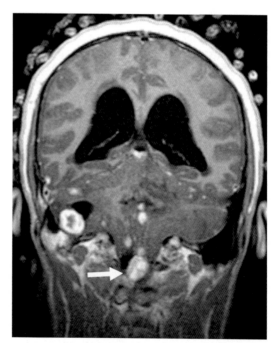

Fig. 5. 16-year-old boy with VHL disease. Coronal T1 postcontrast image demonstrates numerous hemangioblastomas within the cerebellum and in the cervicomedullary junction (*arrow*).

with superficial heterogeneous enhancement. Peritumoral vasogenic edema is typically mild. In VHL, multiple lesions may occur simultaneously. Additional lesions may be present along the spinal cord. Imaging of the entire neural axis is consequently advised. The lesion may mimic a pilocytic astrocytoma. The clinical findings usually allow differentiation. In addition, hemangioblastomas are typically characterized by the prominent vascular signal voids. Finally, hemangioblastomas may hemorrhage into the subarachnoid space with resultant hemosiderosis due to their high vascular nature and close proximity to the subarachnoid space. Endolymphatic sac tumors are, with a prevalence of up to 16%, a component of VHL disease. Contrast-enhanced MR imaging of the petrous bone must be part of annual surveillance.[34]

Affected children may present with a history of minor neurologic symptoms, such as occipital or frontal headaches or imbalance. Significant neurologic deficit may result from development of obstructive hydrocephalus, tonsillar herniation, and brainstem compression, requiring immediate neurosurgical intervention.[35]

NEUROCUTANEOUS MELANOSIS

Neurocutaneous melanosis (NCM; OMIM 249400) is a rare NCS characterized by congenital melanocytic nevi (CMN) associated with CNS involvement.[36] CMN can be single or multiple and are present at birth or arise within the first few weeks of life. It has recently been found to be caused by mosaicism for heterozygous somatic mutations in the NRAS codon 61 of a progenitor cell within the neuroectoderm.[37] NCM is characterized by excessive proliferation of melanocytes in the leptomeninges and brain parenchyma, and is considered an embryologic abnormality of the developing neuroectoderm. MR imaging of the entire neural axis is the modality of choice in children with 2 or more CMN at birth, and performed in the first year of life (ideally within the first 6 months due to progressing myelination, which may obscure the signal of melanin).[36]

Seizures represent the most common initial neurologic symptom in children.[38] Neurodevelopmental delay and increasing intracranial pressure from hydrocephalus are other neurologic symptoms in NCM. Progressive leptomeningeal melanocytosis and/or melanoma of the brain and spine are associated with a poor prognosis. Proliferating leptomeningeal deposits are associated with communicating hydrocephalus and/or increasing intracranial pressure.

The most common neuroimaging abnormality on MR imaging is isolated intraparenchymal melanosis (foci of melanin-containing cells in the brain parenchyma), which was previously considered to be secondary only to overlying invasive leptomeningeal disease.[36] The typical location for melanin deposition with T1-hyperintensity and/or T2 hypointensity is in the anterior regions of the temporal lobes (amygdala), cerebellum, pons, and leptomeningeal surface.[38] In addition to T1-hyperintensity (melanin) on the precontrast images, diffuse nodular enhancement may be present postcontrast with progressive leptomeningeal melanocytosis. Diffuse leptomeningeal melanoma may develop and is biopsy proven.

Intraparenchymal melanosis with T1-hyperintense lesions may affect the cerebellum (Fig. 6A). Cerebellar hypoplasia may be associated with NCM (Fig. 6B).

GÓMEZ-LÓPEZ-HERNÁNDEZ SYNDROME

Gómez-López-Hernández (GLH) syndrome (OMIM 601853) also known as cerebello-trigeminal-dermal dysplasia is a rare NCS comprising the triad of rhombencephalosynapsis (RS) (Fig. 7A, B), parietal alopecia (Fig. 7C), and trigeminal anesthesia.[39] The cause remains unknown. No chromosomal abnormalities have been reported to date. The clinical signs of GLH (alopecia, trigeminal anesthesia, ataxia, and head stereotypies) can be very mild and easily missed.[39] In GLH, there is a broad range of cognitive impairment but cognition can even be normal.[39]

Neuroimaging plays a key role in establishing RS, which is a key feature of GLH and, hence, is needed for the diagnosis of GLH. RS is characterized by dorsal continuity of the cerebellar hemispheres, agenesis, or hypogenesis of the vermis, and fusion of the dentate nuclei and superior cerebellar peduncles.[39] Recently, the absence of trigeminal nerves and foramina rotunda bilaterally has been shown in GLH, suggesting a possible structural basis for trigeminal anesthesia.[40]

ENCEPHALOCRANIOCUTANEOUS LIPOMATOSIS

Encephalocraniocutaneous lipomatosis (ECCL; OMIM 613001) is a sporadic NCS characterized by ocular anomalies, skin lesions, and CNS anomalies.[41] The CNS anomalies in ECCL are most likely caused by a mesenchymal and neural crest defect affecting the tissue surrounding the brain and the vessels.[41]

Typical findings include eye anomalies (mainly choristomas) and skin lesions (nonscarring alopecia, nevus psiloliparus, subcutaneous fatty masses, nodular skin tags, or aplastic scalp

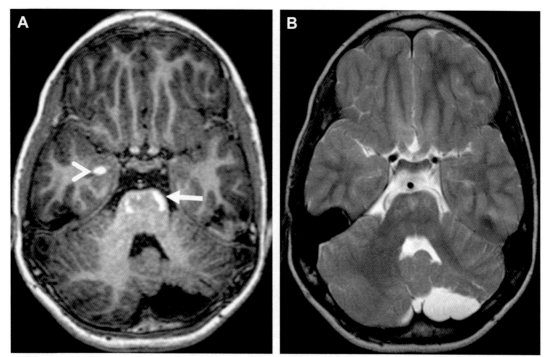

Fig. 6. NCM. (*A*) Axial T1-weighted image demonstrates hyperintense signal in the anterior aspect of the pons (*arrow*) and right mesial temporal lobe (*arrowhead*) consistent with NCM. Cerebellar hypoplasia is shown on the left. (*B*) Axial T2-weighted image showing cerebellar hypoplasia on the left with volume loss in a normal-sized posterior fossa.

defects), which may be unilateral or bilateral.[42] Children with ECCL may present with developmental delay, intellectual disability, and/or seizures. Neurodevelopmental delay is not related to the severity of neuroimaging findings.

Neuroimaging plays an important role in identifying the CNS anomalies. Posterior fossa involvement in ECCL may include DWM, cerebellar

hypoplasia (**Fig. 8**A, B), arachnoid cysts, and mega cisterna magna. The common CNS anomalies include (1) intracranial lipomas (predominantly cerebello-pontine angle in location) (**Fig. 8**C), (2) spinal lipomas (**Fig. 8**D), (3) arachnoid cysts, (4) intracranial vessel anomalies, (5) unilateral ventriculomegaly, and (6) widening of subarachnoid spaces. Lipomas may be characterized by the

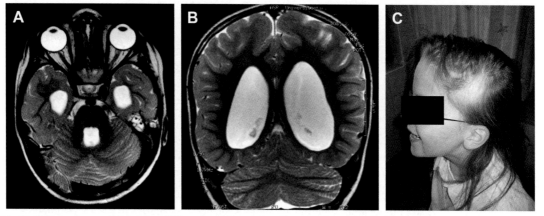

Fig. 7. GLH syndrome. (*A*) Axial and (*B*) coronal T2-weighted images showing RS with keyhole appearance of fourth ventricle, fusion of the cerebellar hemispheres without an intervening vermis, as well as fusion of the dentate nuclei and superior cerebellar peduncles. (*C*) 10-year-old girl with GLH syndrome showing alopecia in the left scalp.

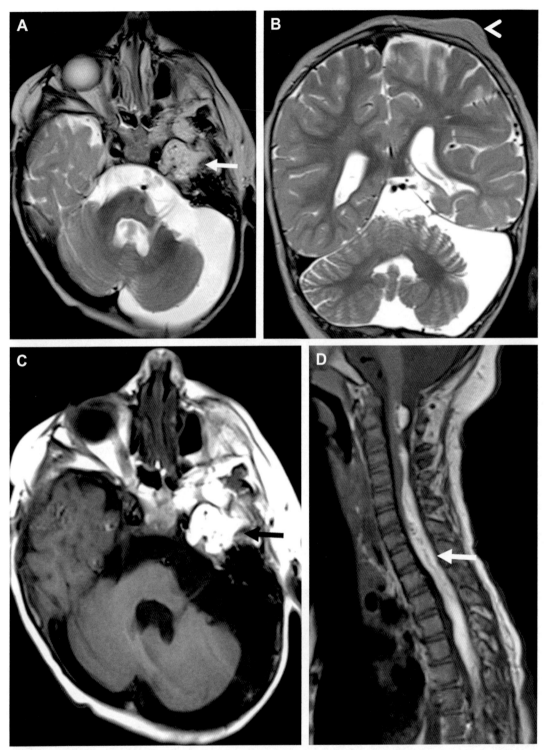

Fig. 8. ECCL. Axial and coronal T2-weighted images showing left cerebellar hypoplasia with prominent CSF space subjacent to left cerebellar hemisphere. (*A*) Intracranial lipoma infiltrating the left petrous temporal bone (*arrow*) and (*B*) scalp lesion (*arrowhead*). (*C*) Axial T1-weighted image demonstrates left cerebellar hypoplasia and T1 bright lipoma (*black arrow*) infiltrating the left petrous temporal bone. (*D*) Sagittal T1-weighted image of the cervical spine showing epidural location of intraspinal lipoma (*arrow*).

presence and suppression of fat signal on T1-weighted with and without fat suppression, respectively.

OCULOCEREBROCUTANEOUS SYNDROME

Oculocerebrocutaneous syndrome (OCCS; OMIM 164180), also known as Delleman Oorthuys syndrome is a rare sporadic NCS characterized by the triad of eye, brain, and skin malformations.[43] There is a male preponderance. The cause is unknown.

The typical eye findings include orbital cyst, microphthalmia or anophthalmia, and eyelid coloboma. Cutaneous lesions described in OCCS are skin appendages, focal dermal hypoplasia or aplasia, punch-like defects, and crescent-shaped hypoplasia.[43]

Neuroimaging demonstrates a forebrain malformation consisting of frontal predominant polymicrogyria; periventricular nodular heterotopia, located beneath the polymicrogyria; complete or partial agenesis of the corpus callosum, sometimes associated with interhemispheric cysts; and supratentorial ventriculomegaly. Moog and colleagues[43] described a novel mid-hindbrain malformation consisting of a giant dysplastic tectum and absent vermis. The midbrain is angled more forward than normal, leading to a short, horizontal aqueduct, enlarging prematurely into the fourth ventricle. The combination of a giant dysplastic tectum and absent vermis is pathognomonic for OCCS (**Fig. 9**). In addition, the cerebellar hemispheres are hypoplastic with a dysplastic foliar pattern. The absence of the vermis and cerebellar hypoplasia leads to wide communication of the fourth ventricle with a posterior fossa cerebrospinal fluid (CSF) space.

EPIDERMAL NEVUS SYNDROME

Epidermal nevus syndrome (ENS) includes a heterogeneous group of primary sporadic NCS characterized by the presence of epidermal nevi that follow the lines of Blaschko and are associated with systemic involvement.[44] ENS are neurocristopathies due to defective neural crest development. The incidence of ENS is unknown.

The principal manifestations of ENS are epilepsy, developmental delay, intellectual disability, and focal motor deficits. Hemimegalencephaly (HME) is the primary cause of epilepsy in all forms of ENS but often is unrecognized.[44] HME is present in more than 50% of children with ENSs and neurologic symptoms. MR imaging is the neuroimaging tool of choice for evaluation of HME. The typical MR imaging appearance of HME includes a moderate to marked enlargement of the affected cerebral hemisphere with midline shift, a thickened cortex with broad gyri, shallow sulci and blurring of the cortical-white matter junction, cortical thickening, an increased volume and T2-hyperintense signal of the white matter, and enlarged lateral ventricle with straightening of the frontal horn and/or unilateral colpocephaly.[45] Ipsilateral enlargement of the cerebellum and brain stem is referred to as total HME (**Fig. 10**) and has been reported in several cases of ENS.[46]

PTEN HAMARTOMA TUMOR SYNDROME

PTEN hamartoma tumor syndrome (PHTS) is an autosomal dominant cancer-predisposition syndrome caused by mutations in the tumor suppressor gene *PTEN* on chromosome 10q23.31.[47] PHTS includes Cowden syndrome, Bannayan–Riley–Ruvalcaba syndrome, Proteus syndrome, and Proteus-like syndrome. These allelic disorders are associated with unregulated cellular proliferation leading to the formation of hamartomas. Children and adults with PHTS are at increased risk for benign and malignant tumors of various organs, including the thyroid, breast, endometrium, skin, kidneys, CNS, and gastrointestinal tract.

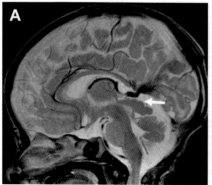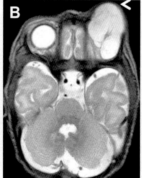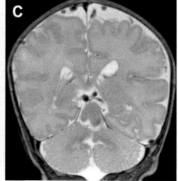

Fig. 9. OCCS. Sagittal, axial, and coronal T2-weighted images showing (*A*) giant dysplastic tectum (*arrow*), (*B*) left orbital cyst (*arrowhead*), and (*C*) absent vermis.

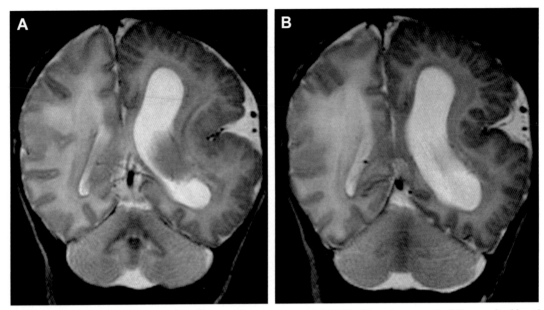

Fig. 10. ENS. (*A*, *B*) Coronal T2-weighted images demonstrate total HME with enlargement of the cerebral hemisphere and ipsilateral cerebellar hemisphere. The enlarged cerebral hemisphere shows a thickened cortex with broad gyri, shallow sulci with blurring of the cortical-white matter junction, and T2-hyperintense signal of the white matter.

Although most tumors occur only in adulthood, tumors have been reported in children.[47]

Macrocephaly is a consistent finding. Intellectual and developmental disability is a common finding in children with PTEN mutations. A child with developmental concerns, who exhibits any finding of PHTS (eg, macrocephaly, pigmented penile macules, lipomas, vascular malformations) at any age should be suspected of having PHTS.[47]

Lhermitte-Duclos disease (LDD) is a rare overgrowth of hamartoma arising from the cerebellar cortex characterized by abnormal ganglion cells, absence of Purkinje cells, and hypertrophy of granular cell layer.[48] LDD is commonly sporadic but can also be familial if associated with Cowden syndrome.[49] LDD typically manifests during the third and fourth decades of life but may also present in childhood. Clinical manifestations of a posterior fossa mass include headaches, cerebellar ataxia, and perturbed vision.

Neuroimaging pattern of multifocal static white matter abnormalities and dilated perivascular spaces should suggest the possibility of a PHTS in a child with macrocephaly and developmental delay and/or autism spectrum disorder.[50,51]

Typical MR imaging findings of LDD are a discrete stable, nonprogressive cerebellar mass lesion with a striated corduroy or tiger-striped folia pattern. The central T2-hyperintense and T1-hypointense regions relative to gray matter correspond to the unmyelinated white matter, widened granular cell layer, and the inner portions of the dysplastic molecular layer. The outer T1- and T2-isointense to hypointense regions relative to gray matter correspond to the outer molecular layer and leptomeninges (**Fig. 11**).[52] Expansion of the cortex, infiltration of the brain stem, and a space-occupying mass are typical imaging findings of LDD. LDD typically does not show enhancement postcontrast; however, several exceptional cases have been reported.[53]

BASAL CELL NEVUS SYNDROME

Basal cell nevus syndrome (BCNS; OMIM 109400), also known as Gorlin-Goltz syndrome, is an autosomal dominant disorder characterized by multiple basal cell carcinomas, jaw cysts, palmar or plantar pits, calcification of the falx cerebri, and spine and rib anomalies.[54] The estimated prevalence of BCNS is 1 in 56,000 to 256,000.[55] There is no gender or ethnic predilection. BCNS originates from a heterozygous germline mutation in the Patched homolog 1 is a transmembrane glycoprotein that is encoded by the gene *PTCH1* on chromosome 9q22 to 31 and serves as a tumor suppressor of the sonic Hedgehog signaling pathway.[55]

The clinical hallmarks of the disease include multiple basal cell carcinomas of the skin, medulloblastoma, and odontogenic keratocysts (OKCs)

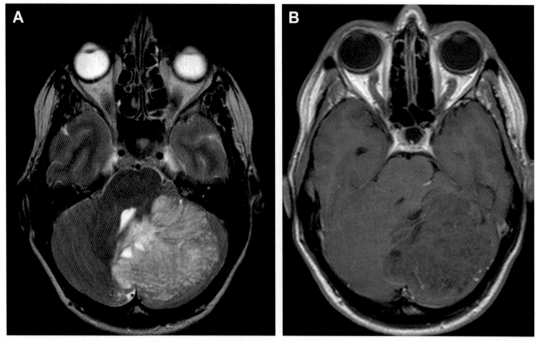

Fig. 11. LDD. (*A*) Axial T2-and (*B*) axial T1 postcontrast images showing a left cerebellar hemisphere mass with a striated corduroy or tiger-striped folia pattern. Striated pattern consists of central T2-hyperintense and T1-hypointense regions as well as peripheral T1- and T2-isointense to hypointense regions relative to gray matter. Mass effect on the fourth ventricle and no significant postcontrast enhancement is shown.

of the oral cavity.[56] Children with BCNS have a predisposition for secondary tumors after exposure to both ionizing and ultraviolet radiation.[57] Medulloblastoma treatment usually includes radiation therapy to the posterior fossa, and management of OKCs keratocysts may require sequential computed tomography (CT) imaging studies. It is important to make a diagnosis of BCNS as early as possible to avoid unnecessary exposures to ionizing radiation.[56]

OKCs can be seen in the maxilla and mandible of children. Initial diagnosis of OKC is typically made on maxillofacial CT and follow-up examination with MR imaging is recommended due to the sensitivity of BCNS children to ionizing radiation. Osseous bridging of the sella turcica is rare in the general population but represents an important imaging clue for the diagnosis of BCNS. Macrocephaly is often provided as part of the patients clinical history as the indication for brain imaging. Hence, in the context of macrocephaly, it is important to evaluate for ectopic calcifications, bony bridging of the sella, or other clinical features compatible with BCNS.[56]

Medulloblastoma is frequently the first manifestation of BCNS. The median age of presentation in BCNS (2 years) is much earlier

than in the sporadic presentation (6.9 years). Desmoplastic medulloblastoma (DMB) variant and medulloblastoma with extensive nodularity (MBEN) are histologic variants associated with BCNS.[58,59] DMB is typically more laterally situated within the cerebellar hemispheres and is frequently associated with meningeal enhancement. DMB and MBEN are considered to have favorable prognosis, an important consideration when the diagnosis of BCNS coexists and radiation therapy is omitted.[56]

COCKAYNE SYNDROME

Cockayne syndrome (OMIM 216400) is an autosomal recessive multisystem NCS characterized by developmental delay, microcephaly, severe growth failure, cutaneous photosensitivity, dental decay, and pigmentary retinopathy. Cockayne syndrome is caused by mutations in *ERCC6* (CSB) in 65% of patients and *ERCC8* (CSA) in the remainder.[60] The CSA and CSB proteins are involved in nucleotide excision repair, which is closely related to the basal transcription machinery and preferentially targets DNA lesions in actively transcribed genes.[61] There is lack of recovery of RNA synthesis in cultured skin fibroblasts after ultraviolet irradiation, which may explain the cutaneous manifestations.

Cockayne syndrome is a progressive disorder and there is a spectrum of symptom severity. The cardinal neuroimaging features of Cockayne syndrome include cerebral and cerebellar atrophy, calcifications, and white matter anomalies (Fig. 12).[61] Cerebral white matter loss and ventricular dilation are the earliest signs on MR imaging. Calcifications are typically bilateral and symmetric, most frequently seen in the putamen. Progressive cerebellar atrophy is a common feature and contributes to the diagnosis. Dysmetria and action tremor progress over time with progressive cerebellar atrophy.[61]

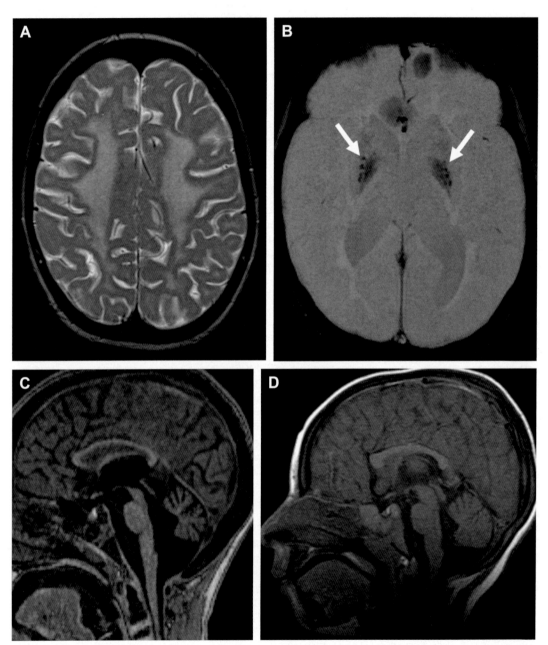

Fig. 12. 9-year-old girl with Cockayne syndrome. (*A*) Axial T2-weighted image shows confluent abnormal hyperintense signal in the supratentorial white matter. (*B*) Axial SWI image shows hypointense signal in bilateral globi pallidi (*arrows*) consistent with calcifications. (*C*) and (*D*) Sagittal T1-weighted images at 9-years and 2-years of age, respectively, showing progressive cerebellar atrophy. (*From* Wagner MW, Poretti A, Wang T, et al. Susceptibility-weighted imaging for calcification in Cockayne syndrome. J Pediatr 2014;165(2):416; with permission.)

TRICHOTHIODYSTROPHY

Trichothiodystrophy (TTD) is a rare, autosomal recessive NCS, characterized by brittle, sulfur-deficient hair and multisystem abnormalities.[62] TTD results from defective repair of nucleotide errors in DNA. It is caused by mutations of *XPD*, rarely of *XPB*, *TTDA*, and*TTDN1*; the latter 2 are not associated with photosensitivity.[63]

Skin findings of photosensitivity and/or ichthyosis were reported in 70% of these patients. Neurologic abnormalities (86%) were frequently reported, manifesting most commonly as developmental delay, intellectual impairment, microcephaly, impaired motor control, or psychomotor retardation.[62] Neurologic abnormalities seem to be mainly related to impaired development and maturation of the nervous system.[64]

The most common neuroimaging abnormalities are white matter anomalies, cerebellar atrophy, and ventriculomegaly (**Fig. 13**).[62]

COSTELLO SYNDROME

Costello syndrome (CoS; OMIM 218040) is an autosomal dominant disorder caused by heterozygous germline mutations in proto-oncogene *HRAS*. Prolonged activation of the HRAS protein results in dysregulation of the Ras/mitogen-activated protein kinase pathway. Ras/mitogen activated-protein kinase pathway determines cell proliferation and differentiation, and its dysregulation affects cardiac and brain development.[65]

CoS can be diagnosed clinically in the older child with a characteristic facial appearance of curly or fine hair, prominent epicanthal folds, long eyelashes, full nasal tip, fleshy ear lobes, and a wide mouth with full lips.[65] Infants demonstrate hypotonia, irritability, developmental delay, and nystagmus with delayed visual maturation improving with age. Macrocephaly is a typical finding and likely reflects brain overgrowth.[66]

Disproportionate cerebellar size due to brain overgrowth and a normal-sized posterior fossa results in crowding of the posterior fossa. Gripp and colleagues[66] showed posterior fossa crowding with cerebellar tonsillar herniation in 96% of subjects and 59% of subjects with serial studies showed progression of posterior fossa crowding. Ventriculomegaly may be seen. Severely affected individuals with cerebellar tonsillar herniation had known complications of hydrocephalus requiring shunt or ventriculostomy, Chiari 1 malformation, and syrinx formation (**Fig. 14**).[66] Neurologic symptoms secondary to cerebellar tonsillar herniation

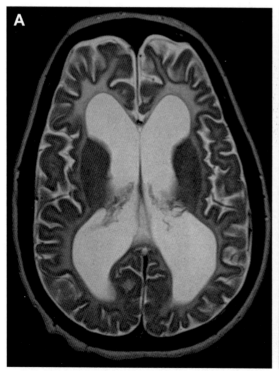
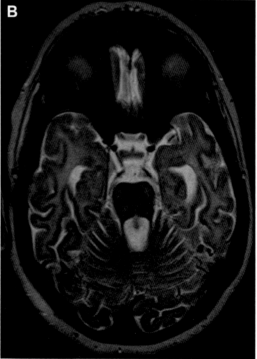

Fig. 13. 14-year-old boy with TTD. (*A*) and (*B*) Axial T2-weighted images show diffuse abnormal T2-hyperintense signal of the supratentorial white matter, ventriculomegaly, and cerebellar atrophy.

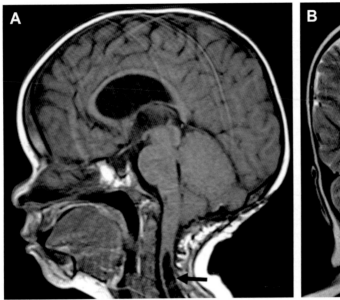
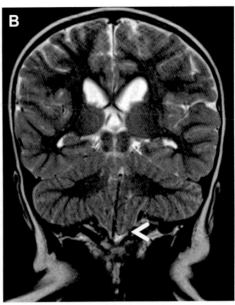

Fig. 14. 6-year-old boy with CoS status post cervicomedullary decompression. (A) Sagittal T1-weighted image shows inferior descent of the cerebellar tonsils, postsurgical changes associated with decompression, and a cervical region syringohydromyelia (*arrow*). (B) Coronal T2-weighted image shows inferior descent of the cerebellar tonsils (*arrowhead*).

may be present and require neurosurgical posterior fossa decompression.

SUMMARY

The cerebellum is affected in a wide number of NCS. Neuroimaging plays an important role in the recognition of cerebellar involvement. Accurate recognition and characterization of cerebellar involvement in NCS allows the clinician to: (1) establish the diagnosis, (2) predict the prognosis, (3) support clinical findings/diagnosis, and (4) determine its influence on neurocognitive outcome.

REFERENCES

1. Williams VC, Lucas J, Babcock MA, et al. Neurofibromatosis type 1 revisited. Pediatrics 2009;123: 124–33.
2. Ferner RE. The neurofibromatoses. Pract Neurol 2010;10:82–93.
3. Ferner RE, Gutmann DH. Neurofibromatosis type 1 (NF1): diagnosis and management. Handb Clin Neurol 2013;115:939–55.
4. Nandigam K, Mechtler LL, Smirniotopoulos JG. Neuroimaging of neurocutaneous diseases. Neurol Clin 2014;32:159–92.
5. Ertan G, Zan E, Yousem DM, et al. Diffusion tensor imaging of neurofibromatosis bright objects in children with neurofibromatosis type 1. Neuroradiol J 2014;27:616–26.
6. Pascual-Castroviejo I, Pascual-Pascual SI, Viano J, et al. Posterior fossa tumors in children with neurofibromatosis type 1 (NF1). Childs Nerv Syst 2010;26: 1599–603.
7. Vinchon M, Soto-Ares G, Ruchoux MM, et al. Cerebellar gliomas in children with NF1: pathology and surgery. Childs Nerv Syst 2000; 16:417–20.
8. Piscitelli O, Digilio MC, Capolino R, et al. Neurofibromatosis type 1 and cerebellar T2-hyperintensities: the relationship to cognitive functioning. Dev Med Child Neurol 2012;54:49–51.
9. Toelle SP, Poretti A, Weber P, et al. Cerebellar hypoplasia and dysmorphia in neurofibromatosis type 1. Cerebellum 2015;14(6):642–9.
10. Curatolo P, Maria BL. Tuberous sclerosis. Handb Clin Neurol 2013;111:323–31.
11. Northrup H, Krueger DA. International tuberous sclerosis complex consensus G. Tuberous sclerosis complex diagnostic criteria update: recommendations of the 2012 International Tuberous Sclerosis Complex Consensus Conference. Pediatr Neurol 2013;49:243–54.
12. van Eeghen AM, Ortiz-Teran L, Johnson J, et al. The neuroanatomical phenotype of tuberous sclerosis complex: focus on radial migration lines. Neuroradiology 2013;55:1007–14.
13. Daghistani R, Rutka J, Widjaja E. MRI characteristics of cerebellar tubers and their longitudinal changes in children with tuberous sclerosis complex. Childs Nerv Syst 2015;31:109–13.

14. Vaughn J, Hagiwara M, Katz J, et al. MRI characterization and longitudinal study of focal cerebellar lesions in a young tuberous sclerosis cohort. AJNR Am J Neuroradiol 2013;34:655–9.

15. Ertan G, Arulrajah S, Tekes A, et al. Cerebellar abnormality in children and young adults with tuberous sclerosis complex: MR and diffusion weighted imaging findings. J Neuroradiol 2010;37:231–8.

16. Weber AM, Egelhoff JC, McKellop JM, et al. Autism and the cerebellum: evidence from tuberous sclerosis. J Autism Dev Disord 2000;30:511–7.

17. Weisenfeld NI, Peters JM, Tsai PT, et al. A magnetic resonance imaging study of cerebellar volume in tuberous sclerosis complex. Pediatr Neurol 2013;48: 105–10.

18. Tsai PT, Hull C, Chu Y, et al. Autistic-like behaviour and cerebellar dysfunction in Purkinje cell Tsc1 mutant mice. Nature 2012;488:647–51.

19. Nabbout R, Juhasz C. Sturge-Weber syndrome. Handb Clin Neurol 2013;111:315–21.

20. Shirley MD, Tang H, Gallione CJ, et al. Sturge-Weber syndrome and port-wine stains caused by somatic mutation in GNAQ. N Engl J Med 2013;368:1971–9.

21. Parsa CF. Focal venous hypertension as a pathophysiologic mechanism for tissue hypertrophy, port-wine stains, the Sturge-Weber syndrome, and related disorders: proof of concept with novel hypothesis for underlying etiological cause (an American Ophthalmological Society thesis). Trans Am Ophthalmol Soc 2013;111:180–215.

22. Vezina G. Neuroimaging of phakomatoses: overview and advances. Pediatr Radiol 2015;45(Suppl 3): 433–42.

23. Sudarsanam A, Ardern-Holmes SL. Sturge-Weber syndrome: from the past to the present. Eur J Paediatr Neurol 2014;18:257–66.

24. Griffiths PD, Coley SC, Romanowski CA, et al. Contrast-enhanced fluid-attenuated inversion recovery imaging for leptomeningeal disease in children. AJNR Am J Neuroradiol 2003;24:719–23.

25. Hu J, Yu Y, Juhasz C, et al. MR susceptibility weighted imaging (SWI) complements conventional contrast enhanced T1-MRI in characterizing brain abnormalities of Sturge-Weber Syndrome. J Magn Reson Imaging 2008;28:300–7.

26. Arulrajah S, Ertan G, M Comi A, et al. MRI with diffusion-weighted imaging in children and young adults with simultaneous supra- and infratentorial manifestations of Sturge-Weber syndrome. J Neuroradiol 2010;37:51–9.

27. Metry D, Heyer G, Hess C, et al. Consensus statement on diagnostic criteria for PHACE syndrome. Pediatrics 2009;124:1447–56.

28. Hess CP, Fullerton HJ, Metry DW, et al. Cervical and intracranial arterial anomalies in 70 patients with PHACE syndrome. AJNR Am J Neuroradiol 2010; 31:1980–6.

29. Bracken J, Robinson I, Snow A, et al. PHACE syndrome: MRI of intracerebral vascular anomalies and clinical findings in a series of 12 patients. Pediatr Radiol 2011;41:1129–38.

30. Metry DW, Haggstrom AN, Drolet BA, et al. A prospective study of PHACE syndrome in infantile hemangiomas: demographic features, clinical findings, and complications. Am J Med Genet A 2006; 140:975–86.

31. Monsalve J, Kapur J, Malkin D, et al. Imaging of cancer predisposition syndromes in children. Radiographics 2011;31:263–80.

32. Kanno H, Kuratsu J, Nishikawa R, et al. Clinical features of patients bearing central nervous system hemangioblastoma in von Hippel-Lindau disease. Acta Neurochir (Wien) 2013;155:1–7.

33. Lin DD, Barker PB. Neuroimaging of phakomatoses. Semin Pediatr Neurol 2006;13:48–62.

34. Bausch B, Wellner U, Peyre M, et al. Characterization of endolymphatic sac tumors and von Hippel-Lindau disease in the International Endolymphatic Sac Tumor Registry. Head Neck 2016. [Epub ahead of print].

35. Vortmeyer AO, Falke EA, Glasker S, et al. Nervous system involvement in von Hippel-Lindau disease: pathology and mechanisms. Acta Neuropathol 2013;125:333–50.

36. Waelchli R, Aylett SE, Atherton D, et al. Classification of neurological abnormalities in children with congenital melanocytic naevus syndrome identifies MRI as the best predictor of clinical outcome. Br J Dermatol 2015;173(3):739–50.

37. Kinsler VA, Thomas AC, Ishida M, et al. Multiple congenital melanocytic nevi and neurocutaneous melanosis are caused by postzygotic mutations in codon 61 of NRAS. J Invest Dermatol 2013;133: 2229–36.

38. Ramaswamy V, Delaney H, Haque S, et al. Spectrum of central nervous system abnormalities in neurocutaneous melanocytosis. Dev Med Child Neurol 2012; 54:563–8.

39. Poretti A, Bartholdi D, Gobara S, et al. Gomez-Lopez-Hernandez syndrome: an easily missed diagnosis. Eur J Med Genet 2008;51:197–208.

40. Choudhri AF, Patel RM, Wilroy RS, et al. Trigeminal nerve agenesis with absence of foramina rotunda in Gomez-Lopez-Hernandez syndrome. Am J Med Genet A 2015;167A:238–42.

41. Moog U, Jones MC, Viskochil DH, et al. Brain anomalies in encephalocraniocutaneous lipomatosis. Am J Med Genet A 2007;143A:2963–72.

42. Moog U. Encephalocraniocutaneous lipomatosis. J Med Genet 2009;46:721–9.

43. Moog U, Jones MC, Bird LM, et al. Oculocerebrocutaneous syndrome: the brain malformation defines a core phenotype. J Med Genet 2005;42: 913–21.

44. Laura FS. Epidermal nevus syndrome. Handb Clin Neurol 2013;111:349–68.

45. Flores-Sarnat L. Hemimegalencephaly: part 1. Genetic, clinical, and imaging aspects. J Child Neurol 2002;17:373–84 [discussion: 84].

46. Sato N, Yagishita A, Oba H, et al. Hemimegalencephaly: a study of abnormalities occurring outside the involved hemisphere. AJNR Am J Neuroradiol 2007;28:678–82.

47. Smpokou P, Fox VL, Tan WH. PTEN hamartoma tumour syndrome: early tumour development in children. Arch Dis Child 2015;100:34–7.

48. Meltzer CC, Smirniotopoulos JG, Jones RV. The striated cerebellum: an MR imaging sign in Lhermitte-Duclos disease (dysplastic gangliocytoma). Radiology 1995;194:699–703.

49. Chen XY, Lu F, Wang YM, et al. PTEN inactivation by germline/somatic c.950_953delTACT mutation in patients with Lhermitte-Duclos disease manifesting progressive phenotypes. Clin Genet 2014;86: 349–54.

50. Bhargava R, Au Yong KJ, Leonard N. Bannayan-Riley-Ruvalcaba syndrome: MRI neuroimaging features in a series of 7 patients. AJNR Am J Neuroradiol 2014;35:402–6.

51. Vanderver A, Tonduti D, Kahn I, et al. Characteristic brain magnetic resonance imaging pattern in patients with macrocephaly and PTEN mutations. Am J Med Genet A 2014;164A:627–33.

52. Thomas B, Krishnamoorthy T, Radhakrishnan VV, et al. Advanced MR imaging in Lhermitte-Duclos disease: moving closer to pathology and pathophysiology. Neuroradiology 2007;49:733–8.

53. Kulkantrakorn K, Awwad EE, Levy B, et al. MRI in Lhermitte-Duclos disease. Neurology 1997;48: 725–31.

54. Kimonis VE, Mehta SG, Digiovanna JJ, et al. Radiological features in 82 patients with nevoid basal cell carcinoma (NBCC or Gorlin) syndrome. Genet Med 2004;6:495–502.

55. John AM, Schwartz RA. Basal cell nevus syndrome: an update on genetics and treatment. Br J Dermatol 2016;174(1):68–76.

56. Sartip K, Kaplan A, Obeid G, et al. Neuroimaging of nevoid basal cell carcinoma syndrome (NBCCS) in children. Pediatr Radiol 2013;43:620–7.

57. Choudry Q, Patel HC, Gurusinghe NT, et al. Radiation-induced brain tumours in nevoid basal cell carcinoma syndrome: implications for treatment and surveillance. Childs Nerv Syst 2007;23:133–6.

58. Amlashi SF, Riffaud L, Brassier G, et al. Nevoid basal cell carcinoma syndrome: relation with desmoplastic medulloblastoma in infancy. A population-based study and review of the literature. Cancer 2003;98: 618–24.

59. Garre ML, Cama A, Bagnasco F, et al. Medulloblastoma variants: age-dependent occurrence and relation to Gorlin syndrome–a new clinical perspective. Clin Cancer Res 2009;15:2463–71.

60. Laugel V. Cockayne syndrome: the expanding clinical and mutational spectrum. Mech Ageing Dev 2013;134:161–70.

61. Koob M, Laugel V, Durand M, et al. Neuroimaging in Cockayne syndrome. AJNR Am J Neuroradiol 2010; 31:1623–30.

62. Faghri S, Tamura D, Kraemer KH, et al. Trichothiodystrophy: a systematic review of 112 published cases characterises a wide spectrum of clinical manifestations. J Med Genet 2008;45:609–21.

63. Rapin I. Disorders of nucleotide excision repair. Handb Clin Neurol 2013;113:1637–50.

64. Kraemer KH, Patronas NJ, Schiffmann R, et al. Xeroderma pigmentosum, trichothiodystrophy and Cockayne syndrome: a complex genotype-phenotype relationship. Neuroscience 2007;145: 1388–96.

65. Gripp KW, Lin AE. Costello syndrome: a Ras/mitogen activated protein kinase pathway syndrome (rasopathy) resulting from HRAS germline mutations. Genet Med 2012;14:285–92.

66. Gripp KW, Hopkins E, Doyle D, et al. High incidence of progressive postnatal cerebellar enlargement in Costello syndrome: brain overgrowth associated with HRAS mutations as the likely cause of structural brain and spinal cord abnormalities. Am J Med Genet A 2010;152A:1161–8.

Vascular Disorders of the Cerebellum in Children

Reade A. De Leacy, MBBS, BSc, FRANZCR[a,b,]*, Alejandro Berenstein, MD[b,c,d],
Thomas P. Naidich, MD[e,f,g]

KEYWORDS

- Cerebellum • Cerebral vascular embryology • Cavernous malformations
- Developmental venous anomalies • Capillary telangiectasia • Cerebral arteriovenous malformations
- Cerebral arteriovenous fistulae • Intracranial arterial aneurysms

KEY POINTS

- An understanding of the embryologic development of the intracranial vascular system helps to explain the common and uncommon variations in normal vertebrobasilar vascular anatomy.
- There are key differences in the etiology, clinical presentation, and imaging characteristics of vascular lesions in children as compared with adults.
- Cross-sectional imaging with computed tomography (CT) and MR imaging aids the clinician in planning proper interventional and operative therapies for the lesions displayed.
- Dedicated thin section CT angiography (CTA) or time-of-flight and time-resolved MR angiography (MRA) help to characterize arteriovenous malformations, arteriovenous fistulae, and intracranial arterial aneurysms.
- Catheter angiography remains the gold standard for lesion morphology, hemodynamic characterization, and therapeutic decision making.

INTRODUCTION

Neurovascular disease that involve the posterior fossa in the pediatric population include cavernous malformations, developmental venous anomalies (DVAs), capillary telangiectasias, intracranial aneurysms, and both arteriovenous (AV) malformations (AVM) and AV fistulae (AVF). Despite these conditions being uncommon, they can be associated with significant morbidity and mortality. In the case of intracranial aneurysms and posterior fossa AVMs/AVFs, their pathogenesis, clinical course, and angioarchitecture often differs significantly from the same condition in the adult population. An understanding of the epidemiology and pathogenesis as well as the clinical and imaging findings is crucial to accurately diagnose these lesions and to assess for,

Disclosure Statement: The authors have nothing to disclose.
[a] Department of Neurosurgery, Cerebrovascular Center, Mount Sinai Hospital, Mount Sinai Medical Center, KCC 1-North, 1450 Madison Avenue, New York, NY 10029, USA; [b] Department of Radiology, Cerebrovascular Center, Mount Sinai Hospital, Mount Sinai Medical Center, KCC 1-North, 1450 Madison Avenue, New York, NY 10029, USA; [c] Pediatric Cerebrovascular Program, Department of Neurosurgery, Cerebrovascular Center, Mount Sinai Hospital, Mount Sinai Medical Center, KCC 1-North, 1450 Madison Avenue, New York, NY 10029, USA; [d] Department of Pediatrics, Cerebrovascular Center, Mount Sinai Hospital, Mount Sinai Medical Center, KCC 1-North, 1450 Madison Avenue, New York, NY 10029, USA; [e] Department of Radiology, Mount Sinai Medical Center, Box 1234, One Gustave Levy Place, New York, NY 10029, USA; [f] Department of Neurosurgery, Mount Sinai Medical Center, One Gustave Levy Place, New York, NY 10029, USA; [g] Department of Pediatrics, Mount Sinai Medical Center, One Gustave Levy Place, New York, NY 10029, USA
* Corresponding author. Cerebrovascular Center, Mount Sinai Hospital, KCC 1-North, 1450 Madison Avenue, New York, NY 10029.
E-mail address: reade.deleacy@mountsinai.org

Neuroimag Clin N Am 26 (2016) 435–458
http://dx.doi.org/10.1016/j.nic.2016.03.009
1052-5149/16/$ – see front matter © 2016 Elsevier Inc. All rights reserved.

neuroimaging.theclinics.com

or exclude the presence of, any affiliated disease processes. Additionally, the variation in vascular anatomy provides insight into neurovascular embryogenesis. The study of these variations may also provide guidance for treatment of malformations that may result from dysembryogenesis.

In this article, we provide a synopsis of the early development of the posterior fossa vasculature and its variations and review the clinical and imaging findings associated with neurovascular disorders of the posterior fossa in the pediatric population.

DEVELOPMENT OF THE CEREBELLAR AND BRAINSTEM ARTERIAL SUPPLY

Much of our understanding of the embryologenesis of the cranial vascular system is based on the work of Dorkas Paget and George Streeter in the first half of the twentieth century.[1–3] In brief, the intracranial arterial vascular network develops in response to changing metabolic and hemodynamic demands within the developing brain. As the primitive brain enlarges, it no longer receives adequate nourishment by diffusion from the amniotic fluid.[4] Increasing metabolic demands then initiate sequential—and broadly overlapping—changes that are conceptualized as a "4-step model" for the development of the cerebral arterial system[2–4]:

1. During the first 2 to 4 weeks, the exposed neural groove, neural plate and the open neural tube are fed by diffusion from the amniotic fluid.
2. At week 4, the neural tube is closed and is covered by a dense connective tissue called the *meninx primitiva,* the precursor of the future meningeal coverings of the brain. The meninx primitiva contains a vascular plexus that supplies the neural tube during weeks 5 to 7 via the primitive dorsal aorta and the cardinal veins.
3. Between weeks 5 and 7, the primary brain vesicles enlarge and differentiate. The meninx primitiva invaginates into the developing neural tube to create the primordial choroid plexus and the associated choroidal vasculature, including the choroidal arteries.
4. With further enlargement, the neural tube becomes too thick to be supplied by diffusion alone. Intrinsic capillaries then develop from the vascular plexus of the meninx primitiva, first at the areas of highest metabolic demand (the ventricular/subventricular proliferative germinal zone), and then everywhere.

In greater detail, Dorkas Paget defined 7 stages in the development of the cerebral arterial system from the early (undifferentiated) stage to the morphologically mature pattern.[2] These were summarized by Dr. Charles Raybaud in 2010.[4]

1. During stage 1 (4–5 mm, embryonic day 28–29), the blood supply to the developing forebrain is provided by the primitive carotid arteries. The developing hindbrain is supplied by 4 transient caroticovertebral connections arising from the developing carotid arteries. These connections comprise 3 presegmental branches (named trigeminal, otic, and hypoglossal for their association with the 5th, 8th, and 12th cranial nerves, respectively) and 1 intersegmental arterial branch (the proatlantal artery). The trigeminal artery and the otic artery are thought to arise from the proximal developing internal carotid artery (although the existence of the otic artery is debated). The hypoglossal artery and the proatlantal artery (first intersegmental cervical C1 artery) arise from the paired dorsal aortae.[4] These 4 primitive caroticovertebral connections supply the hindbrain via the paired ventral longitudinal neural arteries. The ventral longitudinal neural arteries are the precursors to the basilar artery during this stage of development.
2. During stage 2 (5–6 mm, embryonic day 29), the posterior communicating arteries are formed. The primitive internal carotid arteries extend caudally to join the bilateral longitudinal neural arteries to form the posterior communicating arteries. During this stage, both the trigeminal and hypoglossal arteries start to involute at their carotid origins. The longitudinal neural arteries begin to fuse in the midline to form the primitive basilar artery. However, the developing hindbrain still relies heavily on the caudal supply derived from the first intersegmental (proatlantal) arteries.[4]
3. During stage 3 (7–12 mm, embryonic day 32), the basilar and vertebral arteries are completed. A mesencephalic artery now extends toward the midbrain from the caudal end of the developing posterior communicating arteries. The basilar artery is better developed and the paired vertebral arteries are in the process of forming bilateral paired longitudinal anastomoses that link the intersegmental cervical arteries between C1 and C7. The trigeminal arteries have

typically disappeared, and the anterior superior cerebellar arteries become evident (Fig. 1).[4]

4. During stage 4 (12–14 mm, embryonic day 35), the morphology of the cerebellar arterial system becomes more mature. The basilar and vertebral arteries develop further, and early branches supplying the rhombencephalon now become recognizable (Fig. 2).[4]

5. During stage 5 (16–18 mm, embryonic day 40), the arterial system has a nearly adult morphology. During this stage primitive lateral, third and fourth ventricles form by invagination of the meninx primitiva. The mesencephalic artery, which develops from the primitive posterior communicating arteries, forms a rich vascular plexus over the tectal plate (Fig. 3).[4]

6. and 7. During stages 6 (20–24 mm, embryonic day 44) and 7 (40 mm, embryonic day 52), the circle of Willis is completed and the vertebrobasilar arteries now supply the posterior cerebral hemispheres. The anterior inferior and posterior inferior cerebellar arteries become better developed and play a larger role in supplying the caudal hindbrain (Fig. 4).[4]

Anatomic Variations

Normal variations in the vertebrobasilar arteries are understood best as variations in the pattern by which the early arterial plexus condenses into mature vascular channels.[4] Because arteries develop in response to the increasing metabolic demands of specific tissues, there are few variations in patterns of the smaller, distal "end territory" vessels. That is, the distal, intraparenchymal vasculature is more nearly constant. Because the proximal portions of the early vascular plexus may receive adequate supply through many different routes, successful embryogenesis tolerates far greater variation in the pattern of the larger, proximal vessels that feed into the developing networks.[2,4–6] This process explains the development ("tolerance") of fenestrations, anomalous origins of defined vessels, absence or duplications of the major cerebellar arterial branches and interruption, partial fusion, or duplication of the basilar artery (Fig. 5).[7]

Persistent Caroticovertebral Connections

The existence of persistent trigeminal, hypoglossal, and proatlantal arteries is well-documented, as are variations among them (Figs. 6–9).[8–13] The existence of a persistent otic artery is debated.[14,15] Some authors suggest that the "otic artery" is simply a variant form of persistent trigeminal artery that arises unusually caudally. The "otic" artery has no homologue in other species, whereas the other presegmental and intersegmental arteries do, further fueling contention about the existence of a real persistent otic artery.[16]

VENOUS DEVELOPMENT AND DRAINAGE OF THE CEREBELLUM AND BRAINSTEM

The ventral mesencephalic vein is the most prominent venous structure within the posterior fossa of the developing 60 to 80 mm embryo.[1] This vessel drains the ventral aspect of the developing brainstem and cerebellar plate, and is the precursor of the petrosal vein and superior petrosal sinus.

Slightly later, before the cerebellar plate forms the cerebellar hemispheres, a conspicuous dorsal mesencephalic vein begins to drain the dorsal aspect of the developing cerebellum. Once present, the dorsal mesencephalic vein drains into the straight and lateral sinuses via the primitive tentorial venous plexi. This flow from the superior surface of the cerebellum is then captured by the Galenic venous system.[1]

The veins draining the posterior fossa have been classified in diverse ways. In 1 system, these veins are divided into 3 major groups: (1) the superior or "Galenic" group, (2) the posterior or "tentorial" group and (3) the anterior or "petrosal" group. In a second system, the veins of the posterior fossa may be classified, instead, into 4 separate groups, designated: (1) superficial veins that drain the cortical surfaces of the cerebellum, (2) deep veins that drain the tissue within the depths of the cerebellar folds, (3) veins of the brainstem, and (4) bridging veins that cross the subarachnoid space and dura to drain the parenchyma into the dural venous sinuses.

Superficial Veins of the Cerebellum

The superficial veins drain the cortical surfaces of the cerebellum. They are named for the specific surfaces they drain, as superior (synonym: tentorial), anterior (synonym: petrosal), and posterior (synonym: suboccipital) veins. These superficial veins are then subclassified by whether they drain the vermis or the cerebellar hemispheres.[17]

Superior (tentorial) veins drain through the superior vermian and the superior hemispheric veins. Superior vermian veins that are situated anteriorly drain to the vein of Galen. Superior vermian veins that are situated posteriorly drain to the torcular. Superior hemispheric veins are considered in

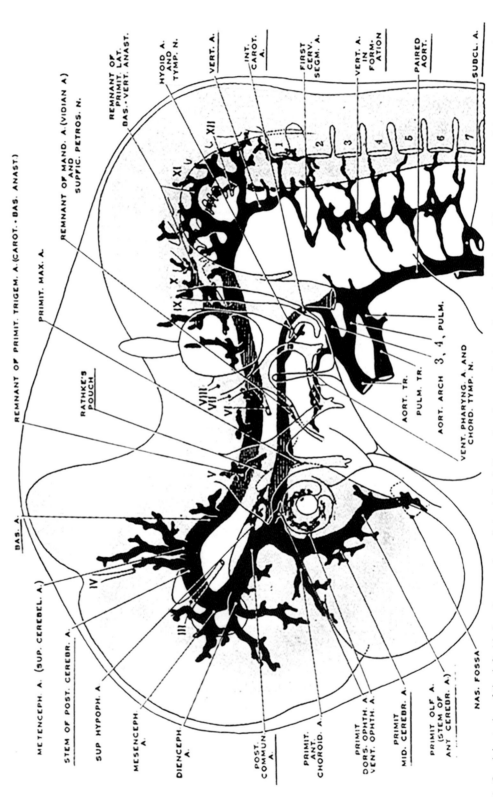

Fig. 1. Cranial arteries of the left side in a 9 mm embryo (lateral view). Note that the vertebral arteries are being formed from elements of the upper cervical segments. (*From* Padget DH. The development of the cranial arteries in the human embryo. Contrib Embryol 1948;12(pub no: 575):205–61.)

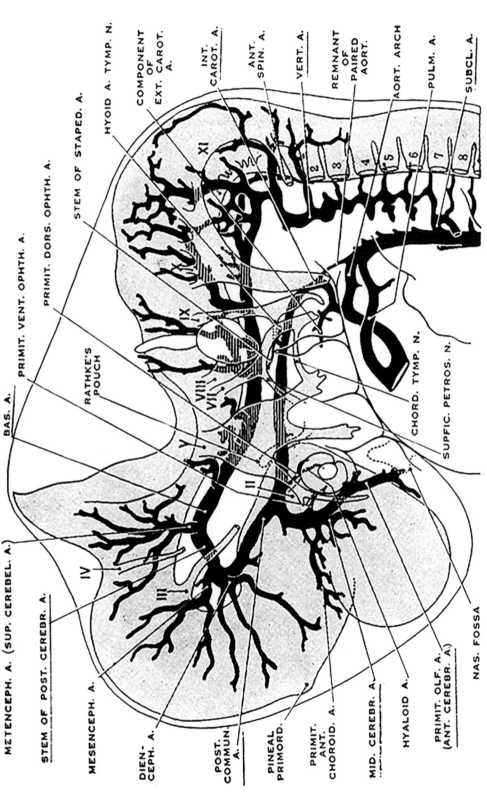

Fig. 2. Cranial arteries in an 12.5-mm embryo. The developing vertebral arteries have a more advanced conformation. (*From* Padget DH. The development of the cranial arteries in the human embryo. Contrib Embryol 1948;12(pub no: 575):205–61.)

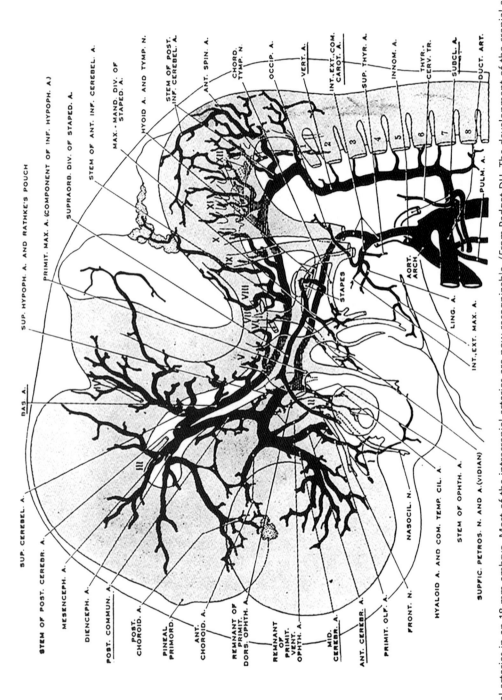

Fig. 3. Cranial arteries in an 18-mm embryo. Most of the intracranial arteries are now recognizable. (*From* Padget DH. The development of the cranial arteries in the human embryo. Contrib Embryol 1948;12(pub no: 575):205–61.)

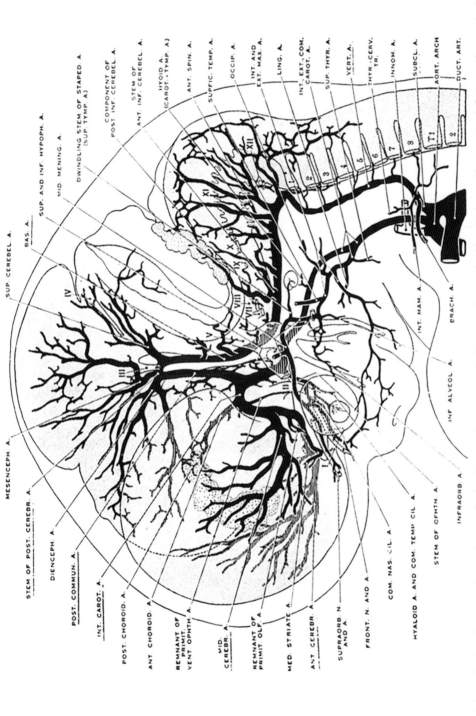

Fig. 4. Cranial arteries in a 24-mm embryo. The anterior inferior and posterior inferior cerebellar arteries now supply the posterior cerebral hemispheres. The vertebrobasilar arteries now supply the posterior cerebral hemispheres. The vertebrobasilar arteries are better developed. (*From* Padget DH. The development of the cranial arteries in the human embryo. Contrib Embryol 1948;12(pub no: 575):205–61.)

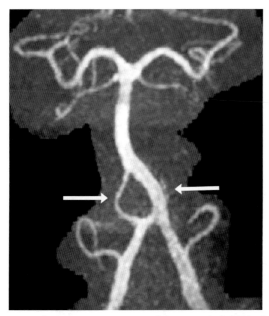

Fig. 5. (*Arrows*) Fenestration of the proximal third of the basilar artery.

anterior, posterior, and lateral groups. The anterior superior hemispheric veins typically drain the anterior tentorial surface of the cerebellum. The posterior superior hemispheric veins typically form a common trunk with the inferior hemispheric veins from the suboccipital surface and drain together into the adjacent sinuses.[17] The lateral superior hemispheric veins typically drain the lateral aspect of the tentorial surface of the cerebellum.

Anterior (petrosal) surface veins are subdivided into superior, middle, and inferior groups. These converge in the region of the flocculus to form the vein of the cerebellopontine fissure, which then drains into the superior petrosal sinus.[17]

Posterior (suboccipital) surface veins include the paired groups of superficial tonsillar veins, the paired inferior vermian veins, and the paired groups of inferior hemispheric veins. The superficial tonsillar veins from the medial, lateral, and posterior surfaces of the tonsil converge into retro-tonsillar veins that give rise to the more caudal inferior vermian veins.[17] The paired inferior vermian veins drain the tonsils and the surface of the vermis into the torcular or medial portions of the transverse sinuses. The paired groups of inferior hemispheric veins run transversely to drain to the tentorial sinuses or longitudinally to drain into the inferior vermian veins.

Deep Veins of the Cerebellum

The deep veins of the cerebellum are divided into (1) fissural veins that course longitudinally within the cerebellomesencephalic, cerebellopontine, and cerebellomedullary fissures, and (2) peduncular veins that course along the superior, inferior, and middle cerebellar peduncles.[17]

Veins of the Brainstem

The veins of the brainstem are named for the territories they drain and the direction in which they course. Veins coursing along the brainstem are called longitudinal veins and are considered to belong to the midline and lateral groups. The direction of venous flow within these veins may be superior or inferior.[17] Veins coursing across the brainstem, perpendicular to the longitudinal veins, are called transverse veins. From cranial to caudal, the transverse veins are designated peduncular veins, transverse pontine veins, pontomedullary sulcal veins, and transverse medullary veins.

Bridging Veins

The bridging veins cross the subarachnoid space and dura to drain the brainstem and cerebellum into the dural venous sinuses. In the posterior fossa, these veins drain superiorly to the vein of Galen, laterally to the transverse petrosal vein and superior petrosal sinus, and posterosuperiorly to the torcular and tentorial sinuses.[17]

VASCULAR LESIONS OF THE CEREBELLUM AND BRAINSTEM
Cavernous Malformations

Cavernous malformations (cavernomas) account for approximately 20% to 25% of vascular malformations within the central nervous system in children.[18] Posterior fossa cavernomas represent between 8% and 36% of all cases, with the vast majority being located within the brainstem.[19] Histologically, cavernomas are rounded collections of cavernous or sinusoidal vascular spaces of variable size, with no intervening brain parenchyma. The malformations are formed by dilated and hypertrophied capillary beds, which contain regions of both clotted and liquid blood.[20] The different states of blood within the malformation account for their characteristic signal and susceptibility on MR imaging scans. Most cavernous malformations are supratentorial (~80%), but they can be found anywhere within the brain and may be distributed throughout the brainstem and cerebellar tissue (**Figs. 10** and **11**). Cavernomas may be solitary or multiple, "eloquent," or often clinically silent. These lesions are typically seen in adults, but may be associated with familial syndromes and are seen both in children and adolescents.[21]

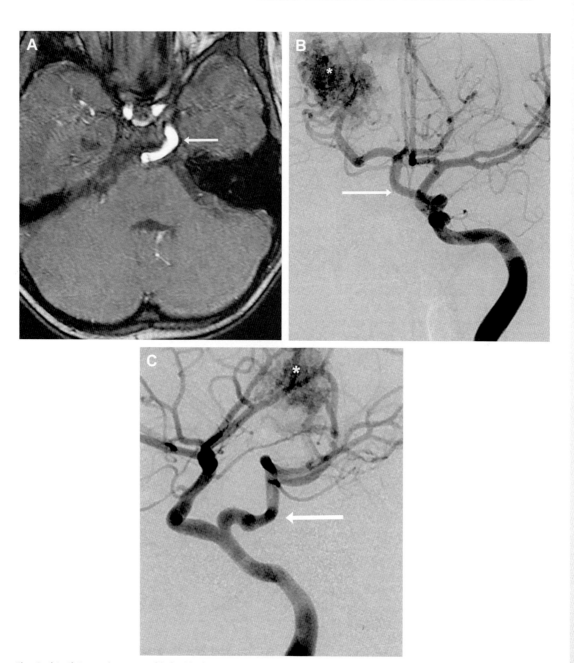

Fig. 6. (*A–C*) Lateral course of left sided persistent trigeminal artery. A 6-year-old boy with known right thalamic arteriovenous malformation (AVM) and persistent left trigeminal artery. (*A*) Axial time of flight MR angiography shows the lateral variant of a persistent left trigeminal artery (*arrow*). (*B, C*) Frontal and lateral left internal carotid artery injection catheter angiogram shows the persistent caroticobasilar connection (*arrow*) and a compact right thalamic AVM (*asterisk*).

Unlike AVMs, cavernomas show no AV shunting. For that reason, the supplying arteries and draining veins have normal caliber. Cavernomas are often associated with both DVAs and capillary telangiectasias.[22,23] At least 40% of sporadic cavernous malformations are reported to develop a DVA in their vicinity (see **Fig. 10D**). However, recent research suggests that DVAs are less likely to be associated with patients who have familial cavernous malformations.[24]

Cavernomas are commonly multiple and have familial associations with 3 causative genes: KRIT1 (CCM1), CCM2/malcavernin, and PDCD10 (CCM3).[24–26] When familial, cavernomas are

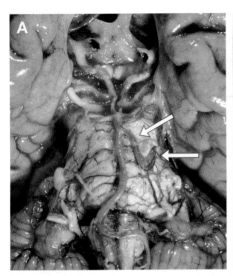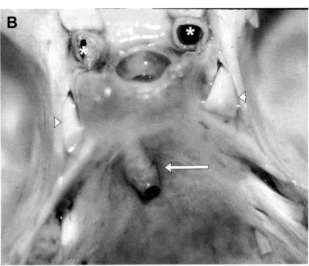

Fig. 7. (*A*, *B*) Anatomic specimen (*A*) shows the basilar arterial attachment of a left-sided trigeminal artery (*arrows*). Anatomic specimen (*B*) shows cut end of a medial variant trigeminal artery (*arrows*). The optic nerves (*arrow heads*) and supraclinoid internal carotid arteries (*asterisk*) are also visible. (*Courtesy of* Dr John Deck, Toronto, CA.)

inherited in an autosomal dominant pattern with incomplete penetrance and are more often associated with an aggressive clinical time course.[18]

Asymptomatic cavernomas are typically identified incidentally. Symptomatic cavernomas usually present with signs and symptoms related to hemorrhage and the localized mass effect from blood products.[21] The clinical signs and symptoms often resolve or improve as the edema and mass effect related to the acute bleed diminish and the blood products are absorbed gradually. In the posterior fossa, the clinical presentation relates to the location of the lesion and the volume of hemorrhage. Cavernous malformations of the brainstem may present acutely with cranial nerve deficits, hemiparesis, and sensory changes, as well as changes in level of consciousness. Lesions within the cerebellar hemispheres may manifest with hemorrhage or mass effect. These malformations should not be mistaken for neoplasms. The possibility of a cavernoma should always be considered when a child or adolescent presents with a small, typically a less than 3-cm intraparenchymal hemorrhage in the posterior fossa.[21]

Radiotherapy remains an integral part of therapy in pediatric neurooncology. Cavernous malformations may be seen several years after radiation therapy and of importance the incidence does not seem to be related to either the dose of radiation delivered or the type of underlying malignancy. However, children who underwent cranial radiation therapy before the age of 10 are at higher risk for developing subsequent cavernous malformations within the treated field.[27,28]

Imaging findings

Computed tomography Cavernomas are often occult on computed tomography (CT) scans unless they are relatively large, have recently bled, or have associated macrocalcification. If visible, cavernous malformations appear as a hyperdense or mixed density lesion with little if any mass effect. They typically show no appreciable contrast enhancement, but may occasionally exhibit mild enhancement.[21] It is critical to distinguish cavernous malformations from low-grade neoplasms, because both diseases may have a similar appearance on precontrast and postcontrast CT studies.

MR imaging MR imaging is the modality of choice and the gold standard for imaging cavernous malformations. Lesions not associated with acute hemorrhage are seen as a well-demarcated, lobulated mass with no or little adjacent edema or significant mass effect.[21] Intralesional signal is variable on T1-weighted, T2-weighted, and fluid attenuated inversion recovery sequences owing to the presence of blood products of varying ages. T2*-weighted gradient echo/susceptibility weighted imaging (SWI) shows characteristic "blooming" artifact owing to the ferromagnetic properties of the aging blood products. SWI has proven to be far superior to the T1- and T2-weighted sequences for the identification of

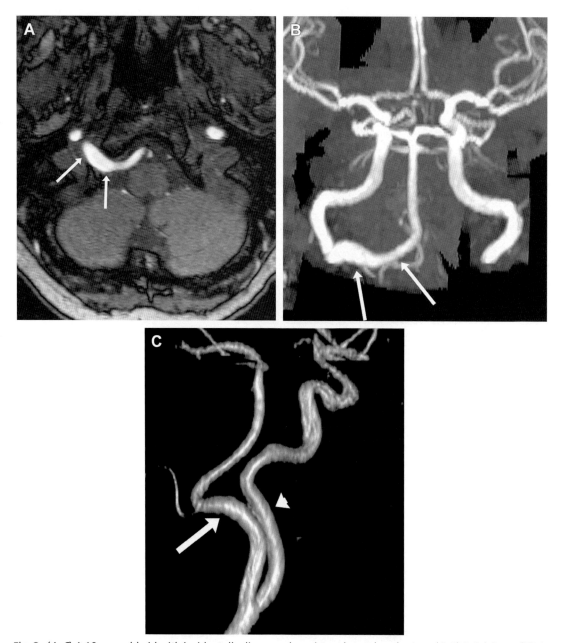

Fig. 8. (A–C) A 16-year-old girl with incidentally diagnosed persistent hypoglossal artery. (A–C) Axial time of flight MR angiography with rotational minimal intensity projection and 3-dimensional (3D) reconstructions shows the anomalous caroticovertebral anastomosis (*arrows*). The 3D study also shows the relationship to the ipsilateral internal carotid artery (*arrow head*).

cavernomas. If contrast is administered, an associated DVA may be identified.[22] Identifying and localizing associated DVA's is important for planning safe resection of a cavernoma.[22]

Developmental Venous Anomalies

DVAs have also been called venous angiomas. They are considered to be a nonpathologic variation of normal venous drainage. Supratentorial DVAs may be situated both superficial and deep with the brain parenchyma. Infratentorial DVAs are more frequently situated superficially within the brainstem and cerebellum. Isolated DVAs are thought to arise only where the parenchyma contains tectal derivatives. For that reason, isolated DVAs may be found in the telencephalon, mesencephalon, and rhombencephalon, but not

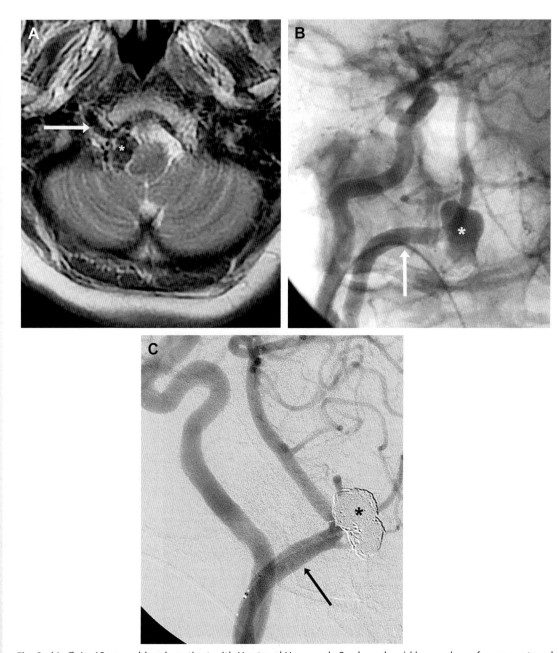

Fig. 9. (*A–C*) An 18-year-old male patient with Hunt and Hess grade 2 subarachnoid hemorrhage from a ruptured right hypoglossal artery/posterior inferior cerebellar artery origin aneurysm. (*A*) Axial T2-weighted image shows a persistent right hypoglossal artery within the hypoglossal canal (*arrow*) with an associated intracranial aneurysm (*asterisk*). (*B, C*) Angiographic images of the ruptured aneurysm (*asterisk*) arising at the distal hypoglossal artery (*arrow*) before and after coil embolization.

within the diencephalon, lower brainstem, or spinal cord.[29]

DVAs are characterized by a collection of medullary and subcortical veins that are arranged radially with normal brain tissue interposed between the individual tributary channels. The smaller channels converge onto a single dilated venous pedicle that may drain superficially to the cortical surface or deeply to the deep venous system. Importantly, AV shunting is absent, so dilated arteries are not seen in association with DVA, and the lesions are most often clinically silent.[21] Rarely, DVAs have been associated with headache, focal neurologic deficit, and seizure. In such cases, the

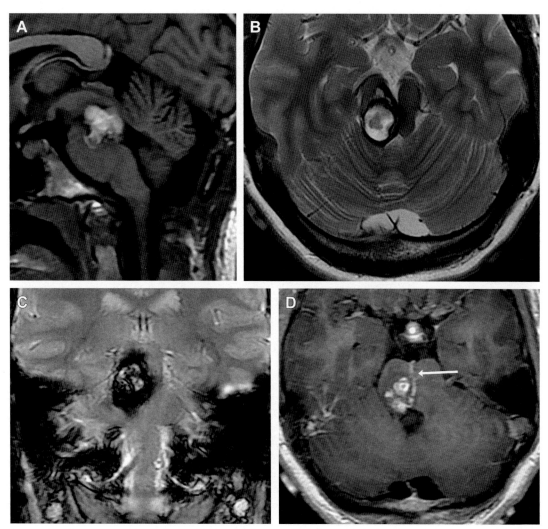

Fig. 10. (A–D) Pontomesencephalic cavernous malformation with associated developmental venous anomalies (DVA). A 15-year-old male patient who presented with cranial nerve deficits. (A, B) Sagittal T1- and axial T2-weighted images demonstrate a lobulated heterogeneous but predominantly hyperintense mass within the dorsal aspect of the pontomesencephalic junction with some distortion of the normal anatomy. The characteristic lobulated margin and "chocolate-covered popcorn" appearance with mixed internal signal is presented consistent with blood products of varying ages. (C) Coronal gradient echo image through the lesion demonstrates characteristic blooming secondary to the susceptibility effects of hemosiderin. (D) Postcontrast axial and sagittal T1-weighted images of the lesion demonstrate an associated midline DVA (arrow) draining ventrally.

symptoms have been attributed to stenosis/narrowing of the venous pedicle at its confluence with a draining dural sinus.[30,31]

When DVAs are found in association with a hemorrhage, a cavernous malformation or other vascular malformation should be excluded. In cases with concurrent cavernous malformations, the DVAs should be identified and preserved during surgery, because injury to them will interrupt the normal venous drainage and lead to venous infarction/hemorrhage.[22]

In children, DVAs have been described in association with maxillofacial venous malformations, maxillofacial lymphatic malformations, sinus pericranii, schizencephaly, pachygyria, microgyria, cavernous malformations, dural sinus malformations, and multiple mucocutaneous venous malformations.

Imaging findings
The cross-sectional imaging features of are identical in children and adults. The characteristic imaging feature is a "caput medusa" of smaller draining veins that converge onto a main venous pedicle that most often drains to an adjacent venous sinus or occasionally the deep venous system.

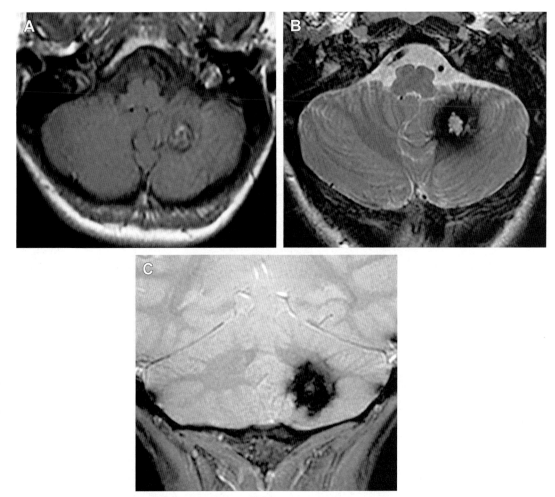

Fig. 11. (A–C) Left inferior cerebellar hemisphere cavernous malformation. A 16-year-old girl who presented with seizures. (A–C) Axial T1-weighted, T2-weighted, and coronal susceptibility weighted imaging (SWI) images show lobulated mixed signal intensity mass within the left cerebellar hemisphere with blooming on SWI consistent with a cavernous malformation.

Computed tomography On CT, the draining pedicle can sometimes be identified on a noncontrast study owing to the slow intravascular flow. The lesion can be confirmed on venous/delayed phase postcontrast studies and appears as a linear or curvilinear enhancing structure.

MR Imaging On MR imaging, these lesions are seen on most sequences but are best demonstrated on postcontrast T1-weighted and SWI sequences. Again the lesion appears as a linear or curvilinear vascular structure with characteristic tuft of small veins converging onto a larger pedicle. Even a substantial venous angioma may not be detectable on routine noncontrast MR imaging, although it is easily visualized after contrast administration.

Catheter angiography On angiography, these lesions are seen in the venous phase and importantly have no associated AV shunting. Importantly, any associated cavernoma may remain undetected on catheter angiography because of the inherent hemodynamic/contrast enhancement characteristics.

Posterior Fossa Capillary Telangiectasias

Capillary telangiectasias are a form of vascular malformation that occurs most commonly within the pons, temporal lobe, and medulla. They are typically asymptomatic and associated with a benign clinical course. Uncommonly, a capillary telangiectasia may manifest with seizures, cranial nerve dysfunction, confusion, dizziness, visual changes, and vertigo, tinnitus, or progressive spastic paresis.[32] Prior case reports have implicated hemorrhage, direct pressure on adjacent normal structures, and hypoperfusion/hypoxic injury secondary to capillary dilation and stasis in the uncommon symptomatic capillary telangiectasias.[33] Histopathologically, capillary telangiectasias are characterized by a collection of dilated capillaries/small vascular channels with normal intervening brain parenchyma (**Fig. 12A**).[21,32]

Imaging findings

Computed tomography Capillary telangiectasias are usually occult on routine CT scans, even with contrast enhancement.[34]

MR Imaging On MR imaging, capillary telangiectasias are typically nearly undetectable with standard noncontrast T1-weighted, T2-weighted, fluid attenuated inversion recovery, and diffusion weighted imaging sequences. On occasion, contrast-enhanced T1-weighted sequences may display the malformation as a faintly enhancing lesion with a "brush"-like appearance (see **Fig. 12**).[35] In up to two-thirds of lesions, there may be an enlarged vessel adjacent to the telangiectasia. This vessel is thought to be a prominent draining vein.[32,36] SWI successfully displays capillary telangiectasias, especially in MR imaging performed at higher field strengths (3T and higher; **Fig. 13**). The stagnant blood in low-flow capillaries/venous channels increases local deoxyhemoglobin, increasing lesion conspicuity.[37] True SWI has been shown to be more effective than T2*-weighted gradient echo sequences in demonstrating capillary telangiectasias.[34,37]

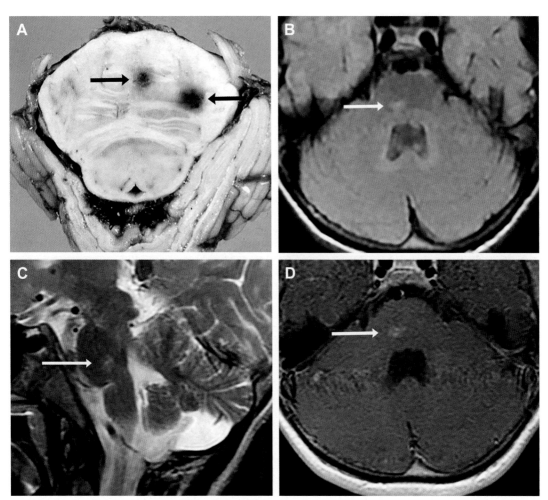

Fig. 12. (*A–D*) Pontine capillary telangiectasias. (*A*) Anatomic specimen sectioned at the mid-pons shows 2 adjacent capillary telangiectasia (*arrows*) exhibiting the characteristic dark brown staining seen after fixation. (*B–D*) A 13-year-old boy for whom MR imaging was performed to investigate seizures. Axial fluid attenuated inversion recovery and sagittal T2-weighted images show a poorly demarcated, faintly hyperintense lesion within the right pons (*arrow*). The lesion shows "brushlike" enhancement on the postcontrast T1-weighted image consistent with a capillary telangiectasia.

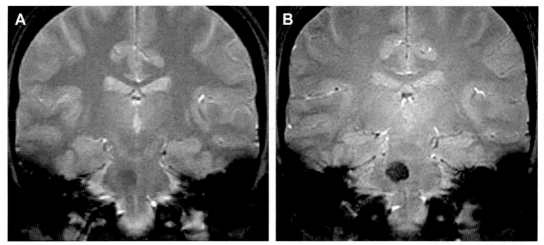

Fig. 13. (*A, B*) Right pontine capillary telangiectasia. Coronal gradient echo image at 1.5 T (*A*) and 3 T (*B*). The conspicuity of capillary telangiectasias on T2-weighted gradient echo and susceptibility weighted imaging is greatly increased at higher field strengths. (*Courtesy of* Dr Bradley Delman, New York, NY.)

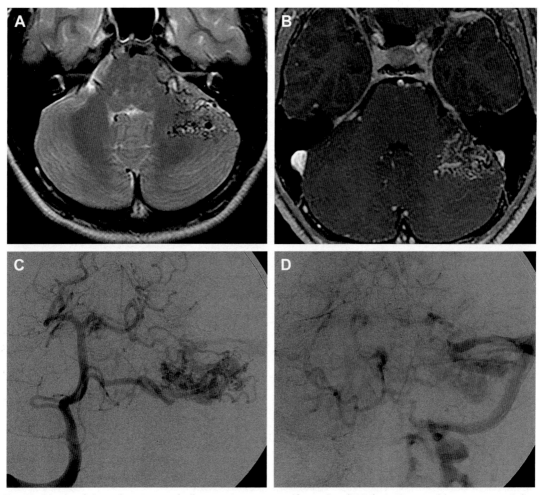

Fig. 14. (*A–D*) Left lateral aspect cerebellar arteriovenous malformation (AVM). A 15-year-old, asymptomatic boy who underwent MR imaging and catheter angiogram for investigation of abnormality seen on computed tomography study performed for trauma. (*A, B*) Axial T2-and postcontrast T1-weighted images show an AVM located within the lateral left cerebellar hemisphere. The lesion has a compact nidus and superficial drainage to the adjacent transverse/sigmoid junction. (*C, D*) Right vertebral artery injection from the corresponding catheter angiogram shows dual arterial supply from enlarged left anterior inferior and superior cerebellar arteries. Single vessel venous drainage laterally to the junction of the left transverse and sigmoid sinuses.

Posterior Fossa Arteriovenous Malformations and Arteriovenous Fistulae

In children, AV shunts often have very different characteristics than they do in adults. The pediatric population is more likely to have multifocal lesions, induced remote AV shunts, large venous ectasias, high flow lesions, and single AVF.[29] In addition, systemic phenomena associated with high flow shunts, such as congestive cardiac failure, renal and hepatic failure, and failure to thrive, often complicates treatment.[29] Vascular steal and increased venous pressures with consequently reduced blood flow may lead to atrophy of large portions of the brain, venous thromboses, and venous infarctions/hemorrhages. Conversely, children less commonly show flow related aneurysms and high flow-related angiopathic changes.[29]

Cerebral AVMs are vascular lesions characterized by an abnormal connection between a cerebral artery and a cerebral vein through an intervening "nidus" that is located typically within the subpial meningeal space.[29] The AVM may lie within the superficial, subcortical, deep, or subependymal portions of the hemispheres (**Figs. 14** and **15**).

Cerebral AVF are characterized by direct communication between a pial artery and a cerebral vein with no intervening nidus (**Figs. 16** and **17**). They are distinct from cerebral AVMs and show distinctly different angioarchitecture.

Posterior fossa AVMs are as common as cerebral hemispheric AVMs, when their incidence is normalized for the volume of tissue affected. The clinical presentation and natural history of childhood AVMs is different from that of adults. In older children, concurrent hemorrhage is likely related to bleeding from the nidus itself. In neonates and younger children, concurrent hemorrhage is more likely to be the result of venous infarction.[29]

Imaging features
Computed tomography, MR imaging, and catheter angiography Imaging workup for cerebral vascular malformations or cerebral AVF most often includes CT, MR imaging, and static/dynamic MR angiography (MRA). Catheter angiography remains the gold standard and is the method of choice for delineation of the angioarchitecture and determining the most appropriate therapy, be that embolization, radiosurgery, surgical

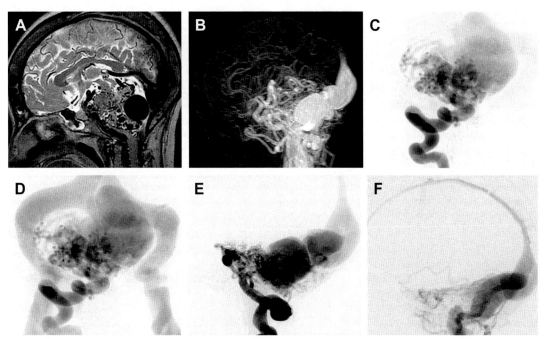

Fig. 15. (*A–F*) High flow pontomedullary arteriovenous malformation (AVM) with varicoid venous drainage and marked cerebral venous hypertension. A 15-year-old girl with seizures and developmental delay. (*A, B*) Sagittal T2-weighted image and reconstructed contrast-enhanced time resolved MR angiography shows a diffuse vascular lesion throughout the brainstem with large varicoid vermian draining vein and extensive supratentorial and infratentorial venous congestion. (*C–F*) Right vertebral catheter angiogram in frontal and lateral projections demonstrates a high flow compact pontine AVM without intranidal aneurysm or outlet venous stenosis. Marked arteriovenous shunting with antegrade and retrograde flow through the dural venous sinuses and cortical venous reflux.

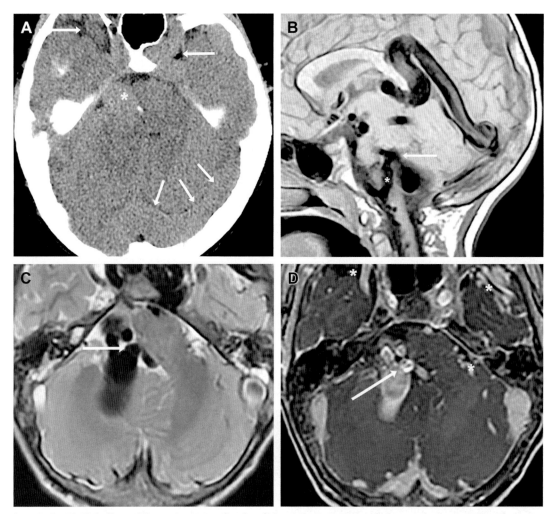

Fig. 16. (*A–D*) High-flow pial arteriovenous fistula of the right posterior inferior cerebellar artery with venous congestion/hypertension. A 4-year-old boy with seizures and developmental delay. (*A*) Noncontrast computed tomography study shows an isodense lesion in the superior margin of the right cerebellopontine angle (*asterisk*) and prominence of the left cavernous sinus, right middle cerebral vein, and left transverse sinuses (*arrows*), suggesting venous hypertension. (*B*) Midline sagittal T1-weighted image shows enlarged perimedullary segment of the right posterior inferior cerebellar artery (*asterisk*) and fistulous connection (*arrow*). (*C, D*) Axial T2-weighted and postcontrast T1-weighted images reveal the site of the arteriovenous connection (*arrows*). (*D*) Marked venous congestion/hypertension noted with multiple dilated cortical veins (*asterisk*).

resection, or a combination of these modalities. Imaging should be used to identify the distribution and number of supplying arteries, nidal position and size, the presence or absence of intranidal aneurysms and/or draining venous stenoses, the number and distribution of draining veins (superficial or deep), the presence of any sinus occlusions, and the extent and distribution cortical venous reflux/venous hypertension.[29,38] Dynamic cross-sectional CT angiography and MRA techniques allow the radiologist to determine of the extent of AV shunting. This information is especially important in young children, who are at risk for high-output cardiac failure. Determining eloquence of the adjacent tissue is difficult in infants with developing brains. Adult experience is not directly applicable to the pediatric patient, especially for the supratentorial brain.[29]

In the acute setting, noncontrast CT scans may show a mass or curvilinear lesion with associated hyperdense components representing either hemorrhage or calcification. Adjacent gliosis may be present as a result of a prior hemorrhage or steal phenomenon.

Surface or pial lesions that have ruptured are often associated with subarachnoid hemorrhage.

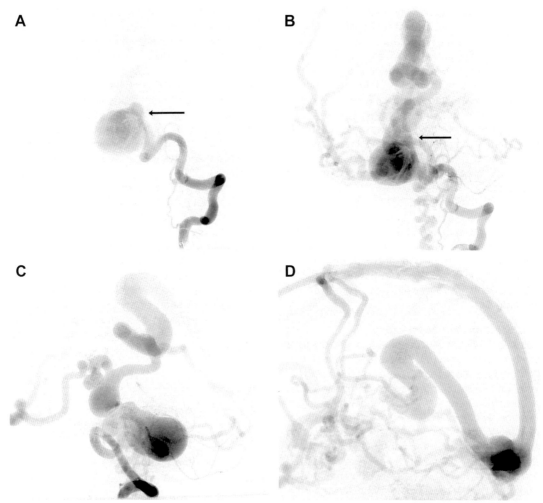

Fig. 17. (*A–D*) High-flow pial arteriovenous fistula of the right posterior inferior cerebellar artery with marked venous congestion/hypertension. (*A, B*) Frontal and lateral (*C, D*) images of a left vertebral catheter angiogram from patient in **Fig. 7**. The fistula can be identified clearly without an intervening nidus (*arrows*) (in contrast with an arteriovenous malformation). The true extent of the venous congestion is appreciated with chronic occlusions of the sigmoid sinuses and retrograde venous drainage through the sagittal sinus and supratentorial and infratentorial cortical veins.

Subependymal lesions may show intraventricular hemorrhage. Over the ensuing weeks, the hemorrhage will display the expected imaging evolution of aging blood, becoming progressively more isodense to hypodense on CT. The mass effect of the AVM from any associated hematoma will decrease, and the underlying angioarchitecture of the AVM will become visible with both noninvasive and minimally invasive vascular imaging techniques. Any intervention in the early stage after a bleed focuses on treatment of the sequelae of large volume or symptomatic subarachnoid, intraventricular, or intraparenchymal hemorrhage. This management may involve supportive care or more invasive measures, such as placement of a

ventriculostomy or cranial decompression. Any endovascular intervention in the acute phase is reserved to superselective-targeted embolization if a causative lesion such as a nidal aneurysm is visualized.[29]

MR imaging is the noninvasive imaging modality of choice for AVMs and AVFs. In children, this technique may require sedation or general anesthesia. MR imaging provides excellent spatial resolution in multiple planes to determine nidal size, nidal position, and often the nidal architecture. High-flow intraluminal blood appears as regions of signal loss or "flow voids" on T2-weighted sequences. Slowly flowing intraluminal blood or thrombosed vessels can be delineated on

T1-weighted sequences as higher intraluminal signal. T2-weighted sequences display the nidus as a tangle of serpiginous flow voids that may be compact or diffuse. Hemorrhage may be reliably identified. The age of the hemorrhage may be determined from its relative intensity on T1-weighted, T2-weighted, and diffusion weighted imaging sequences, unless surgical intervention or other therapy disturbs the oxygen gradients in the parenchyma. Residual hemosiderin from a prior hemorrhage may be identified using T2*-weighted gradient echo imaging or SWI techniques.

MRA is an excellent tool for identifying the number and morphology of the feeding arteries and draining veins and for confirming nidal size and to a degree the intranidal architecture. Newer time resolved CT angiography and MRA techniques also make it possible to temporally determine patterns of flow and the extent of AV shunting.

Considerations and associations

Multifocal niduses Multifocal AVMs are up to 2 times more common in the pediatric population than in adults. To date, there are no convincing reports of familial occurrence of cerebral AVMs. However, intracranial AVMs are one of the most common findings associated with cerebrofacial AV metameric syndromes.[29] These rare conditions allow insight into the segmental structure of the developing vasculature of the brain and face. Of 3 described subtypes, cerebrofacial AV metameric syndrome type 3 is associated with AVMs of the cerebellum and pons.[29]

Diseases affecting collagen have been associated with diverse forms of cerebral AV shunts. These conditions include neurofibromatosis type 1 and Ehlers-Danlos syndrome. However, the location of the lesion within the brain is not specific for these diseases, and the relationship between these diseases and the development of AV shunts is still unclear. Uncommonly, cerebral AVMs may also be associated with other vascular lesions such as cavernous malformations and DVAs.[29]

Up to 25% of pial AVFs occur in association with hereditary hemorrhagic telangiectasia.[35,39]

Posterior Fossa Aneurysms in Children

Aneurysms are rare in children, accounting for less than 5% of treated aneurysms as reported in the literature by various academic neurovascular centers.[40–42] Population-based epidemiologic studies have shown that aneurysmal subarachnoid hemorrhage accounts for 10% to 15% of hemorrhagic strokes in patients less than 20 years of age.[43]

Much of the data available for the pediatric population are now older. One recent systematic review collated the available epidemiologic data in the pediatric population and compared it with that of the available data from adult studies.[42] It confirmed key differences between the 2 groups. In children, aneurysms were more commonly identified in males than females. There was a higher proportion of posterior circulation aneurysms ($3\times$) in children and a higher proportion of complex aneurysms (fusiform/dissecting) in children.[29,42,44,45]

Conditions such as smoking and hypertension that are more often associated with aneurysm development in adults are not present in children. **Box 1** lists a wide variety of disorders that are associated with intracranial aneurysms in children. There is a clear association between childhood aneurysms and disease processes that weaken the matrix of the blood vessel wall.[16] There is an increased incidence of mycotic, dissecting, and traumatic aneurysms in children, suggesting that blood vessels in this population are more susceptible to damage from an extrinsic cause.

Box 1
Congenital conditions associated with pediatric intracranial aneurysms and vasculopathy

Alpha-1 antitrypsin deficiency

Alpha-glucosidase deficiency

Alport syndrome (type IV collagenopathy)

Aortic coarctation

Autosomal-dominant polycystic kidney disease

Cystic fibrosis

Congenital absence of the carotid artery

Ehlers–Danlos syndrome (vascular subtype)

Klipel–Trenaunay–Weber syndrome

Loeys–Dietz syndrome type 1

Marfan syndrome

Neurofibromatosis type 1

Osler–Weber–Rendu disease

Osteogenesis imperfecta

Parry–Romberg syndrome

Posterior fossa malformations–hemangiomas–arterial anomalies–cardiac defects–eye abnormalities–sternal cleft and supraumbilical raphe (PHACES) syndrome

Tuberous sclerosis

3-M syndrome

Conversely, the arterial wall is more capable of a healing response, with multiple case reports documenting aneurysms that showed spontaneous thrombosis in the pediatric population.[29] Ultimately, however, the majority of pediatric aneurysms seem to be sporadic and cannot be linked to an underlying systemic disorder.

The differences between the adult and pediatric populations are most pronounced in early childhood and become less marked through adolescence. In general, dissecting aneurysms are dominant in the age group less than 5 years with saccular aneurysms occurring between the ages of 6 and 15 years (**Fig. 18**). Multiple aneurysms are less common in the pediatric population,

unless seen in the setting of an infectious cause or an underlying arteriopathy. Young children also have a higher frequency of giant and fusiform aneurysms (**Fig. 19**).[41,43,45]

Aneurysm location

In a recent systematic review that collated data on a total of 480 aneurysms, 25% were identified in the posterior circulation (including the posterior cerebral arteries). The majority (8%) of posterior fossa aneurysms were located at the basilar apex followed by the posterior cerebral arteries (7%), intracranial vertebral arteries (5%), posterior inferior cerebellar arteries (3%), anterior inferior cerebellar arteries (1%) and the superior cerebellar arteries (1%).[42]

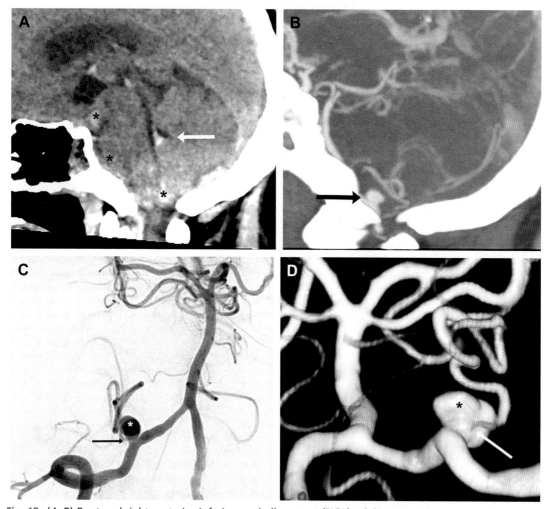

Fig. 18. (*A–D*) Ruptured right posterior inferior cerebellar artery (PICA) origin aneurysm. A 15-year-old girl presented with Hunt and Hess grade 2 subarachnoid hemorrhage (SAH). (*A*) Noncontrast computed tomography scan in sagittal reformat shows the SAH surrounding the brainstem (*asterisk*) and within the fourth ventricle (*arrow*). (*B*) Reconstructed sagittal limited volume minimal intensity projection demonstrates a saccular aneurysm in the region of the right PICA origin (*arrow*). Right vertebral artery catheter angiogram (*C*) and 3-dimensional reconstruction (*D*) confirms the presence of a saccular aneurysm (*asterisk*) at the right PICA origin (*arrow*) incorporating the parent vessel.

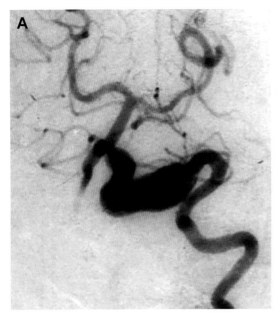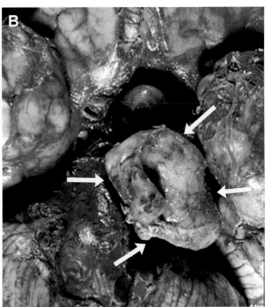

Fig. 19. (*A*, *B*) Ruptured fusiform left vertebral artery aneurysm in a 2-year-old girl. (*A*) Left vertebral injection catheter angiogram shows a large fusiform vertebral artery aneurysm extending from the region of the left posterior inferior cerebellar artery to the vertebrobasilar junction. (*B*) Post mortem specimen photograph of the same patient shows the aneurysm seen on angiography (*arrows*). Note the extensive deep brown staining subarachnoid hemorrhage throughout the basilar cisterns and left temporal pole.

Imaging characteristics

Computed tomography, MR imaging, magnetic resonance angiography, and catheter angiography For patients presenting with clinical suspicion of subarachnoid hemorrhage, a noncontrast CT scan is often the first imaging modality used. Modern dose reduction techniques minimize radiation exposure to the patient without significantly affecting diagnostic efficacy.[46–48]

There is significant overlap in the imaging appearances among the pathogenetic subtypes of intracranial aneurysms in children (**Table 1**). In certain cases, however, specific imaging findings may help to identify a specific subtype. Pediatric patients rarely exhibit multiple aneurysms unless there is an underlying arteriopathy or systemic infection. As in adults, mycotic aneurysms tend to be saccular in morphology, often multiple and involve the distal cortical branches. Idiopathic aneurysms or aneurysms associated with an underlying vasculopathy or arteriopathy tend to be fusiform and involve the proximal vasculature.

Table 1
Etiologic subtypes of pediatric intracranial aneurysms

Idiopathic	By exclusion of other causes
Familial	Aneurysms in sibling or ≥3 first-degree relatives
Traumatic	Resulting from head trauma
Infectious	Secondary to infection of the arterial wall with secondary inflammatory response
Noninfectious inflammatory	Secondary to inflammatory arteriopathies
Vasculopathic	Underlying structural deficiencies within the arterial wall that predisposes to aneurysm development
Oncotic	Secondary to tumor infiltration
Related to hemodynamic stress or increased flow	Secondary to increased or abnormal hemodynamic stress and shear forces (hypertension, high flow arteriovenous shunts, sickle cell disease, etc)

The presence of a skull base fracture, extraaxial collection, or other sequelae of trauma naturally suggests a traumatic aneurysm, although there can be the question as to whether the trauma caused the aneurysm or vice versa. In general, calcifications are unlikely to be associated with pediatric intracranial aneurysms.

SUMMARY

Key differences exist in the epidemiology, pathophysiology, and clinical presentation of cerebellar vascular lesions between the pediatric and adult population. An understanding of these differences and the imaging features aid in predicting lesion etiology and help to direct child specific treatment strategies. The development of the arterial system of the posterior fossa, as with the rest of the primitive brain occurs as a response to hemodynamic and metabolic demand. The process by which the adult vascular morphology is formed allows radiologists to understand and predict variant anatomy.

REFERENCES

1. Padget DH. The cranial venous system in man in reference to development, adult configuration, and relation to the arteries. Am J Anat 1956; 98(3):307–55.
2. Padget DH. The development of the cranial arteries in the human embryo. Contrib Embryol 1948;12(pub no: 575):205–61.
3. GL S. The developmental alteration sin the vascular system of the brain of the human embryo. Contrib Embryol 1918;8:5–38.
4. Raybaud C. Normal and abnormal embryology and development of the intracranial vascular system. Neurosurg Clin N Am 2010;21(3):399–426.
5. Moffat DB. The embryology of the arteries of the brain. Ann R Coll Surg Engl 1962;30:368–82.
6. Kathuria S, Gregg L, Chen J, et al. Normal cerebral arterial development and variations. Semin Ultrasound CT MR 2011;32(3):242–51.
7. Akgun V, Battal B, Bozkurt Y, et al. Normal anatomical features and variations of the vertebrobasilar circulation and its branches: an analysis with 64-detector row CT and 3T MR angiographies. ScientificWorldJournal 2013;2013:620162.
8. Arraez-Aybar LA, Fuentes-Redondo T, Millan JM. Persistent trigeminal artery: a cross-sectional study based on over 3 years conventional angiography, CT angiography and MR angiography images. Surg Radiol Anat 2015. [Epub ahead of print].
9. Mulder M, Lycklama ANGJ, Dinkelaar W, et al. Thrombectomy in posterior circulation stroke through persistent primitive trigeminal artery: a case report. Interv Neuroradiol 2015;21(6):715–8.
10. Kageyama H, Toyooka T, Osada H, et al. Infratentorial arteriovenous malformation associated with persistent primitive hypoglossal artery. Surg Neurol Int 2015;6:71.
11. Silva CF, Hou SY, Kuhn AL, et al. Double embolic protection during carotid artery stenting with persistent hypoglossal artery. J Neurointerv Surg 2014;6(3):e23.
12. Uchino A. Persistent hypoglossal artery versus type I proatlantal artery. Surg Radiol Anat 2016;38(2):273.
13. Teraa M, Toorop RJ, Moll FL. Preserved distal flow in a proximally occluded internal carotid artery due to a persistent proatlantal artery. J Vasc Surg 2014; 59(2):527.
14. Zhang CW, Xie XD, Yang ZG, et al. Giant cavernous aneurysm associated with a persistent trigeminal artery and persistent otic artery. Korean J Radiol 2009; 10(5):519–22.
15. Matsushita A, Yanaka K, Hyodo A, et al. Persistent primitive otic artery with IC-cavernous aneurysm. J Clin Neurosci 2003;10(1):113–5.
16. Lasjaunias PBA, ter Brugge K, editors. Surgical neuroangiography. 2nd edition. Berlin: Springer-Verlag; 2001.
17. Krings TG, S Cruz JP, terBrugge K. Neurovascular anatomy in interventional neuroradiology. A case-based approach. In: Krings T, editor. New York: Thieme; 2015. p. 193–7.
18. Vanaman MJ, Hervey-Jumper SL, Maher CO. Pediatric and inherited neurovascular diseases. Neurosurg Clin N Am 2010;21(3):427–41.
19. de Oliveira JG, Rassi-Neto A, Ferraz FA, et al. Neurosurgical management of cerebellar cavernous malformations. Neurosurg Focus 2006;21(1):e11.
20. Gross BA, Du R, Orbach DB, et al. The natural history of cerebral cavernous malformations in children. J Neurosurg Pediatr 2016;17:123–8.
21. Meyers PM, Halback VV, Barkovich AJ. Pediatric neuroimaging. In: Barkovich ARC, editor. Anomalies of the cerebral vasculature: diagnostic and endovascular considerations. 5th edition. Philadelphia: Lippincott, Williams & Wilkins; Wolters Kluwer; 2012. p. 1051–101.
22. Goulao A, Alvarez H, Garcia Monaco R, et al. Venous anomalies and abnormalities of the posterior fossa. Neuroradiology 1990;31(6):476–82.
23. Lee RR, Becher MW, Benson ML, et al. Brain capillary telangiectasia: MR imaging appearance and clinicohistopathologic findings. Radiology 1997; 205(3):797–805.
24. Petersen TA, Morrison LA, Schrader RM, et al. Familial versus sporadic cavernous malformations: differences in developmental venous anomaly association and lesion phenotype. AJNR Am J Neuroradiol 2010;31(2):377–82.
25. Denier C, Labauge P, Bergametti F, et al. Genotype-phenotype correlations in cerebral cavernous malformations patients. Ann Neurol 2006;60(5):550–6.

26. Polymeropoulos MH, Hurko O, Hsu F, et al. Linkage of the locus for cerebral cavernous hemangiomas to human chromosome 7q in four families of Mexican-American descent. Neurology 1997;48(3):752–7.

27. Strenger V, Sovinz P, Lackner H, et al. Intracerebral cavernous hemangioma after cranial irradiation in childhood. Incidence and risk factors. Strahlenther Onkol 2008;184(5):276–80.

28. Larson JJ, Ball WS, Bove KE, et al. Formation of intracerebral cavernous malformations after radiation treatment for central nervous system neoplasia in children. J Neurosurg 1998;88(1):51–6.

29. Lasjaunias P, Berenstein A, ter Brugge K. Surgical neuroangiography. 2nd edition. Berlin: Springer; 2001. p. 2006.

30. Naff NJ, Wemmer J, Hoenig-Rigamonti K, et al. A longitudinal study of patients with venous malformations: documentation of a negligible hemorrhage risk and benign natural history. Neurology 1998; 50(6):1709–14.

31. Field LR, Russell EJ. Spontaneous hemorrhage from a cerebral venous malformation related to thrombosis of the central draining vein: demonstration with angiography and serial MR. AJNR Am J Neuroradiol 1995;16(9):1885–8.

32. Sayama CM, Osborn AG, Chin SS, et al. Capillary telangiectasias: clinical, radiographic, and histopathological features. Clinical article. J Neurosurg 2010;113(4):709–14.

33. Tang SC, Jeng JS, Liu HM, et al. Diffuse capillary telangiectasia of the brain manifested as a slowly progressive course. Cerebrovasc Dis 2003;15(1–2): 140–2.

34. Gelal F, Karakas L, Sarsilmaz A, et al. Capillary telangiectasia of the brain: imaging with various magnetic resonance techniques. JBR-BTR 2014;97(4): 233–8.

35. Castillo M, Morrison T, Shaw JA, et al. MR imaging and histologic features of capillary telangiectasia of the basal ganglia. AJNR Am J Neuroradiol 2001; 22(8):1553–5.

36. Barr RM, Dillon WP, Wilson CB. Slow-flow vascular malformations of the pons: capillary telangiectasias? AJNR Am J Neuroradiol 1996;17(1):71–8.

37. Chaudhry US, De Bruin DE, Policeni BA. Susceptibility-weighted MR imaging: a better technique in the detection of capillary telangiectasia compared with T2* gradient-echo. AJNR Am J Neuroradiol 2014;35(12):2302–5.

38. Toulgoat F, Lasjaunias P. Vascular malformations of the brain. Handb Clin Neurol 2013;112:1043–51.

39. Walcott BP, Smith ER, Scott RM, et al. Pial arteriovenous fistulae in pediatric patients: associated syndromes and treatment outcome. J Neurointerv Surg 2013;5(1):10–4.

40. Ostergaard JR, Voldby B. Intracranial arterial aneurysms in children and adolescents. J Neurosurg 1983;58(6):832–7.

41. Garg K, Singh PK, Sharma BS, et al. Pediatric intracranial aneurysms–our experience and review of literature. Childs Nerv Syst 2014;30(5):873–83.

42. Beez T, Steiger HJ, Hanggi D. Evolution of management of intracranial aneurysms in children: a systematic review of the modern literature. J Child Neurol 2015. [Epub ahead of print].

43. Aeron G, Abruzzo TA, Jones BV. Clinical and imaging features of intracranial arterial aneurysms in the pediatric population. Radiographics 2012;32(3): 667–81.

44. Buis DR, van Ouwerkerk WJ, Takahata H, et al. Intracranial aneurysms in children under 1 year of age: a systematic review of the literature. Childs Nerv Syst 2006;22(11):1395–409.

45. Sorteberg A, Dahlberg D. Intracranial non-traumatic aneurysms in children and adolescents. Curr Pediatr Rev 2013;9(4):343–52.

46. Ledenius K, Gustavsson M, Johansson S, et al. Effect of tube current on diagnostic image quality in paediatric cerebral multidetector CT images. Br J Radiol 2009;82(976):313–20.

47. Ledenius K, Stalhammar F, Wiklund LM, et al. Evaluation of image-enhanced paediatric computed tomography brain examinations. Radiat Prot Dosimetry 2010;139(1–3):287–92.

48. Sulagaesuan C, Saksobhavivat N, Asavaphatiboon S, et al. Reducing emergency CT radiation doses with simple techniques: A quality initiative project. J Med Imaging Radiat Oncol 2016;60(1):23–34.

Pediatric Cerebellar Tumors
Emerging Imaging Techniques and Advances in Understanding of Genetic Features

Asim F. Choudhri, MD[a,b,c,d,*], Adeel Siddiqui, MD[a,d], Paul Klimo Jr, MD, MPH[b,d,e,f]

KEYWORDS

- Pediatric radiology • Neuroradiology • Brain tumor • Cerebellum • Medulloblastoma
- Pilocytic astrocytoma • Ependymoma

KEY POINTS

- Cerebellar tumors are the most common solid neoplasms in children, with the 3 most common entities including pilocytic astrocytoma, medulloblastoma, and ependymoma.
- Diffusion-weighted/tensor imaging plays a key role in preoperative characterization of pediatric cerebellar tumors, with lower apparent diffusion coefficient values correlating with higher-grade tumors.
- Genetic characterization is resulting in new understanding of medulloblastoma.
- The previous 4 histologic categories are in the process of being supplanted with 4 genetic groupings, in particular based on analysis of the WNT and Sonic Hedgehog pathway genes.
- This genetic characterization has allowed therapeutic options targeted to the specific tumor and improved prediction of tumor aggressiveness compared with histologic categorization.

INTRODUCTION

Cerebellar tumors are among the most common central nervous system (CNS) neoplasms, not to mention solid neoplasms, in children.[1] These tumors include benign and malignant entities, tumors that have slow local spread, and others with leptomeningeal dissemination. Although there are a small number of tumor types that account for most of these tumors, recent work on the genetic origins of these lesions has created an understanding of a much broader landscape of tumors.[2]

The newer understanding of genetic origins has the potential for targeted therapy, and imaging features that may help determine the tumor type (or even subtype) take on an increasingly critical role.

TUMOR TYPES

Pediatric cerebellar tumors most commonly involve four entities. Pilocytic astrocytomas (PAs), ependymomas, and medulloblastomas are the key players, with atypical teratoid rhabdoid tumor (ATRT)

Disclosures: none.
[a] Department of Radiology, University of Tennessee Health Science Center, 848 Adams Ave, Memphis, TN 38103, USA; [b] Department of Neurosurgery, University of Tennessee Health Science Center, 847 Monroe Avenue, Memphis, TN 38163, USA; [c] Department of Ophthalmology, University of Tennessee Health Science Center, 930 Madison Avenue, Memphis, TN 38163, USA; [d] Le Bonheur Neuroscience Institute, Le Bonheur Children's Hospital, 848 Adams Avenue, Memphis, TN 38103, USA; [e] Division of Neurosurgery, St. Jude's Children's Hospital, 262 Danny Thomas Place, Memphis, TN 38105, USA; [f] Semmes Murphey Neurologic & Spine Institute, 6325 Humphreys Boulevard, Memphis, TN 38120, USA
* Corresponding author. Department of Radiology, Le Bonheur Children's Hospital, 848 Adams Avenue–G216, Memphis, TN 38103.
E-mail address: achoudhri@uthsc.edu

Neuroimag Clin N Am 26 (2016) 459–469
http://dx.doi.org/10.1016/j.nic.2016.03.010
1052-5149/16/$ – see front matter © 2016 Elsevier Inc. All rights reserved.

representing a high-grade embryonal tumor most common in the first year or two of life. Initial clinical presentation for all of these lesions is typically due to mass effect, including headaches, nausea and emesis, cranial neuropathies, and obstructive hydrocephalus.

PILOCYTIC ASTROCYTOMA

PAs, sometimes referred to as juvenile PAs, are benign neoplasms, classified as World Health Organization (WHO) grade I tumors. They account for more than two-thirds of all cerebellar astrocytomas and can be seen from birth to about 15 years of age. Other more aggressive astrocytomas, such as anaplastic astrocytomas and glioblastomas, are rare and usually seen in older children. There is an equal incidence of PA in boys and girls. PA of the cerebellum can arise from nearly any location in the cerebellum, including the hemispheres and vermis. PA of the cerebellum most classically has an imaging appearance of a cystic lesion with a mural nodule (Fig. 1). The solid portions of the tumor have a large volume of interstitial space with a high water content, which results in a somewhat hyperintense appearance on T2-weighted (T2W) imaging, and results in facilitated diffusion. The solid portion of PAs typically has diffusion characteristics of greater than 1300×10^{-6} mm^2/s (or 1.3×10^{-3} mm^2/s).[3] The solid portions will

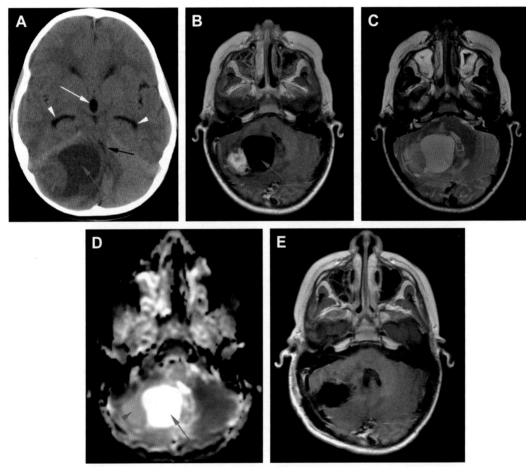

Fig. 1. PA. (A) Axial–computed tomography image in a 6-year-old boy shows a mass in the right cerebellar hemisphere that has a cystic component (*red arrow*) and a solid component (*red arrowhead*). There is near-complete effacement of the fourth ventricle (*black arrow*) with signs of obstructive hydrocephalus in the third ventricle (*white arrow*) and temporal horns of the lateral ventricles (*white arrowheads*). (B) Axial T1W + C image shows enhancement of the solid nodule (*red arrowhead*) but not of the cystic component (*red arrow*). (C) Axial T2W image shows intermediate hyperintense signal for the solid nodule (*red arrowhead*), suggesting a high water content, and fluidlike signal in the cystic component (*red arrow*). (D) ADC map shows facilitated diffusion in the solid nodule (*red arrowhead*), with diffusion characteristics of 1570×10^{-6} mm^2/s. The diffusion characteristics of the cystic component (*red arrow*) were greater than 3000×10^{-6} mm^2/s. (E) Axial T1W + C MR imaging after surgical resection shows gross total resection. This lesion was confirmed to be a PA. T1W + C, T1 + contrast.

usually enhance after contrast administration because of leaky capillaries. Accordingly, there is delayed accumulation of gadolinium within the interstitial space, and the lesions will enhance more on delayed imaging. The contrast enhancement is *not* due to increased vascularity, as would be the case for a hemangioblastoma.

The cyst walls of a PA may or may not enhance. If the enhancement is thin and smooth, this is likely due to leaky capillaries as a result of the pressure from the cyst and not due to neoplasm. If the enhancement is irregular and nodular, then neoplasm is more likely. Inspection of the inside of the cyst under microscopic magnification and illumination will usually allow the surgeon to distinguish whether the wall of the cyst is neoplastic or not. Many PAs are amenable to gross-total resection (GTR) with appropriate surgical planning, but these can be challenging lesions. These tumors can be difficult to distinguish from normal adjacent cerebral tissue, and there can be a transition zone of tumor infiltration. When GTR is achieved, no adjuvant chemotherapy or radiation is typically indicated and patients will undergo imaging surveillance. A recurrence along the margins of the resection cavity may undergo continued surveillance, repeat surgical resection, or (if not amenable to resection) focal irradiation. If surgery is performed and there is a small focus of residual tumor, the neuro-oncologic team may still advocate for observation over radiation, especially if patients are young. Chemotherapy is typically reserved for young children with unresectable residual or recurrent disease, although it is less effective at achieving local disease control than radiation.

PAs tend to have local growth, both of the initial lesion and recurrences. Distant cerebral spinal fluid (CSF) dissemination of the disease, either intracranially or to the spine, is much less common than the other lesions discussed, seen in as little as 2% of these lesions.[4] The 25-year survival rate of cerebellar PA is greater than 90%, and the 25-year survival rate of solid cerebellar astrocytomas is approximately 40%[4,5] but may be improved with more recent therapy.

Recent work has shown that mutations in the BRAF gene are present in some PAs.[6–8] The BRAF proto-oncogene makes a protein called B-Raf that is involved in the mitogen-activated protein kinase (MAPK)/Extracellular signal regulated kinases signaling pathway, which affects cell division and differentiation. BRAF alterations may be a point mutation (V600E) or various fusions (KIAA 1549); the pattern of such genetic alterations may be tumor location specific.[9–11] MAPK (eg, tranetinib) and BRAF inhibitors (eg, dabrafenib and vemurafinib in patients who are V600E positive) are under investigation as a treatment option for PA. Interestingly, the initial studies with these inhibitors were done in patients with melanoma.[12]

MEDULLOBLASTOMA

Medulloblastoma is a malignant tumor classified as WHO grade IV, which most commonly arises from the superior medullary velum in young children and cerebellar hemispheres in adolescents. Medulloblastomas are the most common posterior fossa tumor and the most common brain tumor overall in the 6- to 11-year age group. The median age at diagnosis is 6 years, and boys are affected more than girls. This highly cellular tumor is a small, round, blue cell tumor with 4 histologic subtypes, as defined by the 2007 WHO criteria: classic medulloblastoma, large cell, anaplastic, and nodular desmoplastic[13] (**Fig. 2**). Nodular desmoplastic medulloblastomas tend to occur in older patients, adolescents, and young adults and occur in the cerebellar hemispheres[14] (**Fig. 3**). Based on histologic criteria, medulloblastoma has been considered to be a subtype of a primitive neuroectodermal tumor (PNET) and is sometimes referred to as medulloblastoma-PNET to reflect this relationship.

Beyond histologic characteristics, molecular analysis has given rise to 4 subtypes.[15,16] The Sonic Hedgehog pathway (SHH) and WNT pathway, in particular, correlate with the site of origin of these tumors, and importantly with treatment response and outcome. WNT medulloblastomas are thought to arise from the lower rhombic lip of the brainstem, whereas SHH tumors arise from the external granular layer and are found within the cerebellar hemispheres (overlapping with the histologic category of nodular desmoplastic). Given the different genetic origins and biological behavior, different therapeutic options exist for these tumors. Accordingly, active investigations are underway to determine clinical and imaging biomarkers to help stratify these tumors.[17–19]

Because of the highly cellular nature of these tumors, there are low apparent diffusion coefficient (ADC) values, typically lower than 800×10^{-6} mm^2/s.[3] ADC has not yet been shown to correspond to the genetic subtype of medulloblastoma or treatment responsiveness. Medulloblastomas usually demonstrate postcontrast enhancement, and approximately half of lesions show signs of calcification. The high nuclear to cytoplasmic ratio results in a high-density appearance on computed tomography (CT), even in the absence of calcifications, and a relative hypointense appearance on T2W imaging. Unlike ependymomas,

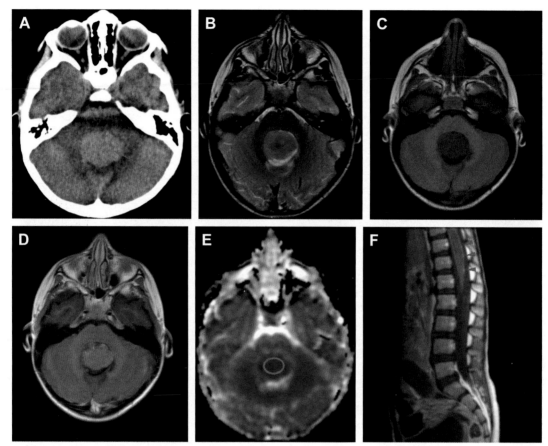

Fig. 2. Medulloblastoma. (*A*) Axial–computed tomography image of the posterior fossa in a 4-year-old girl shows a high-density lesion within the fourth ventricle (*red arrow*). (*B*) Axial T2W image shows the lesion demonstrates intermediate hypointense signal characteristics. (*C*) Axial T1W image shows the lesion demonstrates intermediate signal characteristics. (*D*) Axial T1W + C image shows the lesion demonstrates diffuse postcontrast enhancement. (*E*) Apparent diffusion coefficient maps show the lesion demonstrates restricted diffusion, with diffusivity of 655×10^{-6} mm^2/s as measured within the red oval region of interest. (*F*) Sagittal T1W + C image of the lumbar spine shows irregular enhancement along the posterior aspect of the conus medullaris and thoracolumbar cord (*red arrowheads*), consistent with leptomeningeal metastatic deposits. This lesion was confirmed to be medulloblastoma with intracranial and spinal metastatic disease.

medulloblastomas tend to displace rather than conform to margins and are described as being more spherical. This feature also explains why patients with medulloblastoma have a relatively short clinical history and come to medical attention more quickly than their ependymoma counterparts. Spinal metastatic disease is more common with medulloblastoma than ependymoma.

Like ependymoma, optimal management is multimodal, including maximal cytoreductive surgery in nonmetastatic patients, followed by chemotherapy and depending, on the extent of disease and age of patients, radiation.

EPENDYMOMA

Ependymomas are of 2 types: well differentiated (WHO grade II) and anaplastic (WHO grade III).

Anatomically, posterior fossa ependymomas can be thought of as either midline or lateral in origin (**Fig. 4**). They have a bimodal age distribution, the first between 1 and 5 years of age and the second much later during the fourth decade of life. They account for up to one-fifth of the posterior fossa tumors in children with a slight increase incidence in boys.

Ependymomas are histologically defined by perivascular and ependymal pseudorosettes, among other features.[20] Recent work suggests that the exact cell of origin of ependymoma and genetic origin may vary in lesions of different locations.[21–25] The tumors that are predominantly midline, typically filling the fourth ventricle, represent the most commonly described location for posterior fossa ependymomas. Lateral ependymomas arise from the inferior margin of the middle

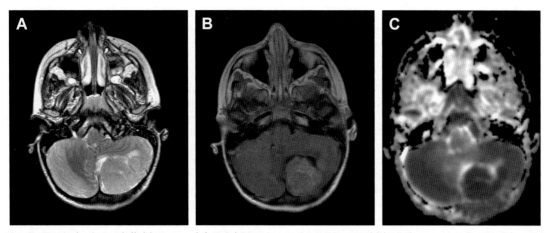

Fig. 3. Hemispheric medulloblastoma. (*A*) Axial T2W image in an 8-year-old boy shows a predominantly solid lesion in the periphery of the left cerebellar hemisphere, with smaller cystic components. The lesion is intermediate hypointense on T2W images. (*B*) Axial T1W + C image shows mild heterogeneous enhancement of the solid component of the tumor. (*C*) Apparent diffusion coefficient map shows the solid portion demonstrates restricted diffusion, with a diffusivity of 655×10^{-6} mm^2/s. This lesion was a nodular-desmoplastic medulloblastoma.

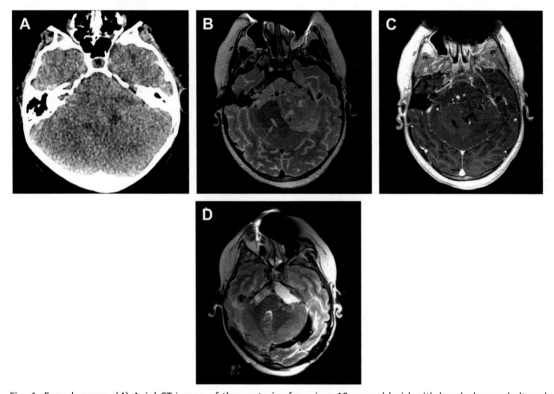

Fig. 4. Ependymoma. (*A*) Axial CT image of the posterior fossa in a 10-year-old girl with headaches and altered mental status shows a paucity of CSF space as well as rightward and posterior displacement of the fourth ventricle (*red arrow*) and internal cystic areas (*red arrowhead*) within a suspected mass. (*B*) Axial T2W image shows a mass in the left cerebellopontine angle with internal cystic changes pushing on the left middle cerebellar peduncle, reconfirmation of the mass effect on the fourth ventricle (*red arrow*). There is extension across midline in the prepontine cistern and encasement of vascular structures including the basilar artery (*red arrowhead*). (*C*) Axial T1W + C image shows only minimal heterogeneous enhancement within the lesion. (*D*) Axial T2W image from intraoperative MR imaging shows resection of this component of the lesion and significantly decreased mass effect on the brainstem. This lesion was confirmed to be an ependymoma.

cerebellar peduncle and can project into the cerebellopontine and medullary angles as well as through the foramen of Luschka into the fourth ventricle. Lateral ependymomas have a higher incidence of recurrence owing to the increased difficulty of achieving a gross total resection.[24]

Ependymomas have a tendency to spread along subarachnoid planes, such as the foramina of Luschka and Magendie around the brainstem and into the cervical spine, encasing vessels and cranial nerves thereby earning the title of "plastic ependymoma."[26] This pattern of growth explains why ependymoma patients typically have a long clinical history of vague symptoms before coming to clinical attention.

Ependymomas have intermediate diffusion characteristics in the range of approximately 1000 to 1300 $\times$ 10^{-6} mm^2/sec, with ADC values lower than that of PAs but higher than that of medulloblastomas. Ependymomas may not enhance, complicating evaluation of metastatic deposits. Small internal cystic components are common, and approximately half of all lesions show signs of calcification.

Outcomes from ependymoma are best when a gross total resection is achieved. Therefore, characterization of metastatic deposits and tumor extent is critical. Ependymomas are not typically responsive to chemotherapy; radiation is critical in achieving long-term local disease control.

ATYPICAL TERATOID RHABDOID TUMOR

ATRT is a malignant tumor classified as WHO grade IV, which can be located in the fourth ventricle, cerebellum, basal cisterns (cerebellopontine and medullary cisterns), and, rarely, in the brainstem. This tumor is primarily identified in the first year or two of life, with the median age at diagnosis being 2 to 4 years. However, ATRT can be seen throughout early childhood. This tumor is another small, blue, cell embryonal tumor and on imaging follows many features of medulloblastoma. ATRT is a highly cellular tumor with low ADC values, typically lower than 700 $\times$ 10^{-6} mm^2/s. ATRT may present with obstructive hydrocephalus and is prone to CSF dissemination of disease. Unlike medulloblastomas, ATRT does not usually respond to chemotherapy and, therefore, overall has a poorer prognosis.

OTHER ENTITIES
Ganglioglioma

Gangliogliomas can occur in the cerebellum as well as within the brainstem with extension into the cerebellum. Cerebellar gangliogliomas accounted for less than 1% of cerebellar tumors in a large series.[27] Cerebellar, brainstem, and cervicomedullary junction gangliogliomas tend to be more infiltrating and less discrete than supratentorial gangliogliomas.[28] The cerebellar component is often within the middle and inferior cerebellar peduncles and the region of the dentate nuclei. They are often calcified, with indistinct margins and a characteristic flame-shape enhancement pattern. Although these lesions may not be amenable to gross total resection because of their infiltrating nature and involvement of more central structures, as opposed to the more peripheral nature of most of the other cerebellar tumors, the unresectable components may be well controlled by adjunct therapy in many cases.

Infiltrating Glioma

Infiltrating gliomas, including fibrillary astrocytomas, anaplastic astrocytoma, and glioblastoma, can occur in the cerebellum. The imaging appearance matches that of their supratentorial counterparts, including expansile areas of T2 hyperintense signal. More high-grade lesions have variable heterogeneous areas of enhancement, diffusion restriction, cystic changes, and hemorrhagic changes. When these lesions are encountered, careful analysis of the clinical history and imaging features are required to differentiate from inflammatory processes such as acute disseminated encephalomyelitis (ADEM), vasculitis, and rhombencephalitis. Advanced imaging techniques, such as diffusion-weighted imaging (DWI) and diffusion tensor imaging (DTI), perfusion imaging, and spectroscopy, can be used; however, lumbar puncture analysis and short-term follow-up imaging may be the most helpful.

Radiation-Induced Glioma

In patients with a history of a radiation therapy to the posterior cranial fossa, radiation-induced gliomas may occur, most commonly at least 5 years after treatment.[29] These lesions will appear ill defined and infiltrating and will not have the same imaging appearance of the original tumor. Differentiating radiation-induced glioma from late radiation necrosis may be aided by PET scan, perfusion imaging, and magnetic resonance (MR) spectroscopy[30–32]; however, ultimately biopsy may be required (**Fig. 5**). In patients with a tumor predisposition condition, a secondary glioma may be a part of the underlying disease process and may or may not be solely related to radiation.

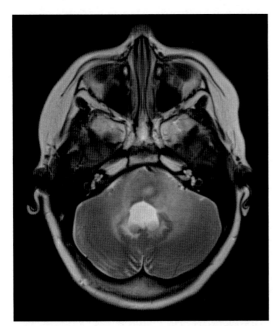

Fig. 5. Secondary glioma. Axial T2W image in a 7-year-old girl with a history of fourth ventricular ependymoma shows an infiltrating slightly expansile lesion in the brainstem as well as the middle cerebellar peduncles and deep cerebellar white matter, left greater than right. This finding did not match the appearance of her original tumor, and biopsy was performed to differentiate an infiltrating glioma versus late radiation necrosis. Biopsy confirmed this to be an infiltrating high-grade glioma without any features to suggest ependymoma.

Metastatic Disease

Intracranial metastatic disease from extracranial primary tumors is exceedingly rare in children, which is very different compared with adults. This disease may be considered in children with known primary tumors, other sites of metastatic disease, and a new cerebellar lesion. This finding is a diagnosis of exclusion and may require biopsy for confirmation. Cerebellar leptomeningeal metastatic disease from known intracranial tumors is a common occurrence.

Syndromic-Associated Tumors

Syndromic-associated cerebellar tumors in children are rare; however, of these, the most common is PA with neurofibromatosis type I (von Recklinghausen disease).[33] Hemangioblastomas are cystic lesions with enhancing nodules that have imaging overlap with PA and are located in the cerebellar hemispheres. Hemangioblastomas in children and adolescents are rarely found without von Hippel Lindau syndrome. A rare but characteristic posterior fossa lesion is dysplastic gangliocytoma, also known as Lhermitte-Duclos disease, a nonenhancing hamartomatous lesion that has a "cerebellum within a cerebellum" appearance. Dysplastic gangliocytomas are commonly associated with Cowden syndrome, which is a syndrome resulting in development of multiple tumors and hamartomas due to mutations in the PTEN gene.[34] Medulloblastomas may occur in association with 2 different inherited cancer syndromes: Gorlin and Turcot, the latter also known as nevoid basal cell carcinoma syndrome.

Tumor Mimicking Conditions

An enhancing and/or edematous lesion in the cerebellum does not always represent tumor. Infectious rhombencephalitis can look like a tumor. In the developed world, the most common infectious rhombencephalitis is related to Listeria, however globally it is due to tuberculosis. Noninfectious inflammatory conditions, such as ADEM, vasculitis, and multiple sclerosis all can overlap with tumors. Radiation necrosis and treatment induced so-called pseudoprogression can also have an aggressive appearance, including changes after proton beam therapy.[35] Appropriate recognition of potential mimicking conditions can help direct prompt and appropriate therapy, and may help prevent unnecessary surgery.

Imaging Considerations

For any patient with a known posterior fossa mass, the MR imaging protocol should be carefully prescribed. Thin-slice T2W and T1-weighted imaging should be performed to rule out foraminal or internal auditory canal invasion, including evaluation in multiple planes. Cranial nerve and vessel involvement may be misleading on sequences with greater than a 2-mm slice thickness. Volumetric image acquisition allows images to be reformatted into any imaging plane, including oblique planes.

Staging requires imaging of the entire neural axis, the brain, and complete spine. Spine imaging should extend to include the caudal most aspect of the thecal sac, often at approximately the S2 level, as CSF dissemination of disease can result in metastatic deposits in the dependent-most portion of the thecal sac. This point is important to be aware of because adult degenerative spine imaging protocols do not always extend below the superior end plate of S1 and could miss metastatic deposits. This point is most important for ependymomas, medulloblastomas, and ATRT, whereas leptomeningeal metastatic disease is less common in PAs. When possible, the spine imaging should take place before surgical resection of the primary lesion to prevent postoperative changes, namely, blood products, confounding the imaging. Postcontrast T2–fluid-attenuated inversion recovery imaging of the brain may provide increased sensitivity to detect leptomeningeal metastatic deposits, however, is subject to artifact and false-positive findings as well.[36]

DWI plays a critical role in characterization of pediatric brain tumors. In particular, quantitative analysis of ADC maps can aid in prediction of tumor cellularity and in conjunction with morphologic features can help predict tumor histology.[3,37] Lower ADC values correspond to more cellular tumors, typically more aggressive. Tumors with ADC values less than than 1000×10^{-6} mm^2/s tend to be high grade.

Research has shown that medulloblastomas are more likely to have identification of taurine on MR spectroscopy versus other lesions.[17] Spectroscopy can help differentiate an enhancing edematous demyelinating lesion from a high-grade tumor; however, low-grade tumors and demyelinating lesions can have similar spectroscopic profiles. For practical reasons, MR spectroscopy does not typically play a significant role in the primary characterization of cerebellar tumors.

Advanced physiologic imaging techniques have advanced diagnosis and surgical planning in supratentorial tumors,[38] which have some applicability to cerebellar tumors as well. DTI can evaluate the location of key white matter fiber bundles.[39] Diffusion tensor fiber tracking has been shown to be able to aid differentiation between discrete lesions, which splay white matter fibers and are, thus, more amenable to resection, and infiltrating lesions, which may not be able to be resected without disruption of the encompassed fiber pathways. Perfusion imaging, including dynamic susceptibility of contrast perfusion and arterial spin labeling perfusion, can show increased blood flow and blood volume within high-grade tumors.[40] Dynamic contrast-enhanced (DCE) perfusion can document signs of neovascularity and capillary leakage. DCE perfusion can also show differences in enhancement between the otherwise structurally similar PA and hemangioblastoma, with slow progressive enhancement in PA and rapid arterial enhancement in hemangioblastoma. Task-based functional MR imaging (fMR imaging) and resting-state fMR imaging do not currently play a significant role in diagnosis or surgical planning of cerebellar tumors. Susceptibility-weighted imaging (SWI) is an imaging sequence that is highly sensitive to magnetic field heterogeneity due to diamagnetic and/or paramagnetic substances, such as calcium and some blood products, respectively. This imaging can provide visualization of calcifications, which may be present in prior stroke, infections, and some syndromic conditions as well as within many cerebellar tumors. Identification of hemorrhagic changes on SWI can be a biomarker indicating an aggressive tumor. SWI has also been shown to be helpful in evaluation of vascularity, including characterization of altered perfusion patterns after stroke.[41,42]

PET with fludeoxyglucose F 18 is not widely used in the primary characterization of pediatric cerebellar tumors; however, 11-C-methionine PET has more recently been shown to be a way of differentiating low-grade from high-grade tumors.[43,44] PET and perfusion imaging have been shown to have a role in differentiating posttreatment tumor recurrence versus radiation necrosis or pseudoprogression.[30,45–47] These techniques have been more widely studied in adult supratentorial gliomas than pediatric cerebellar tumors.

Intraoperative MR Imaging

Intraoperative MR imaging (iMR imaging) is a technology that allows immediate imaging evaluation of a resection cavity while patients are in the operating room.[48,49] This technology is especially suited for the evaluation of pediatric brain tumors, whereby gross-total resection (GTR) is the most important determinant of local control and survival in many tumors. In cases whereby the preoperative surgical goal is a GTR, rates of up to 95% have been achieved with the iMR imaging.[48] Recent advances have allowed iMR imaging to be performed in children as young as 4 months of age.[50] Studies to date have not shown MR imaging–related complications or increased infection rates in patients undergoing iMR imaging–guided surgery. Like other new technologies, iMR imaging does have its challenges, including image interpretation and spatial distortion.[51]

TREATMENT AND MANAGEMENT CONSIDERATIONS
Radiation

Radiation therapy, photons or protons, is commonly performed for ependymoma, medulloblastoma, and ATRT and can serve as an excellent alternative for PA. Depending on the type of tumor and the presence or absence of metastatic disease, local radiation to the surgical bed only with a margin may be appropriate. With metastatic disease or with more aggressive tumors, such as medulloblastoma, more extensive treatment, such as whole-brain irradiation or craniospinal irradiation, may be warranted. Adjunct radiation is avoided, when possible, in children younger than 3 years of age because of the profound detrimental effects on neural development.

Posterior Fossa Syndrome

The resection of any midline/fourth ventricular tumor may lead to a constellation of symptoms known as posterior fossa syndrome (PFS). This syndrome typically occurs several days after surgical resection. The sine qua non of PFS is an inability of the child to speak but still able to comprehend (cerebellar mutism). Additional features of PFS include emotional lability, hypotonia, and ataxia.[52] Large tumors within the fourth ventricle, splaying of the peduncles or invasion into the region of the dentate nuclei, obstructive hydrocephalus, young age, male sex, and medulloblastoma tumor are all risk factors for PFS. PFS may be the result of injury to the efferent cerebellar pathway bilaterally, with resultant imaging and physiologic features, including components of bilateral cerebellar diaschisis and bilateral hypertrophic olivary degeneration.[53,54]

SUMMARY

Cerebellar tumors are the most commonly encountered pediatric CNS neoplasms. We have moved well beyond the days of providing the standard 3-part differential: medulloblastoma, ependymoma, and PA. Advanced imaging techniques, in particular quantitative diffusion analysis, in conjunction with morphologic features and location, combined with knowledge of advances in genetic subtyping of these tumors, can maximize the information provided to the neurosurgical and neuro-oncologic teams. Effective use of advanced imaging, including iMR imaging when available, can maximize the possibility of adequate tumor characterization and GTR, which translates to optimal patient outcomes.

REFERENCES

1. Poussaint Tina Y, Panigrahy A, Huisman TA. Pediatric brain tumors. Pediatr Radiol 2015;45(S3):443–53.
2. Gajjar A, Bowers DC, Karajannis MA, et al. Pediatric brain tumors: innovative genomic information is transforming the diagnostic and clinical landscape. J Clin Oncol 2015;33(27):2986–98.
3. Rumboldt Z, Camacho DLA, Lake D, et al. Apparent diffusion coefficients for differentiation of cerebellar tumors in children. AJNR Am J Neuroradiol 2006; 27(6):1362–9.
4. Koeller Kelly K, Rushing Elisabeth J. From the archives of the AFIP. Radiographics 2004;24(6): 1693–708.
5. Gjerris F, Klinken L. Long-term prognosis in children with benign cerebellar astrocytoma. J Neurosurg 1978;49(2):179–84.
6. Jones DT, Kocialkowski S, Liu L, et al. Tandem duplication producing a novel oncogenic BRAF fusion gene defines the majority of pilocytic astrocytomas. Cancer Res 2008;68(21):8673–7.
7. Jones David TW, Gronych J, Lichter P, et al. MAPK pathway activation in pilocytic astrocytoma. Cell Mol Life Sci 2012;69(11):1799–811.
8. Raabe Eric H, Lim KS, Kim JM, et al. BRAF activation induces transformation and then senescence in human neural stem cells: a pilocytic astrocytoma model. Clin Cancer Res 2011;17(11):3590–9.
9. Gierke M, Sperveslage J, Schwab D, et al. Analysis of IDH1-R132 mutation, BRAF V600 mutation and KIAA1549-BRAF fusion transcript status in central nervous system tumors supports pediatric tumor classification. J Cancer Res Clin Oncol 2016; 142(1):89–100.
10. Bergthold G, Bandopadhayay P, Hoshida Y, et al. Expression profiles of 151 pediatric low-grade gliomas reveal molecular differences associated with location and histological subtype. Neuro Oncol 2015;17(11):1486–96.
11. Faulkner C, Ellis HP, Shaw A, et al. BRAF fusion analysis in pilocytic astrocytomas: KIAA1549-BRAF 15-9 fusions are more frequent in the midline than within the cerebellum. J Neuropathol Exp Neurol 2015; 74(9):867–72.
12. Vennepureddy A, Thumallapally N, Motilal Nehru V, et al. Novel drugs and combination therapies for the treatment of metastatic melanoma. J Clin Med Res 2016;8(2):63–75.
13. Louis David N, Ohgaki H, Wiestler Otmar D, et al. The 2007 WHO classification of tumours of the central nervous system. Acta Neuropathol 2007;114(2): 97–109.
14. Levy RA, Blaivas M, Muraszko K, et al. Desmoplastic medulloblastoma: MR findings. AJNR Am J Neuroradiol 1997;18(7):1364–6.
15. Gibson P, Tong Y, Robinson G, et al. Subtypes of medulloblastoma have distinct developmental origins. Nature 2010;468(7327):1095–9.
16. Taylor MD, Northcott PA, Korshunov A, et al. Molecular subgroups of medulloblastoma: the current consensus. Acta Neuropathol 2011;123(4): 465–72.
17. Panigrahy A, Krieger MD, Gonzalez-Gomez I, et al. Quantitative short echo time 1H-MR spectroscopy of untreated pediatric brain tumors: preoperative diagnosis and characterization. AJNR Am J Neuroradiol 2006;27(3):560–72.
18. Patay Z, DeSain LA, Hwang SN, et al. MR imaging characteristics of wingless-type-subgroup pediatric medulloblastoma. AJNR Am J Neuroradiol 2015; 36(12):2386–93.

19. Perreault S, Ramaswamy V, Achrol AS, et al. MRI surrogates for molecular subgroups of medulloblastoma. AJNR Am J Neuroradiol 2014;35(7): 1263–9.

20. Nobuyuki K, Yagishita S, Hara M, et al. Pathologic features of ependymoma: histologic patterns and a review of the literature. Neuropathology 1998; 18(1):1–12.

21. Johnson Robert A, Wright Karen D, Poppleton H, et al. Cross-species genomics matches driver mutations and cell compartments to model ependymoma. Nature 2010;466(7306):632–6.

22. Taylor Michael D, Poppleton H, Fuller C, et al. Radial glia cells are candidate stem cells of ependymoma. Cancer Cell 2005;8(4):323–35.

23. Pajtler Kristian W, Witt H, Sill M, et al. Molecular classification of ependymal tumors across all CNS compartments, histopathological grades, and age groups. Cancer Cell 2015;27(5):728–43.

24. Hendrik W, Mack Stephen C, Ryzhova M, et al. Delineation of two clinically and molecularly distinct subgroups of posterior fossa ependymoma. Cancer Cell 2011;20(2):143–57.

25. Raghunathan A, Wani K, Armstrong Terri S, et al. Histological predictors of outcome in ependymoma are dependent on anatomic site within the central nervous system. Brain Pathol 2013;23(5):584–94.

26. Courville CB, Broussalian SL. Plastic ependymomas of the lateral recess. Report of eight verified cases. J Neurosurg 1961;18:792–9.

27. Chang T, Teng MM, Lirng JF. Posterior cranial fossa tumours in childhood. Neuroradiology 1993;35(4): 274–8.

28. McAbee JH, Modica J, Thompson CJ, et al. Cervicomedullary tumors in children. J Neurosurg Pediatr 2015;16(4):357–66.

29. Klimo P Jr, Nesvick CL, Broniscer A, et al. Malignant brainstem tumors in children, excluding diffuse intrinsic pontine gliomas. J Neurosurg Pediatr 2015;17(1):57–65.

30. Shah R, Vattoth S, Jacob R, et al. Radiation necrosis in the brain: imaging features and differentiation from tumor recurrence. Radiographics 2012;32(5): 1343–59.

31. Kralik SF, Ho CY, Finke W, et al. Radiation necrosis in pediatric patients with brain tumors treated with proton radiotherapy. AJNR Am J Neuroradiol 2015; 36(8):1572–8.

32. Sundgren PC. MR spectroscopy in radiation injury. AJNR Am J Neuroradiol 2009;30(8):1469–76.

33. Collins VP, Jones DTW, Giannini C. Pilocytic astrocytoma: pathology, molecular mechanisms and markers. Acta Neuropathol 2015;129(6):775–88.

34. Pilarski R, Burt R, Kohlman W, et al. Cowden syndrome and the PTEN hamartoma tumor syndrome: systematic review and revised diagnostic criteria. J Natl Cancer Inst 2013;105(21):1607–16.

35. Sabin ND, Merchant TE, Harreld JH, et al. Imaging changes in very young children with brain tumors treated with proton therapy and chemotherapy. AJNR Am J Neuroradiol 2013; 34(2):446–50.

36. Fukuoka H, Hirai T, Okuda T, et al. Comparison of the added value of contrast-enhanced 3D fluid-attenuated inversion recovery and magnetization-prepared rapid acquisition of gradient echo sequences in relation to conventional postcontrast T1-weighted images for the evaluation of leptomeningeal diseases at 3T. AJNR Am J Neuroradiol 2010;31(5):868–73.

37. Poretti A, Meoded A, Cohen KJ, et al. Apparent diffusion coefficient of pediatric cerebellar tumors: a biomarker of tumor grade? Pediatr Blood Cancer 2013;60(12):2036–41.

38. Pillai JJ, Zaca D, Choudhri AF. Clinical impact of integrated physiologic brain tumor imaging. Technol Cancer Res Treat 2010;9(4):359–80.

39. Choudhri AF, Chin EM, Blitz AM, et al. Diffusion tensor imaging of cerebral white matter. Radiol Clin North Am 2014;52(2):413–25.

40. Yeom KW, Mitchell LA, Lober RM, et al. Arterial spin-labeled perfusion of pediatric brain tumors. AJNR Am J Neuroradiol 2014;35(2):395–401.

41. Bosemani T, Poretti A, Huisman TA. Susceptibility-weighted imaging in pediatric neuroimaging. J Magn Reson Imaging 2014;40(3):530–44.

42. Bosemani T, Poretti A, Orman G, et al. Pediatric cerebral stroke: susceptibility-weighted imaging may predict post-ischemic malignant edema. Neuroradiol J 2013;26(5):579–83.

43. Ogawa T, Inugami A, Hatazawa J, et al. Clinical positron emission tomography for brain tumors: comparison of fludeoxyglucose F 18 and L-methyl-11C-methionine. AJNR Am J Neuroradiol 1996; 17(2):345–53.

44. Kato T, Shinoda J, Oka N, et al. Analysis of 11C-methionine uptake in low-grade gliomas and correlation with proliferative activity. AJNR Am J Neuroradiol 2008;29(10):1867–71.

45. Hustinx R, Pourdehnad M, Kaschten B, et al. PET imaging for differentiating recurrent brain tumor from radiation necrosis. Radiol Clin North Am 2005;43(1):35–47.

46. Fatterpekar GM, Galheigo D, Narayana A, et al. Treatment-related change versus tumor recurrence in high-grade gliomas: a diagnostic conundrum—use of dynamic susceptibility contrast-enhanced (DSC) perfusion MRI. Am J Roentgenol 2012; 198(1):19–26.

47. Zach L, Guez D, Last D, et al. Delayed contrast extravasation MRI: a new paradigm in neuro-oncology. Neuro Oncol 2015;17(3):457–65.

48. Choudhri AF, Klimo P, Auschwitz TS, et al. 3T intraoperative MRI for management of pediatric CNS

neoplasms. AJNR Am J Neuroradiol 2014;35(12): 2382–7.

49. Choudhri AF, Siddiqui A, Klimo P Jr, et al. Intraoperative MRI in pediatric brain tumors. Pediatr Radiol 2015;45(3):397–405.

50. Boop FA, Bate B, Choudhri AF, et al. Preliminary experience with an intraoperative MRI-compatible infant headholder: technical note. J Neurosurg Pediatr 2015;15(5):539–43.

51. Choudhri AF, Chin EM, Klimo P, et al. Spatial distortion due to field inhomogeneity in 3.0 Tesla intraoperative MRI. Neuroradiol J 2014;27(4):387–92.

52. Turgut M. Cerebellar mutism. J Neurosurg Pediatr 2008;1(3):262.

53. Miller NG, Reddick WE, Kocak M, et al. Cerebellocerebral diaschisis is the likely mechanism of postsurgical posterior fossa syndrome in pediatric patients with midline cerebellar tumors. AJNR Am J Neuroradiol 2010;31(2):288–94.

54. Patay Z, Enterkin J, Harreld JH, et al. MR imaging evaluation of inferior olivary nuclei: comparison of postoperative subjects with and without posterior fossa syndrome. AJNR Am J Neuroradiol 2014; 35(4):797–802.

Neuroimaging of Infectious and Inflammatory Diseases of the Pediatric Cerebellum and Brainstem

Andrea Rossi, MD*, Carola Martinetti, MD,
Giovanni Morana, MD, PhD, Mariasavina Severino, MD,
Domenico Tortora, MD

KEYWORDS

• Ataxia • Cerebellitis • Cerebellar infections • Rhombencephalitis

KEY POINTS

- Infectious and inflammatory diseases of the cerebellum are rare in the pediatric age group; most patients are previously healthy preschool children presenting with an acute onset of cerebellar ataxia.
- Acute postinfectious cerebellar ataxia (a benign, self-limiting disease) and acute cerebellitis (a serious, potentially life-threatening disease) may represent 2 ends of a spectrum of viral involvement of the cerebellum, typically in the course of varicella infection.
- The cerebellum may be involved in acute disseminated encephalomyelitis, multiple sclerosis, and acute necrotizing encephalopathy, typically in the context of widespread central nervous system disease.
- Cerebellar abscesses are mostly otogenic in the pediatric age group; an associated dural sinus thrombophlebitis must actively be excluded.
- Congenital infections, mainly cytomegalovirus, may impair cerebellar development/maturation, resulting in cerebellar hypoplasia with abnormal foliation.

INTRODUCTION

The rhombencephalon, or hindbrain, is composed of the pons, cerebellum, and medulla oblongata. The term derives from the Greek rhombos, meaning a lozenge-shaped figure, whereas enkephalos means the brain. During early embryogenesis, the primary rhombencephalic vesicle divides into 2 secondary vesicles: the metencephalon (eventually forming the pons and cerebellum) and the myelencephalon (eventually forming the medulla oblongata). Rhombencephalic involvement by infectious-inflammatory conditions is rare in children. Most affected patients present acutely with ataxia, which is defined as the inability to coordinate muscle activity in the execution of voluntary movements. These children are mostly young (typically preschool) and previously healthy, although preexisting prodromal symptoms such as fever or rash, or chronic medical disorders, are sometimes recorded. Clinically, patients

Disclosure: The authors have nothing to disclose.
Neuroradiology Unit, Istituto Giannina Gaslini, Via Gerolamo Gaslini 5, Genoa 16147, Italy
* Corresponding author.
E-mail address: andrearossi@gaslini.org

Neuroimag Clin N Am 26 (2016) 471–487
http://dx.doi.org/10.1016/j.nic.2016.03.011
1052-5149/16/$ – see front matter © 2016 Elsevier Inc. All rights reserved.

complain with broad-based gait, dysmetria, dysdiadochokinesia, intention tremor, dysarthria, and sometimes nystagmus, all of which progress rapidly to a nadir, which is reached within hours to 1 to 2 days of the onset.[1]

In this clinical context, the term cerebellitis is often used loosely by clinicians to indicate that the acute onset of cerebellar ataxia likely results from primary infection or a postinfectious immune-mediated process involving the cerebellum. However, within this broad category several conditions with often different presentation, outcome, and therapeutic implications are included. The term rhombencephalitis (RE) is also often used loosely, mainly to refer to inflammatory diseases that involve primarily the brainstem; the term brainstem encephalitis is often used interchangeably with RE. The differential diagnosis of patients presenting in the emergency department with acute cerebellar ataxia includes a large group of entities, such as vascular, traumatic, metabolic, and neoplastic diseases next to infectious-inflammatory causes.[1] More specific terminology and agreement about the usage of nomenclature is therefore desirable.

The term acute cerebellitis should be used to refer to an infection that directly affects the cerebellum, either unilaterally or bilaterally, often with abnormal magnetic resonance (MR) imaging findings and with symptoms and signs beyond those of a pure cerebellar syndrome. In contrast, the term acute postinfectious cerebellar ataxia (APCA) should be used to indicate a postinfectious (mostly viral) dysfunction, usually presenting with a pure pancerebellar syndrome and with an initially normal MR imaging scan.[2] Despite these attempts at a correct definition, there is considerable overlap between these entities, which may represent a spectrum of disorders ranging from benign, self-limiting disease to marked swelling of the cerebellum and hydrocephalus. Confusion is also generated by other more widespread central nervous system (CNS) inflammatory disorders, such as acute disseminated encephalomyelitis (ADEM) or multiple sclerosis, that can present with predominantly cerebellar clinical findings but with lesions on neuroimaging that are usually widespread.[3] This article reviews the most common infectious and inflammatory conditions involving the cerebellum and brainstem, with a focus on the role of neuroimaging studies, particularly MR imaging scans, in the work-up of affected children.

NEUROIMAGING: GENERAL PRINCIPLES

Children presenting in the emergency department with an acute onset of cerebellar ataxia are typically referred for urgent imaging studies, which may include a computerized tomography (CT) or MR imaging scan depending on several considerations, including the clinical severity, the need for sedation, and organizational issues at the individual facility. Often, the range of differential diagnosis at this initial stage is wide, and includes tumors involving the brainstem or cerebellum and potentially causing hydrocephalus, metabolic disorders, cerebrovascular causes, trauma, and intoxications; thus, the inclusion of neuroimaging studies in the initial work-up of these patients is fully justified.[4,5] Furthermore, the widespread use of varicella and mumps vaccinations has significantly reduced the number of the pediatric cases of APCA.[6] Patients presenting with acute cerebellar ataxia in the postvaccination era may be presumed to harbor significant disorder in a higher proportion of cases. However, children less than 3 years of age and with duration of ataxia of less than 3 days may represent a low-risk group in which neuroimaging can be deferred if contingent on close clinical follow-up and reassessment.[7]

Cranial ultrasonography provides an excellent bedside examination in premature and term newborns and small infants; however, the exploration of the brain is limited to the first months of life in relation to the patency of the acoustic windows, represented by the cranial fontanelles. A recent study in preterm infants showed that the routine use of ultrasonography through the mastoid fontanelle (MF) may allow a better identification of cerebellar hemorrhages than through the anterior fontanelle[8]; this can easily be explained by the closer and better visualization of posterior fossa structures, both on coronal and axial planes, that can be obtained through the MF, particularly in extremely immature newborns. However, the exploration of the cerebellum remains challenging, and there are differences in the diagnosis and interpretation of cranial ultrasonography examinations according to the available ultrasonography technology and expertise.[9]

The authors prefer MR imaging to CT because of its intrinsically higher contrast resolution and sensitivity, particularly for lesions affecting the posterior fossa, a notoriously difficult region for CT despite newer technological advances,[10] as well as for inherent radiation issues. However, when MR imaging is unavailable or unfeasible, CT remains an important imaging modality. A helical acquisition with reformatted images in 3 planes should be obtained, and the whole brain should be studied including the craniocervical junction and cervical spine until C3. Iodinated contrast material administration is not routine, and should be performed only when there is concern for transverse-sigmoid sinus thrombosis; in this situation, only a postcontrast CT scan should be acquired in order to avoid a double dose of ionizing radiation.

MR imaging scans offer an exquisite depiction of posterior fossa structures, without the burden of ionizing radiation, and should therefore be preferred even in urgent situations whenever possible. In children, slice thickness for MR imaging should not exceed 4 mm. Three-dimensional T1-weighted sequences, and T2-weighted sequences, should be obtained along with axial or coronal fluid-attenuated inversion recovery (FLAIR) sequences. Diffusion-weighted imaging (DWI) with corresponding apparent diffusion coefficient (ADC) maps are of paramount importance to pick up signs of acute cytotoxic or vasogenic edema, which may be caused by either inflammation, infection, or ischemia involving the cerebellum, whereas susceptibility-weighted imaging (SWI) is useful to identify hemorrhagic foci. Postcontrast images, obtained after the intravenous injection of 0.2 mL/kg of gadolinium chelate, are useful in the context of a suspected infectious or inflammatory causes to detect areas of blood-brain barrier damage. In addition, MR venography is important to rule out a dural sinus thrombosis.

ACUTE CEREBELLITIS

Acute cerebellitis (AC) represents the most severe end of the spectrum of infectious-inflammatory disorders of the cerebellum, and may cause long-term cognitive and behavioral impairment. The cause is often unknown, although a well-known association with viral infections exists, prominently including varicella and other viruses such as influenza, rotavirus, human herpesvirus 7, and Epstein-Barr virus, as well as with *Mycoplasma pneumoniae*.[3] Pathologic reports are scarce in the literature; available data suggest an edematous process with lymphocytic and eosinophilic infiltration but no evidence of demyelination,[11] which differentiates AC from ADEM. Clinical findings are variable, and depend on the severity of cerebellar involvement. Fulminant cases, causing sudden death from acute cerebellar herniation, have been reported.[12,13] Cerebellar swelling may cause increased intracranial pressure and hydrocephalus, overshadowing the manifestations of cerebellar dysfunction; patients may complain of irritability, headache, photophobia, nuchal rigidity, and vomiting, with ensuing alteration of sensorium, seizures, focal neurologic deficits, and possibly fever.[3] Less severe cases present with either unilateral or bilateral cerebellar symptoms and signs. Cerebrospinal fluid examination may be hazardous because of the risk of cerebellar herniation. When available, findings may include lymphocytic pleocytosis and protein level increase.

MR imaging scans may show unilateral (**Fig. 1**) or bilateral (**Fig. 2**) cerebellar swelling, with T2 and FLAIR hyperintensity of the cerebellar cortex and/or subcortical and deep white matter. There may be pial contrast enhancement along cerebellar folia. In the acute stage, DWI may show increased signal with corresponding hypointensity on ADC maps, consistent with restricted water diffusion (**Fig. 3**). There have been reports on the use of perfusion-weighted imaging, showing decreased relative cerebral blood flow in the

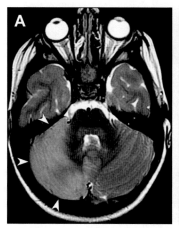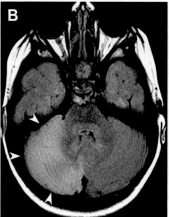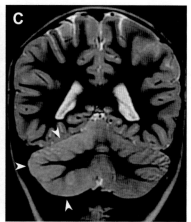

Fig. 1. Hemicerebellitis in a 3-year-old girl with varicella. Axial T2-weighted (*A*) and FLAIR (*B*) images show hyperintense right cerebellar hemisphere (*arrowheads*). The contralateral hemisphere is unaffected. Coronal T2-weighted image (*C*) shows abnormalities involving the cortex and immediate subcortical white matter, whereas the deep white matter is unaffected.

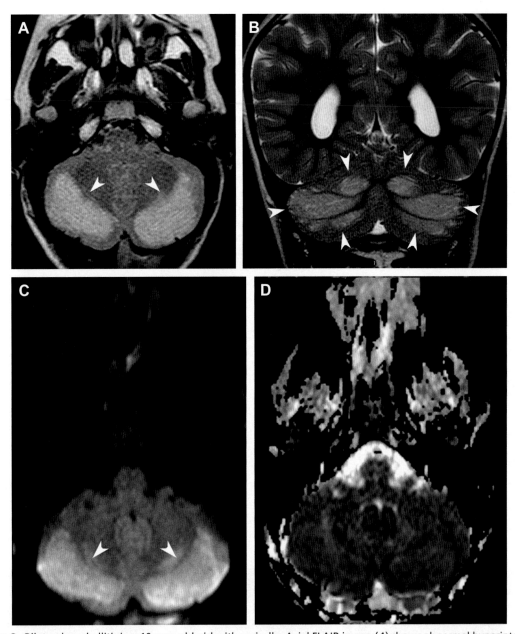

Fig. 2. Bilateral cerebellitis in a 10-year-old girl with varicella. Axial FLAIR image (*A*) shows abnormal hyperintensity of both cerebellar hemispheres posteriorly (*arrowheads*). Coronal T2-weighted image (*B*) shows prevailing involvement of the cerebellar cortex (*arrowheads*), whereas the white matter is unaffected. High signal on the trace diffusion-weighted image (*arrowheads, C*) is not associated with correspondingly low signal on the ADC map (*D*) implicating T2 shine-through.

affected area, and of proton MR spectroscopy (^{1}H-MRS) showing increased choline/creatine (Cho/Cr) and reduced *N*-acetylaspartate/creatine (NAA/Cr) ratios; presence of additional peaks, such as succinate or acetate, has been considered a strong imaging indicator of an infectious cause.[14] In the most severe cases, tonsillar herniation and hydrocephalus with periventricular edema are encountered. Unilateral cerebellar involvement (so-called hemicerebellitis) may be so severe as to mimic tumor.[11,15] In AC, MR imaging signal changes are confined to the cerebellum, unlike other disorders such as ADEM and multiple sclerosis. MR imaging findings may normalize or evolve into cerebellar atrophy on long-term follow-up. CT scan is not sensitive to subtle

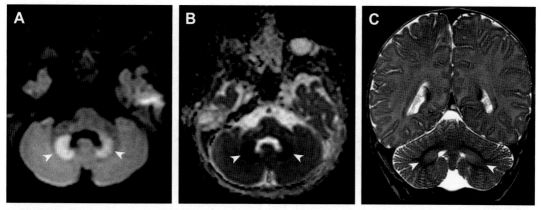

Fig. 3. Cerebellitis in a 6-month-old boy with rotavirus infection. Restricted diffusion (*arrowheads*, A, B) involves the dentate nuclei selectively. Coronal T2-weighted image (*C*) confirms selective involvement of the bilateral dentate nuclei, which appear swollen (*arrowheads*) and surrounded by unaffected white matter. (*Courtesy of* Anna Molinari, MD, Alessandria, Italy.)

alterations in the cerebellum; however, in an acute context it may be useful to display cerebellar swelling, downward tonsillar ectopia, and hydrocephalus if MR imaging is not readily available.

ACUTE POSTINFECTIOUS CEREBELLAR ATAXIA

APCA is the most common cause of acute ataxia in children, accounting for about 30% to 50% of cases. Patients typically present between 2 and 5 years of age with an acute onset of gait alterations and/or inability to perform coordinated movements; these symptoms usually regress within 72 hours. The prognosis is good with a high rate of spontaneous resolution and treatment is rarely indicated.[16] APCA mainly occurs in the aftermath of infection, most notably varicella (about 75% of all cases), mumps, *M pneumoniae*, Epstein-Barr virus, and other nonspecific viral infections, with a latency of a few days to 2 weeks of the prodromal illness.[17]

In patients with APCA, neuroimaging studies including MR imaging with DWI sequences typically show no abnormalities[2,3]; evidence of abnormality involving the cerebellum should redirect classification to AC.[1]

ACUTE DISSEMINATED ENCEPHALOMYELITIS

ADEM is an immunologically mediated inflammatory disease of the CNS involving a first, usually monophasic, episode of inflammatory demyelination with polyfocal neurologic signs implicating involvement of multiple sites of the CNS. Patients present with a rapid onset of encephalopathy and motor and/or sensory deficits with brainstem signs and symptoms and, in most cases, ataxia.

Presence of encephalopathy (defined as altered behavior or consciousness) is a required criterion for ADEM.[18] Most patients with ADEM present in the aftermath (usually 1–3 weeks) of viral infection or, rarely, vaccination.

Unlike AC, ADEM typically is characterized by widespread lesions involving not just the cerebellum but also the supratentorial brain, brainstem, and spinal cord. MR imaging findings typically include multiple, asymmetrically distributed, poorly marginated, hyperintense areas on T2-weighted and FLAIR images, whereas unenhanced T1-weighted images are usually inconspicuous unless the lesions are very large, in which case faint hypointensity is seen. Contrast enhancement is variable and, in our personal experience, extremely uncommon.[19] In typical cases, there are multiple lesions that involve the white matter, the deep gray matter nuclei, and sometimes the cerebral cortex. Involvement of the infratentorial compartment is seen in greater than 50% of cases. The brainstem, middle cerebellar peduncles, and cerebellar white matter may be involved (**Fig. 4**). Especially in the brainstem, lesions may be large and tumefactive, indicating prevalent vasogenic edema as confirmed by increased ADC values on DWI sequences.[20]

MULTIPLE SCLEROSIS

Multiple sclerosis (MS) is a chronic inflammatory demyelinating disease of the CNS characterized by immune-mediated inflammation and progressive neurodegeneration, and causing significant neurologic impairment. Early-onset MS (ie, before 18 years of age) accounts for 2% to 10% of all MS cases.[21] Acute ataxia is a common initial

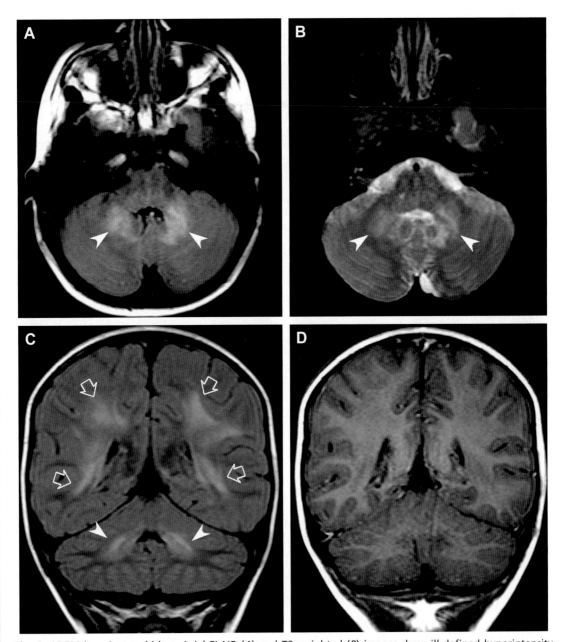

Fig. 4. ADEM in a 4-year-old boy. Axial FLAIR (*A*) and T2-weighted (*B*) images show ill-defined hyperintensity involving the dentate nuclei and adjacent white matter bilaterally (*arrowheads*). (*C*) Coronal FLAIR image shows extensive supratentorial white matter hyperintensity (*open arrows*) other than the dentate nuclei involvement (*arrowheads*). None of the lesions enhance with gadolinium chelate administration (*D*).

manifestation of MS in children younger than 10 years and in adolescents.[22]

The diagnosis of MS in children requires the fulfillment of specific neuroimaging criteria.[18] Infratentorial lesions can involve the brainstem and cerebellum (Fig. 5). In the pediatric age group, the posterior fossa shows a greater incidence and number of T2-weighted lesions on MR imaging compared with adults.[23] It has recently been shown that acquired demyelinating diseases in childhood, including MS and ADEM, lead to impaired age-expected growth of the cerebellum.[24]

ACUTE NECROTIZING ENCEPHALOPATHY

Acute necrotizing encephalopathy (ANE) is a rapidly progressive encephalopathy that can

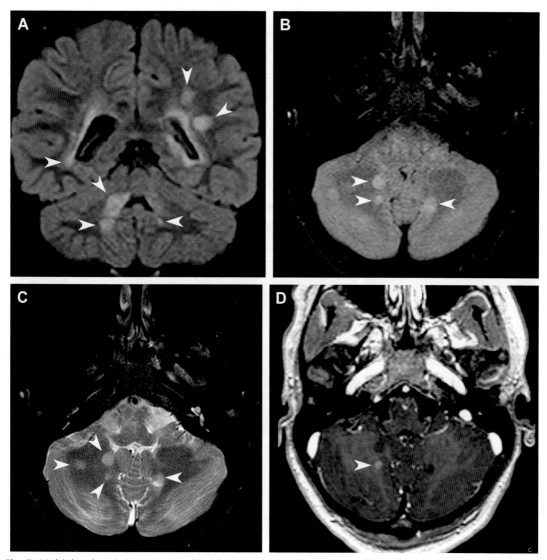

Fig. 5. Multiple sclerosis in a 13-year-old girl. Coronal (*A*) and axial (*B*) FLAIR, and axial T2-weighted (*C*) images show multiple ill-defined hyperintense lesions involving both the periventricular and infratentorial white matter (*arrowheads*), complying with the dissemination in space criteria. Contrast-enhanced axial T1-weighted image (*D*) shows 1 infratentorial lesion that enhances (*arrowhead*), satisfying the criteria for dissemination in time.

occur in otherwise healthy children after common viral infections (eg, influenza) and has a bleak prognosis with increased mortality. Patients present acutely with fever, seizures, and rapid progression to coma after the onset of a viral infection. Most cases are sporadic; however, the observation of multiple cases in the same family with recurrent episodes of ANE led to the identification of a genetic form of the disorder, called ANE1, and to the discovery of the causative mutation in *RANBP2* gene.[25] ANE has been related to intracranial cytokine storms causing blood-brain barrier damage that results in edema and necrosis, without signs of direct viral invasion or parainfectious demyelination.[26]

MR imaging findings involve a characteristic pattern of T2 hyperintense abnormality in the bilateral thalami, which are abnormally swollen; there frequently are accompanying lesions in the brain stem tegmentum, periventricular white matter, putamina, and cerebellum (**Fig. 6**). The abnormalities are characterized by restricted diffusion with variable degrees of enhancement ranging from none to patchy or rimlike on postcontrast scans.[26,27] Involvement of the pons has been shown to be associated with poor outcome.[28]

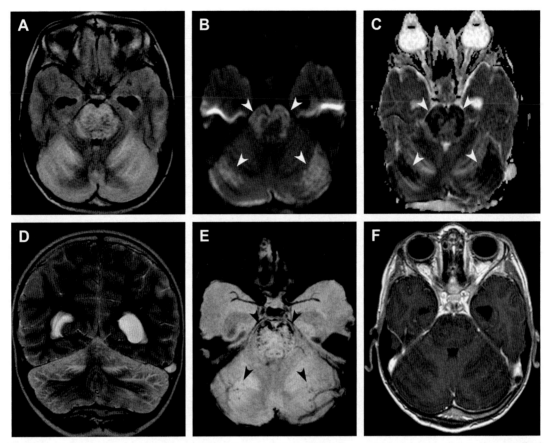

Fig. 6. Acute necrotizing encephalopathy in a 5-year-old boy. This relapse was the fourth of the disease, which started with typical bithalamic involvement at age 1 year (not shown). Axial FLAIR (*A*) and coronal T2-weighted (*D*) images show marked swelling and hyperintensity of the brainstem and cerebellum, with some sparing of the deep white matter. There is restricted diffusion (*arrowheads, B, C*) corresponding with areas with evidence of petechial hemorrhage on the susceptibility-weighted image (*arrowheads, E*), consistent with necrotic-hemorrhagic lesions. On the contrast-enhanced axial T1-weighted image (*F*) there is no enhancement, consistent with a preserved blood-brain barrier in this acute stage.

Follow-up studies may show regression of primary lesions, whereas new lesions appear in different areas during subsequent acute bouts.[25]

OPSOCLONUS-MYOCLONUS SYNDROME

Opsoclonus-myoclonus syndrome (OMS) is a rare autoimmune disorder affecting young children (usually between 1 and 4 years of age) who complain of variable degrees of myoclonus, severe ataxia, opsoclonus (involuntary, chaotic ocular movements), and marked irritability with sleep disturbances.[1,3] OMS presents mainly as a paraneoplastic disorder in patients with neuroblastoma/ganglioneuroma (NB/GM) or in association with various infectious agents. OMS occurs in 2% to 4% of children with NB/GM, and 50% of OMS cases have an NB/GM that may be clinically occult at the time of clinical onset, which mandates chest radiograph; ultrasonography of the neck, abdomen, and pelvis; and a urine test for adrenal metabolites in all children presenting with OMS.[29] The pathophysiology of OMS is thought to be immunologic because of the paraneoplasticity and the symptomatic (although often incomplete) response to immunomodulatory therapies; however, no diagnostic immunologic marker has yet been identified.[30]

Findings on brain MR imaging in the acute phase are normal, whereas cerebellar atrophy that prevailingly involves the vermis and flocculonodular lobe may be found on follow-up scans in about one-third of patients (**Fig. 7**); the severity of atrophy correlates with the persistence of symptoms.[31] MR spectroscopy may reveal reduction of NAA in the affected cerebellar hemispheres.[32]

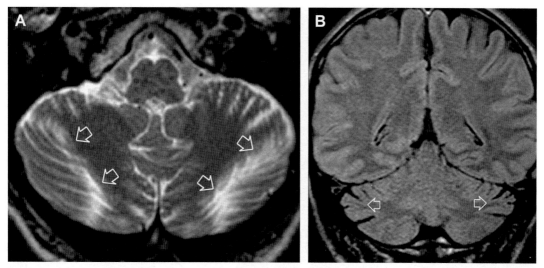

Fig. 7. Opsoclonus-myoclonus syndrome in a 10-year-old boy with prior retroperitoneal neuroblastoma. Axial T2-weighted (A) and coronal FLAIR (B) images show mild cerebellar atrophy with prominent fissures over both cerebellar hemispheres (arrows).

PYOGENIC ABSCESS

Cerebellar abscesses are serious, potentially life-threatening conditions. Almost all are otogenic, and derive from a direct extension of suppurative middle ear infection or mastoiditis and/or through retrograde suppurative thrombophlebitis. Abscesses secondary to dermoid cysts have been reported.[33]

MR imaging is exquisitely sensitive to cerebellar pyogenic abscesses; at the full-blown stage, pyogenic abscesses appear as rounded lesions with a T2-hypointense, strongly enhancing capsule and a necrotic, nonenhancing center that is characterized by restricted diffusion on DWI sequences.[34] This stage is preceded by a cerebritis phase in which there is an ill-defined abnormal signal area with patchy contrast enhancement. Otogenic abscesses are typically located laterally in 1 cerebellar hemisphere, with a typical association with ipsilateral otomastoiditis and transverse-sigmoid sinus thrombosis (Fig. 8) that is exquisitely well seen by MR venography sequences (showing lack of flow signal) or contrast-enhanced CT scans (showing an intraluminal filling defect).[35] In contrast, abscesses originating from an infected dermal sinus or dermoid are typically lodged in or near the midline, in the cisterna magna below the inferior vermis, and are often connected to a dermal sinus tract that courses through the occipital squama and opens into the overlying skin[36] (Fig. 9).

TUBERCULOSIS

Infection of the CNS with *Mycobacterium tuberculosis* (tuberculosis [TB]) is almost always caused by hematogenous spread from a primary focus elsewhere in the body, usually the lungs.[37] Abscesses and tuberculomas may involve the cerebellum in the course of TB. Cerebellar TB abscesses in immunocompetent children are exceptionally rare.[38] Their appearance on contrast-enhanced MR imaging is similar to that of pyogenic abscess in that there is peripheral capsule enhancement with a nonenhancing center; however, T2-weighted images display a characteristic low signal intensity that differentiates them from pyogenic abscesses and is caused by caseated content. Typical basal meningitis is often associated (Fig. 10).

Tuberculomas are firm, avascular, spherical masses containing necrotic areas of caseation in which tubercle bacilli may be found. Most intracranial tuberculomas occur in individuals younger than age 20 years and are often infratentorial.[39] Clinical presentation is usually with fever, headaches, seizures, and signs of increased intracranial pressure. They are characteristically low signal intensity on T2-weighted images and show single or multiple conglomerate ring enhancements after gadolinium chelate administration[40] (Fig. 11). Their size is variable, but they can exceed 5 to 6 cm in largest diameter.[39] Tuberculous lesions uniformly show increased lipid peaks by ^{1}H-MRS, which permits clinicians to discriminate between tuberculous and nontuberculous brain lesions.[41]

FUNGAL INFECTIONS

Fungal CNS infection is uncommon in children. However, the increased number of immunosuppressed patients has led to an increased

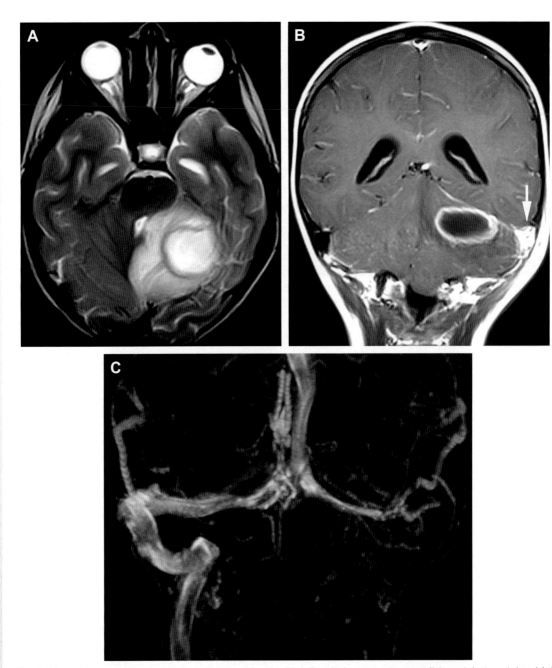

Fig. 8. Pyogenic cerebellar abscess in an 8-year-old girl with left-sided acute otomastoiditis. Axial T2-weighted (*A*) and contrast-enhanced coronal T1-weighted image (*B*) show a rounded lesion with a T2-hypointense, strongly enhancing capsule and necrotic unenhancing center, consistent with a pyogenic abscess; there is marked perifocal edema. Note the enhancing left sigmoid sinus, consistent with thrombophlebitis (*arrow, B*). Coronal maximal intensity projection from an MR venography sequence (*C*) shows complete absence of flow signal in the left sigmoid sinus and internal jugular vein.

frequency of CNS fungal infections in the pediatric age group. *Cryptococcus*, *Candida*, and *Aspergillus* are the main causes in immunodepressed patients, whereas coccidiosis and histoplasmosis are more frequent in the rare immunocompetent children with fungal infection.[42] Meningitis is the most common form of fungal CNS involvement. Meningoencephalitis, thrombophlebitis, and abscesses may occur as well.

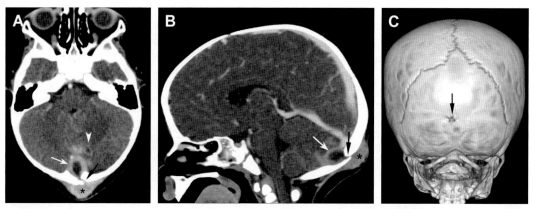

Fig. 9. Infected dermoid in a 1-year-old boy. Contrast-enhanced axial (*A*) and sagittal (*B*) CT scans show soft tissue mass (*asterisk*) overlying a skull defect of the occipital squama (*black arrow*); in the immediate intracranial vicinity there is a ring-enhancing lesion consistent with an abscess (*white arrow*); note the satellite microabscess in the adjacent left cerebellar hemisphere (*arrowhead, A*). (*C*) Three-dimensional skull reformat shows midline ostium in the occipital squama (*arrow*) indicating the intraosseous dermal sinus tract.

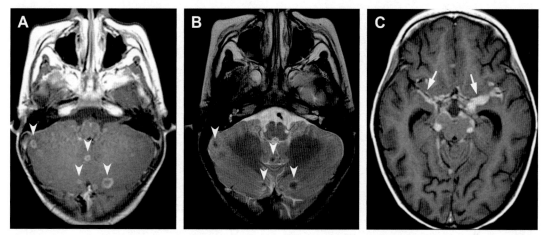

Fig. 10. Tubercular abscesses in a 5-year-old boy. Contrast-enhanced axial T1-weighted image (*A*) shows multiple small ring-enhancing lesions involving the cerebellum bilaterally (*arrowheads*). (*B*) On the corresponding T2-weighted image, the center of the lesions is hypointense (*arrowheads*), consistent with a hydrophobic caseating content. Supratentorially, contrast-enhanced axial T1-weighted image (*C*) shows typical basal meningitis (*arrows*).

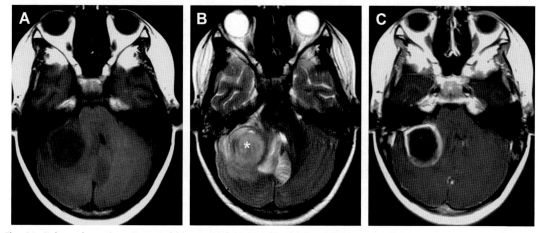

Fig. 11. Tuberculoma in a 7-year-old boy. Axial T1-weighted (*A*) and T2-weighted (*B*) image show rounded mass lesion in the right cerebellar hemisphere; note the low T2 signal intensity of the lesion center (*asterisk*). After contrast material administration (*C*) there is ring enhancement, like that of pyogenic abscesses.

On MR imaging studies, fungal abscesses are similar to pyogenic abscesses, although they are commonly smaller, show a thicker wall, and are often multiple. The content of the abscess is low signal intensity on T2-weighted images. The most common location is the gray-white matter junction.[43] Meningitis is often associated, in which case a thick enhancing exudate is found in the subarachnoid spaces; T2 hypointense granulomas may colonize the infected spaces (**Fig. 12**).

CYSTICERCOSIS

Neurocysticercosis is caused by infection of the CNS by the larval stage (cysticercus) of the tapeworm *Taenia solium*, accidentally ingested by humans from fecal-contaminated substances. The ova are ingested and their coverings are dissolved by gastric secretions. The oncospheres are transported to the bowel, where they penetrate the walls and gain access into the circulatory

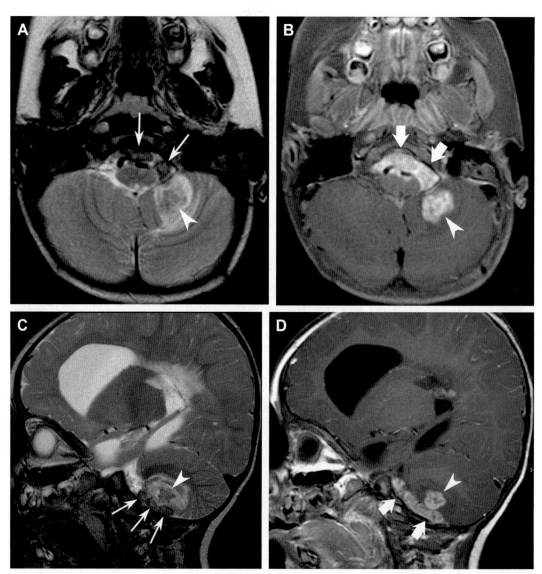

Fig. 12. Fungal infection in a 1-year-old boy with a prior history of hydrocephalus and shunt infection. Axial (*A*) and sagittal (*C*) T2-weighted images show hypointense granulomas involving the inferior surface of the left cerebellar hemispheres (*arrowhead*) and also colonizing the adjacent subarachnoid spaces (*arrows*). On contrast-enhanced axial (*B*) and coronal (*D*) T1-weighted images, there is strong ring enhancement of the cerebellar granuloma (*arrowhead*) as well as diffusely enhancing subarachnoid spaces (*arrows*), consistent with fungal meningitis.

system. They become larva once they lodge in the brain and other organs. CNS involvement occurs in about 60% to 90% of cases, and is now considered the most common parasitic disease of the CNS. Although it is an endemic disease in developing countries, it is becoming a more common health problem in industrialized countries because of immigrant populations. Clinical manifestations of neurocysticercosis are highly variable, and include seizures, hydrocephalus, and headache.[44]

Most cases are diagnosed on imaging at the colloidal vesicular or granular nodular stage, in which there are multiple lesions with ringlike or nodular enhancement located near the gray-white matter junction (**Fig. 13**). The parasite (scolex) is only visible on earlier purely vesicular stages.[45] Because the evolution of cysticercal cysts is a dynamic process, it is possible to observe transitions and overlaps from one stage to another.

CONGENITAL INFECTIONS

Intracranial congenital infections can either be transmitted during intrauterine life by transplacental passage (ie, fetal infection) or during passage through an infected birth canal (ie, parturitional infection). Causal agents include a host of viruses, protozoa, spirochetes, bacteria, and fungi. Postnatal infection may occur as well. The main infections are often designated by the acronym TORCH (toxoplasmosis, others [such as syphilis and human immunodeficiency virus], rubella, cytomegalovirus [CMV], and herpes simplex virus [HSV]). The fetal stage of development

at the time of infection is an important factor in determining the effects of infections to the CNS; this is more important than the nature of the agent.[46] The cerebellum is actively developing during the second and third trimesters of gestation. Varying degrees of cerebellar hypoplasia and abnormal foliation have been reported in congenital CMV.[47]

On imaging studies, patients with congenital CMV infections may have a small cerebellum with coarse foliation, abnormal orientation of individual folia, abnormal cortical thickness, and T2-hyperintense white matter containing calcified deposits. SWI increases visibility of calcifications and may remove the need to perform CT. Other typical manifestations of the disease, such as cortical malformations, temporal pole cysts, and intracranial calcifications, are also typically present. Although less frequently, the authors have seen cases of congenital toxoplasmosis also showing cerebellar foliation abnormalities (**Fig. 14**).

RHOMBENCEPHALITIS (BRAINSTEM ENCEPHALITIS)

The term RE refers to inflammatory diseases of the rhombencephalon; the term brainstem encephalitis often has been used interchangeably with RE.[48] The causal categories of RE include infections, autoimmune diseases (mostly represented by Behçet syndrome), and paraneoplastic syndromes. Listeria is the most common cause of infectious RE, and mostly affects young adults. Enteroviruses are the second most common viral cause and prominently include Enterovirus 71 (EV71), which is associated with outbreaks of

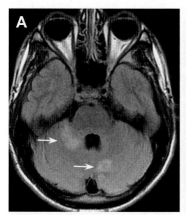
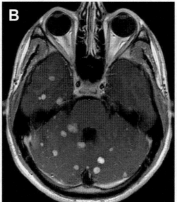
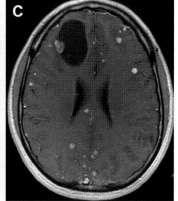

Fig. 13. Cysticercosis in a 13-year-old girl. Axial FLAIR image (*A*) shows few ill-defined lesions involving the cerebellar hemispheres bilaterally (*arrows*). However, contrast-enhanced axial T1-weighted images (*B, C*) show innumerable nodular enhancing lesions, with a larger cystic lesion with a mural enhancing nodule in the right frontal lobe. (*Courtesy of* Dr Beatriz Roedel, MD, Saõ Paulo, Brazil.)

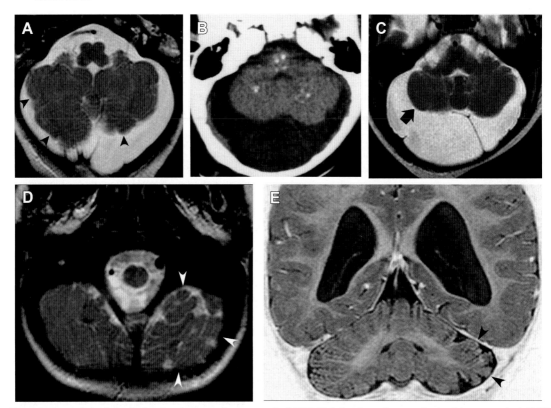

Fig. 14. Examples of cerebellar involvement by congenital TORCH infections. In a patient with congenital CMV infection, axial T2-weighted image (*A*) shows dysplastic appearance of the cerebellar hemispheres with a nodular aspect of the hemispheric surface (*arrowheads*). In a different patient also harboring congenital CMV infection, axial CT scan (*B*) shows calcification involving both cerebellar hemispheres and the brainstem; corresponding axial T2-weighted image (*C*) shows that the right cerebellar hemisphere is hypoplastic (*arrow*); also note the enlarged cisterna magna. In a patient with congenital toxoplasmosis, axial T2-weighted (*D*) and coronal inversion recovery (*E*) images show hypoplastic left cerebellar hemispheres with abnormal foliation (*arrowheads*).

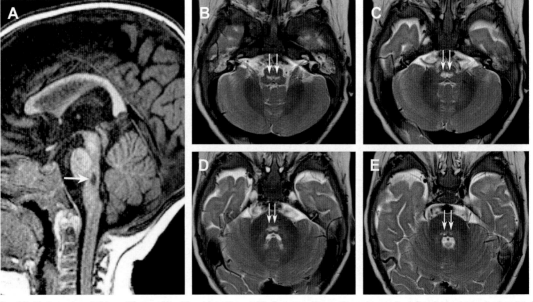

Fig. 15. Enterovirus RE in a 12-month-old presenting with fever, rash, and cerebrospinal fluid pleocytosis. Sagittal T1-weighted image (*A*) shows hypointense area involving the brainstem tegmentum at the pontomedullary junction (*arrow*). Axial T2-weighted images (*B–E*) reveal symmetric hyperintense areas involving the dorsal medulla oblongata and pons (*arrows*). (*Courtesy of* Andrea Poretti, MD, PhD, Thierry Huisman, MD, PhD, Baltimore, MD.)

hand-foot-mouth disease in the Asian south east.[49] HSV is the third most common infectious cause of RE, and about 80% of cases are caused by HSV1 and 20% by HSV2[48]; in 50% of cases, concurrent supratentorial involvement is absent.[50]

MR imaging studies are abnormal in most (>70%) patients with RE[48]; the usual findings are increased signal intensity in the pons, medulla, upper cervical cord, and cerebellum more frequently than the midbrain on T2-weighted and FLAIR MR imaging scans (**Fig. 15**). EV71 encephalitis gives characteristic unilateral or bilateral symmetric patchlike T1-hypointense, T2-hyperintense signal in the posterior brainstem at the pontomedullary junction.[51] HSV1 RE has been described to involve preferentially the cerebellar peduncles[50] (**Fig. 16**).

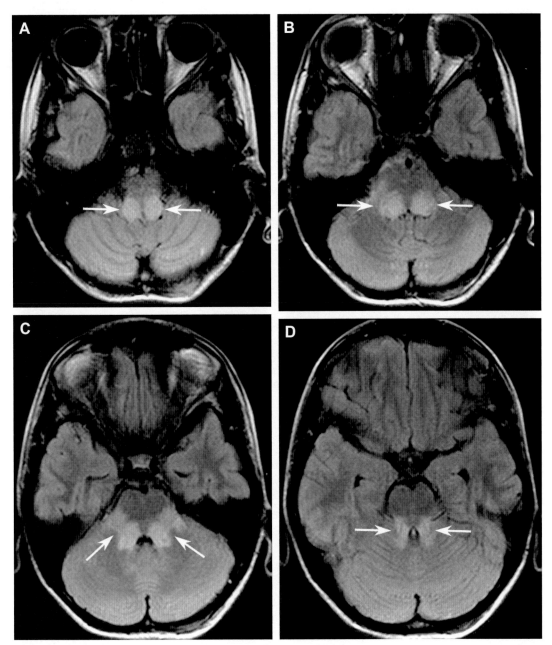

Fig. 16. HSV 1 RE in a 14-year-old boy presenting with fever and sore throat followed by vertigo, nausea, and vomiting. Axial FLAIR images (*A–D*) show swollen, hyperintense inferior, middle, and superior cerebellar peduncles bilaterally (*arrows*). (*Courtesy of* Mirella Maccarini Peruchi, MD, Saõ Paulo, Brazil.)

SUMMARY

Several types of infectious-inflammatory diseases may involve the cerebellum, either primarily or in the context of widespread CNS disease. Patients may present in the emergency department with an acute onset of ataxia, which is often accompanied by a host of other neurologic symptoms and signs. Accurate anamnesis and clinical examination (pure cerebellar syndrome vs presence of additional findings) are helpful in suggesting the correct cause. MR imaging studies play a crucial role in the evaluation of these patients, and should be performed with protocols tailored to the pediatric patient and with a sensible use of available techniques. In the absence of MR imaging, CT may play a role, although its sensitivity to cerebellar lesions is not as high.

REFERENCES

1. Poretti A, Benson JE, Huisman TA, et al. Acute ataxia in children: approach to clinical presentation and role of additional investigations. Neuropediatrics 2013;44:127–41.
2. Pruitt AA. Infections of the cerebellum. Neurol Clin 2014;32:1117–31.
3. Desai J, Mitchell WG. Acute cerebellar ataxia, acute cerebellitis, and opsoclonus-myoclonus syndrome. J Child Neurol 2012;27:1482–8.
4. Javalkar V, Kelley RE, Gonzalez-Toledo E, et al. Acute ataxias: differential diagnosis and treatment approach. Neurol Clin 2014;32:881–91.
5. Fenichel GM. Clinical pediatric neurology: a signs and symptoms approach. 6th edition. Philadelphia: Saunders/Elsevier; 2009.
6. van der Maas NA, Bondt PE, de Melker H, et al. Acute cerebellar ataxia in the Netherlands: a study on the association with vaccinations and varicella zoster infection. Vaccine 2009;27:1970–3.
7. Rudloe T, Prabhu SP, Gorman MP, et al. The yield of neuroimaging in children presenting to the emergency department with acute ataxia in the post-varicella vaccine era. J Child Neurol 2015;30:1333–9.
8. Parodi A, Rossi A, Severino M, et al. Accuracy of ultrasound in assessing cerebellar haemorrhages in very low birthweight babies. Arch Dis Child Fetal Neonatal Ed 2015;100:F289–92.
9. Routine screening cranial ultrasound examinations for the prediction of long term neurodevelopmental outcomes in preterm infants. Paediatr Child Health 2001;6(1):39–52.
10. Paolicchi F, Faggioni L, Bastiani L, et al. Optimizing the balance between radiation dose and image quality in pediatric head CT: findings before and after intensive radiologic staff training. AJR Am J Roentgenol 2014;202:1309–15.
11. Amador N, Scheithauer BW, Giannini C, et al. Acute cerebellitis presenting as tumor: report of two cases. J Neurosurg 2007;107:57–61.
12. Levy EI, Harris AE, Omalu BI, et al. Sudden death from fulminant acute cerebellitis. Pediatr Neurosurg 2001;35:24–8.
13. Kamate M, Chetal V, Hattiholi V. Fulminant cerebellitis: a fatal, clinically isolated syndrome. Pediatr Neurol 2009;41:220–2.
14. Gupta R, Maralani PJ, Chawla S, et al. Advanced neuroimaging findings of pseudotumoral hemicerebellitis in an elderly male requiring surgical decompression. J Neurosurg 2014;120:522–7.
15. Jabbour P, Samaha E, Abi Lahoud G. Hemicerebellitis mimicking a tumour on MRI. Childs Nerv Syst 2003;19:122–5.
16. Naselli A, Pala G, Cresta F, et al. Acute post-infectious cerebellar ataxia due to co-infection of human herpesvirus-6 and adenovirus mimicking myositis. Ital J Pediatr 2014;40:98.
17. Nussinovitch M, Prais D, Volovitz B, et al. Post-infectious acute cerebellar ataxia in children. Clin Pediatr (Phila) 2003;42:581–4.
18. Krupp LB, Tardieu M, Amato MP, et al, International Pediatric Multiple Sclerosis Study Group. International Pediatric Multiple Sclerosis Study Group criteria for pediatric multiple sclerosis and immune-mediated central nervous system demyelinating disorders: revisions to the 2007 definitions. Mult Scler 2013;19:1261–7.
19. Rossi A. Imaging of acute disseminated encephalomyelitis. Neuroimaging Clin N Am 2008;18:149–61.
20. Zuccoli G, Panigrahy A, Sreedher G, et al. Vasogenic edema characterizes pediatric acute disseminated encephalomyelitis. Neuroradiology 2014;56:679–84.
21. Verhey LH, Shroff M, Banwell B. Pediatric multiple sclerosis: pathobiological, clinical, and magnetic resonance imaging features. Neuroimaging Clin N Am 2013;23:227–43.
22. Banwell B, Ghezzi A, Bar-Or A, et al. Multiple sclerosis in children: clinical diagnosis, therapeutic strategies, and future directions. Lancet Neurol 2007;6:887–902.
23. Waubant E, Chabas D, Okuda DT, et al. Difference in disease burden and activity in pediatric patients on brain magnetic resonance imaging at time of multiple sclerosis onset vs adults. Arch Neurol 2009;66:967–71.
24. Weier K, Fonov V, Aubert-Broche B, et al. Impaired growth of the cerebellum in pediatric-onset acquired CNS demyelinating disease. Mult Scler 2015. [Epub ahead of print].
25. Neilson DE, Adams MD, Orr CM, et al. Infection-triggered familial or recurrent cases of acute necrotizing encephalopathy caused by mutations in a

component of the nuclear pore, RANBP2. Am J Hum Genet 2009;84:44–51.

26. Bergamino L, Capra V, Biancheri R, et al. Immuno-modulatory therapy in recurrent acute necrotizing encephalopathy ANE1: is it useful? Brain Dev 2012;34:384–91.

27. Wong AM, Simon EM, Zimmerman RA, et al. Acute necrotizing encephalopathy of childhood: correlation of MR findings and clinical outcome. AJNR Am J Neuroradiol 2006;27:1919–23.

28. Okumura A, Mizuguchi M, Kidokoro H, et al. Outcome of acute necrotizing encephalopathy in relation to treatment with corticosteroids and gammaglobulin. Brain Dev 2009;31:221–7.

29. Pang KK, de Sousa C, Lang B, et al. A prospective study of the presentation and management of dancing eye syndrome/opsoclonus-myoclonus syndrome in the United Kingdom. Eur J Paediatr Neurol 2010;14:156–61.

30. Pike M. Opsoclonus-myoclonus syndrome. Handb Clin Neurol 2013;112:1209–11.

31. Anand G, Bridge H, Rackstraw P, et al. Cerebellar and cortical abnormalities in paediatric opsoclonus-myoclonus syndrome. Dev Med Child Neurol 2015;57:265–72.

32. De Grandis E, Parodi S, Conte M, et al. Long-term follow-up of neuroblastoma-associated opsoclonus-myoclonus-ataxia syndrome. Neuropediatrics 2009;40:103–11.

33. Pandey P, Umesh S, Bhat D, et al. Cerebellar abscesses in children: excision or aspiration? J Neurosurg Pediatr 2008;1:31–4.

34. Ebisu T, Tanaka C, Umeda M, et al. Discrimination of brain abscess from necrotic or cystic tumors by diffusion-weighted echo planar imaging. Magn Reson Imaging 1996;14:1113–6.

35. Tortori-Donati P, Rossi A, Biancheri R. Infectious diseases. In: Tortori-Donati P, Rossi A, editors. Pediatric neuroradiology. Berlin: Springer; 2005. p. 469–542.

36. Yang B, Jin HM, Sun LP, et al. Posterior fossa abscesses secondary to dermal sinus associated with dermoid cyst in children. Neuropediatrics 2008;39:39–42.

37. Chatterjee S. Brain tuberculomas, tubercular meningitis, and post-tubercular hydrocephalus in children. J Pediatr Neurosci 2011;6(Suppl 1):S96–100.

38. Roopesh Kumar VR, Gundamaneni SK, Biswas R, et al. Tuberculous cerebellar abscess in immunocompetent individuals. BMJ Case Rep 2012;2012.

39. Sharma PK, Saikia B, Hussain Z, et al. Isolated cerebellar tuberculoma. Pediatr Neurol 2013;49:296–7.

40. Kim TK, Chang KH, Kim CJ, et al. Intracranial tuberculoma: comparison of MR with pathologic findings. AJNR Am J Neuroradiol 1995;16:1903–8.

41. Santy K, Nan P, Chantana Y, et al. The diagnosis of brain tuberculoma by (1)H-magnetic resonance spectroscopy. Eur J Pediatr 2011;170:379–87.

42. Castillo M, Mukherji SK. Imaging of the pediatric head, neck, and spine. Philadelphia: Lippincott-Raven; 1996.

43. Go JL, Kim PE, Ahmadi J, et al. Fungal infections of the central nervous system. Neuroimaging Clin N Am 2000;10:409–25.

44. Ruiz-Garcia M, Gonzalez-Astiazaran A, Rueda-Franco F. Neurocysticercosis in children. Clinical experience in 122 patients. Childs Nerv Syst 1997; 13:608–12.

45. Dumas JL, Visy JM, Belin C, et al. Parenchymal neurocysticercosis: follow-up and staging by MRI. Neuroradiology 1997;39:12–8.

46. Ressler JA, Nelson M. Central nervous system infections in the pediatric population. Neuroimaging Clin N Am 2000;10:427–43.

47. de Vries LS, Gunardi H, Barth PG, et al. The spectrum of cranial ultrasound and magnetic resonance imaging abnormalities in congenital cytomegalovirus infection. Neuropediatrics 2004;35:113–9.

48. Jubelt B, Mihai C, Li TM, et al. Rhombencephalitis/brainstem encephalitis. Curr Neurol Neurosci Rep 2011;11:543–52.

49. Zeng H, Wen F, Gan Y, et al. MRI and associated clinical characteristics of EV71-induced brainstem encephalitis in children with hand-foot-mouth disease. Neuroradiology 2012;54:623–30.

50. Arita JH, Lin J, Peruchi MM, et al. Herpes simplex type 1 encephalitis restricted to the brainstem in a pediatric patient. Case Rep Med 2010;2010:606584.

51. Chen F, Li J, Liu T, et al. MRI characteristics of brainstem encephalitis in hand-foot-mouth disease induced by enterovirus type 71–will different MRI manifestations be helpful for prognosis? Eur J Paediatr Neurol 2013;17:486–91.

Index

Note: Page numbers of article titles are in **boldface** type.

Neuroimag Clin N Am 26 (2016) 489–492
http://dx.doi.org/10.1016/S1052-5149(16)30041-7
1052-5149/16/$ – see front matter

Moving?

Make sure your subscription moves with you!

To notify us of your new address, find your **Clinics Account Number** (located on your mailing label above your name), and contact customer service at:

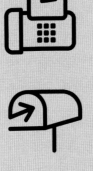

Email: journalscustomerservice-usa@elsevier.com

800-654-2452 (subscribers in the U.S. & Canada)
314-447-8871 (subscribers outside of the U.S. & Canada)

Fax number: 314-447-8029

Elsevier Health Sciences Division
Subscription Customer Service
3251 Riverport Lane
Maryland Heights, MO 63043

*To ensure uninterrupted delivery of your subscription, please notify us at least 4 weeks in advance of move.